Online Course Management

Also available are FREE online companions for facilities using course management systems. The online course management solutions feature all instructor and student online
course materials for this book, such as interactive modules,
electronic test bank, PowerPoint images and text slides,
email and communications and other tools. For more information about adopting an online course management solution to accompany *Informatics for Nurses & Health Care
Professionals, Third Edition,* please contact your Prentice
Hall Health Sales Representative or go online to the appropriate website below and select "Course," then "Nursing"
and search for the book cover and select "Adopt Now" or
"Preview."

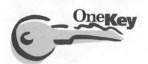

OneKey WebCT:
http://cms.prenhall.com/webct/index.html

**OneKey BlackBoard: http://cms.prenhall.com/black-
board/index.html**

OneKey CourseCompass: www.prenhall.com/onekey

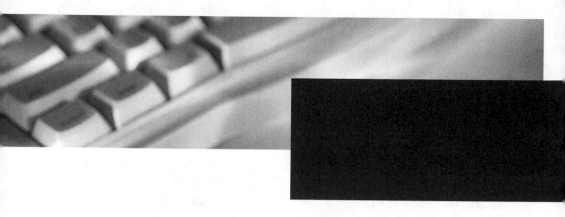

Handbook
of Informatics
for Nurses & Health Care
Professionals

Third Edition

Toni Hebda, RN, MN Ed, PhD, MSIS
Nurse Clinician at the University of Pittsburgh
and
Adjunct Professor
Duquesne University, Pittsburgh, PA

Patricia Czar, RN
Information Systems Consultant
Pittsburgh, PA

Cynthia Mascara, RN, MSN, MBA
Principal Consultant with Siemens
Medical Solutions
Malvern, PA

PEARSON
Prentice
Hall

Upper Saddle River, New Jersey 07458

Library of Congress Cataloging-in-Publication Data

Hebda, Toni.
    Handbook of informatics for nurses & health care professionals / Toni Hebda, Patricia
Czar, Cynthia Mascara.—3rd ed.
        p. ; cm.
    Includes bibliographical references.
    ISBN 0-13-151262-5 (alk. paper)
    1. Nursing informatics—Handbooks, manuals, etc. 2. Medical informatics—Handbooks,
manuals, etc.
        [DNLM: 1. Medical Informatics. 2. Nursing. 3. Allied Health Personnel. WY 26.5 H443h
2005] I. Czar, Patricia. II. Mascara, Cynthia. III. Title.

RT50.5 H43 2005
610.73'0285—dc22   2004007466

Publisher: Julie Levin Alexander
Assistant to the Publisher: Regina Bruno
Editor-in-Chief: Maura Connor
Assistant Editor: Sladjana Repic
Editorial Assistant: Bonnie Bennett-Walker
Media Editor: John J. Jordan
Director of Production & Manufacturing:
Bruce Johnson
Managing Production Editor: Patrick Walsh
Production Liaison: Danielle Newhouse
Production Editor: Emily Bush, Carlisle
Publishers Services
Manufacturing Manager: Ilene Sanford
Manufacturing Buyer: Pat Brown

Design Director: Cheryl Asherman
Design Coordinator: Maria Guglielmo-Walsh
Cover Designer: Mary Siener
Director of Marketing: Karen Allman
Marketing Manager: Nicole Benson
Channel Marketing Manager: Rachele Strober
Marketing Coordinator: Janet Ryerson
Manager of Media Production: Amy Peltier
New Media Project Manager: Stephen Hartner
New Media Production: TSI Graphics
Composition: Carlisle Publishers Services
Cover Printer: Phoenix Color
Printer/Binder: RR Donnelley & Sons

Pearson Education Ltd., *London*
Pearson Education Singapore, Pte. Ltd.
Pearson Education Canada, Ltd., *Toronto*
Pearson Education—Japan, *Tokyo*
Pearson Education Australia Pty., Limited, *Sydney*

Pearson Education North Asia Ltd., *Hong Kong*
Pearson Educación de Mexico, S.A. de C.V.
Pearson Education Malaysia, Pte. Ltd.
Pearson Education, *Upper Saddle River, New Jersey*

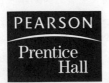

10 9 8 7
ISBN: 0-13-151262-5

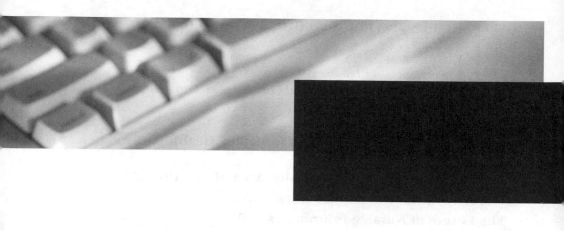

Contents

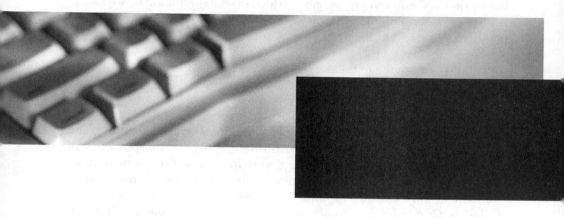

Preface

The original idea for this book came from the realization that there were few comprehensive sources available with practical information about computer applications and information systems in health care. From its inception this book was envisioned as a guide for nurses and other health care professionals who need to learn how to adapt and use computer applications in the workplace. As the outline developed, it became apparent that this book could also serve as an informatics text for students in the health care professions. This third edition contains updates and revisions to reflect changes that have occurred in the rapidly evolving technology of health. Each of the authors has a long-standing interest and involvement in nursing informatics, having worked in the field, been active in informatics groups, and presented nationally and internationally.

ORGANIZATION

The book is divided into three sections. The first section, General Computer Information, reviews information common to all information systems. It assumes no prior knowledge or experience with computers. Chapter 1 introduces the reader to the role of informatics in contemporary health care. Chapter 2 reviews basic information and terminology related to computer hardware and software. The section on the roles of various support personnel has been expanded, with content added on wireless and mobile computing. Chapter 3 emphasizes the importance of maintaining data integrity and suggests some practical steps to ensure current, accurate data in health care information systems. The fourth chapter addresses basic Internet use to support health care. The discussion on search tools has been expanded and content has been added on the evaluation of Web sites. Additional information on Internet use and resources are found in the appendices at the end of the book.

The second section, Health Care Information Systems, covers information and issues related to the use of computers and information systems in health care. This section bridges the gap between the theory and practice of nursing informatics. Chapter 5 covers basic information on health care information systems, including decision support and expert systems. Chapters 6 through 14 discuss all aspects of selecting, implementing, and operating these systems. Chapters 6 through 9 discuss the processes of overall and system strategic planning, system selection, implementation, and training. Chapter 8 contains additional information on testing, system evaluation, and strategies to implement system changes after system installation. Other pertinent topics are addressed in the remaining chapters. Chapter 10 discusses information security and confidentiality; Chapter 11, system integration; and Chapter 12, the Electronic Health Record. Chapter 13, Regulatory and Accreditation Issues, has been updated to reflect the implications of the Health Insurance Portability and Accountability Act (HIPAA) and in particular the impact on nursing informatics and health care professionals. Chapter 14 covers contingency planning and disaster recovery.

Section III covers three specialty applications of computers in health care. Chapter 15 discusses ways that computers can support health care education. It contains content on Web-based education as well as the use of wireless and handheld computers in education. Chapter 16, Telehealth, discusses the applications and issues associated with this area of practice. Chapter 17 looks at ways that computers are being used in nursing and health care research. The major themes of privacy, confidentiality, and information security are woven throughout the book.

Three appendices are included at the end of the book. The first two provide detailed information on getting up and running on the Internet and using the Internet to perform a job search. The third appendix provides suggested answers to the case studies that are found at the end of every chapter.

FEATURES

Each chapter contains pedagogical aids that help the readers learn and apply the information discussed. At the beginning of each chapter, a MediaLink box lists specific content, multiple-choice review questions, case studies, and other interactive exercises that appear on the accompanying Companion Website. The EXPLORE MediaLink sections in each chapter encourage students to use the Companion Website to apply what they have learned in the text in multiple choice questions and discussion questions, and to use additional resources. The purpose of the MediaLink feature is to further enhance the student experience, build on knowledge gained from the textbook, and foster critical thinking.

In each chapter, learning objectives let the readers know what they can expect to learn from the chapter. Case studies at the end of each chapter discuss common, real-life applications, which review and reinforce the concepts presented in the chapter. Each chapter also includes a summary and list of references. The Glossary at the back of the book serves to familiarize readers with the vocabulary used in this book and in health care informatics.

We recognize that health care professionals have varying degrees of computer and informatics knowledge. This book does not assume that the reader has prior knowledge of computers. All computer terms are defined in the chapter, in the Glossary at the end of the book, and on the Companion Website.

HOW TO USE THIS BOOK

This book may be used in the following different ways:

- It may be read from cover to cover for a comprehensive view of nursing informatics.
- Specific chapters may be read according to reader interest or need.
- It may serve as a reference for nurses and other clinicians involved in system design, selection and implementation, and ongoing maintenance.
- It may be useful for the educator or researcher who wants to make better use of information technology.
- It can serve as a review for the American Nurses Association's Informatics Credentialing examination.

RESOURCES

For students, nurses, and health professionals looking for additional background information about the Internet, services that it provides, and various types of Internet resources available, the *Internet Resource Guide for Nurses & Health Care Professionals, 3rd Edition, by Hebda, Mascara & Czar* is a concise guide to online health care environment. This book has been updated and expanded to reflect the rapidly changing issues and trends seen in relation to the Internet. New topics include PDAs, instant messaging, and wireless computing. For more information on adopting this guide, please contact your Prentice Hall Health Sales Representative.

Finally, if you are an educator using this book to introduce nurses or students to the world of nursing informatics, this book does come with FREE online companions available for schools using course management systems. The online course management solutions feature all instructor and student online course materials for this book, such as interactive modules, electronic test bank, PowerPoint images and text slides, email and communication, and other tools. For more information about adopting an online course management solution to accompany *Handbook of Informatics for Nurses & Health Care Professionals*, *3rd edition*, please contact your Prentice Hall Health Sales Representative or go online to the appropriate Web site below and select "Course," then "Nursing," and search for the book cover and select "Adopt Now" or "Preview."

OneKey WebCT: *http://cms.prenhall.com/webct/index.html*

OneKey BlackBoard: *http://cms.prenhall.com/blackboard/index.html*

OneKey CourseCompass: *www.prenhall.com/onekey*

Toni Hebda
Patricia Czar
Cynthia Mascara

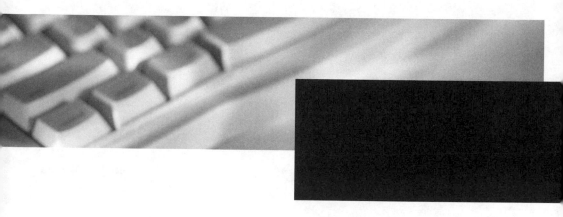

Acknowledgments

We acknowledge our gratitude first and foremost to our families for their support as we wrote and revised this book. We are grateful to our co-workers and professional colleagues who provided encouragement and support throughout the process of conceiving and writing this book. We appreciate the many helpful comments offered by our reviewers and thank our project editor for her efforts. Finally, we thank the staff at Prentice Hall for their encouragement, suggestions, and support as we developed this third edition.

When we started writing together, the three of us knew each other only on a professional basis. As we worked on this book, we found that our varied professional backgrounds, experiences, and personalities complemented each other well and added to the quality of the final product. The best part of this project, however, has been the close friendship that we have developed as we have worked together.

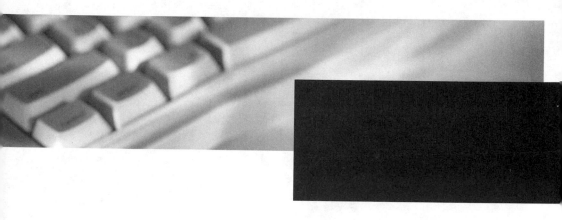

Media Contributors

Mary Boylston, RN, MSN, CCRN
Associate Professor/Informatics Coordinator
Eastern University
St. Davids, Pennsylvania
Companion Web site and PowerPoint Lecture Outlines

Marilyn L. Dickey, EdD (c)
Instructor/Coordinator Information Technology
School of Nursing, Florida A & M University
Tallahassee, Florida
Companion Web site

Cheryl D. Parker, RN, MSN, PhD
Nursing Instructor
Skagit Valley College
Mount Vernon, Washington
Staff Nurse
Providence Everett Medical Center
Test Item File

Denis A Tucker, DSN, RN, CCRN
Associate in Nursing
Florida State University
School of Nursing
Tallahassee, Florida
Test Item File

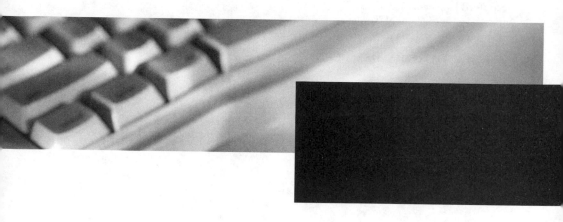

Reviewers

Mary Boylston, RN, MSN, CCRN
Associate Professor/Informatics Coordinator
Eastern University
St. Davids, Pennsylvania

Michael S. Chalambaga
Director of Informatics
Lamar University
Beaumont, Texas

Mary Ruth Hassett, PhD, RN, BC, ARNP-CNS
Chair and Professor of Nursing
Fort Hays State University
Hays, Kansas

Loretta Henry, RN, MS
Assistant Professor
McNeese State University
College of Nursing
Lake Charles, Louisiana

Carol A. Kilmon, PhD, RN
Associate Professor
The University of Texas at Tyler
College of Nursing
Tyler, Texas

Darlene Mathis, MSN, RN, APRN, BC, NP-C, CRNP
Assistant Professor, Family Nurse Practitioner
Samford University
Ida V. Moffett School of Nursing
Birmingham, Alabama

Denise A. Tucker, RN, DSN, CCRN
Associate in Nursing
Florida State University
School of Nursing
Tallahassee, Florida

Bruce Wilson, PhD, RN, BC
Professor
University of Texas-Pan American
Department of Nursing
Edinburg, Texas

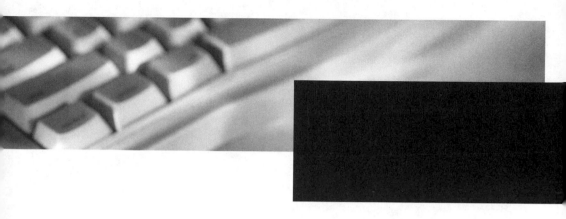

About the Authors

Toni Hebda, RN, PhD, is a nurse clinician at the University of Pittsburgh Medical Center. She has worked as a system analyst and adjunct faculty for Duquesne University School of Nursing, having taught both nursing informatics and clinical courses. Her interest in informatics provided a focus for her dissertation and subsequently led her to help establish a regional nursing informatics support group and obtain a graduate degree in information science and ANCC certification as informatics nurse. She is a reviewer for the *Online Journal of Nursing Informatics.*

 Patricia Czar, RN, is an Information Systems Consultant. She has been active in informatics for more than 25 years, serving as manager of clinical systems at a major medical center where she was responsible for planning, design, implementation, and ongoing support for all of the clinical information systems. She has been an active member of several informatics groups and has presented nationally and internationally. Ms. Czar has served as mentor for nursing and health informatics students and has a Microcomputer Specialist certificate.

 Cynthia Mascara, RN, MSN, MBA, is a Principal Consultant with Siemens Medical Solutions–Health Services. She provides consulting related to clinical systems implementation in the United States and internationally. Ms. Mascara has extensive experience with project management as well as the design and implementation of clinical information systems. She previously served as a nursing informatics specialist at a major medical center and has been an active member and leader in several informatics groups. Ms. Mascara has also presented extensively. She previously served in nursing services and administration at the University of Pittsburgh Medical Center.

One

General Computer Information

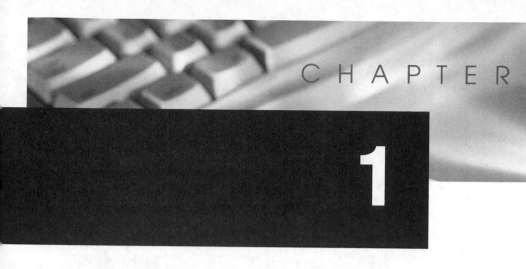

CHAPTER

1

Informatics in the
Health Care Professions

After completing this chapter, you should be able to:

- Define the terms *data*, *information*, and *knowledge*.
- Describe the role of the nurse as knowledge worker.
- Discuss the significance of good information mangement for health care delivery, the health care disciplines, and health care consumers.
- Distinguish between *medical informatics*, *nursing informatics*, and *consumer informatics*.
- Differentiate between *computer* and *information literacy*.
- Identify basic informatics competencies for beginning and experienced

nurses as well as for the nursing informatics specialist.

- Provide specific examples of how nursing informatics can affect the health care consumer as well as professional practice, administration, education, and research.
- Discuss factors in the current health care delivery system that act as incentives for the deployment of information technology in health care.
- Discuss characteristics that define nursing informatics as a specialty area of practice.

 MEDIALINK

Additional resources for this content can be found on the Companion Website at *www.prenhall.com/hebda*. Click on "Chapter 1" to select the activities for this chapter.

Companion Website

- Glossary
- Multiple Choice
- Discussion Points
- Case Study: Introduction to Informatics
- MediaLink Application: American Medical Informatics Association
- Web Hunt: Educating the Nurse Informaticist
- Links to Resources
- Crossword Puzzle

DATA, INFORMATION, AND KNOWLEDGE

During the course of any day, nurses handle large amounts of data and information and apply knowledge. This is true whether the nurse provides direct care or is an administrator, educator, or researcher. Informatics provides tools to help process, store, retrieve, and analyze data and information that have been collected for the purpose of documenting and improving patient care, as well as the creation and support of knowledge that contributes to the scientific foundation for nursing.

Data are a collection of numbers, characters, or facts that are gathered according to some perceived need for analysis and possibly action at a later point in time (Anderson 1992). Examples of data include a client's vital signs. Other examples of data are the length of hospital stay for each client; the client's race, marital, or employment status; and next of kin. Sometimes this type of data may be given a numeric or alphabetic code, as shown in Table 1–1.

A single piece of datum has little meaning. However, a collection of data can be examined for patterns and structure that can be interpreted (Saba and McCormick 1996; Warman 1993). **Information** is data that have been interpreted. For example, individual temperature readings are data. When they are plotted onto a graph, the client's change in temperature over time and comparison with normal values become evident, thus becoming information. Table 1–2 provides examples of data and information. Although it is possible to determine whether individual values (data) fall within the normal range, the collection of several values over time creates a pattern, which in this case demonstrates the presence of a low-grade fever (information).

Data and information are collected when nurses record the following activities:

- Initial client history and allergies
- Initial and ongoing physical assessment

Table 1–1	Example of Coded Data: Employment Status Codes	

Code	Status	Explanation
1	Employed full-time	Individual states that he or she is employed full-time.
2	Employed part-time	Individual states that he or she is employed part-time.
3	Not employed	Individual states that he or she is not employed full-time or part-time.
4	Self-employed	Self-explanatory
5	Retired	Self-explanatory
6	On active military duty	Self-explanatory
7	Unknown	Individual's employment status is unknown.

Table 1–2	Examples of Data and Information		
Time	**Temperature**	**Pulse**	**Respirations**
7 AM	37.8° C	88	24
12 NOON	38.9° C	96	24
4 PM	38° C	84	22
8 PM	37.2° C	83	20

The values in the table above represent data: a client's vital signs over the course of a day. Each individual value is limited in meaning. The pattern of the values represents information, which is more useful to the health care provider.

- Vital signs such as blood pressure and temperature
- Response to treatment
- Client response and comprehension of educational activities

Knowledge is a more complex concept. **Knowledge** is the synthesis of information derived from several sources to produce a single concept or idea. It is based on a logical process of analysis and provides order to thoughts and ideas and decreases uncertainty (Ayer 1966; Engelhardt 1980). Validation of information provides knowledge that can be used again. Historically, nursing has acquired knowledge through tradition, authority, borrowed theory, trial and error, personal experience, role modeling, reasoning, and research. Current demands for safer, cost-effective, quality care require evidence of the best practices supported by research. Computers and information technology provide tools that aid data collection and the analysis associated with research to support the overall work of nurses. **Information technology (IT)** is a general term used to refer to the management and processing of information, generally with the assistance of computers.

An example of knowledge can be seen in the determination of the most effective nursing interventions for the prevention of skin breakdown. If a research study produces data related to the prevention of skin breakdown achieved through specific interventions, these data can be collected and analyzed. The trends or patterns depicted by the data provide information regarding which treatment is more effective than others in preventing skin breakdown. The validation of this information through repeated studies provides knowledge that nurses can use to prevent skin breakdown in their clients.

Large-scale use of data, information, and knowledge requires that it is accessible. Traditionally, client data and information have been handwritten in an unstructured format on paper and placed in the patient record. This process makes the location, abstraction, and comparison of information slow and difficult, limiting the creation of knowledge. Recent demands for improvements in health care call for the ability to use information for health care delivery as well as quality measurement and improvement, research, and education. This can be achieved only through the use of information technology as a means to automate and share information (Institute of Medicine [IOM], 2001). Technology exists to move from paper-based to computer-based records. It is essential that nurses collaborate with technical personnel to plan what information to include, the source of the information, and how it will be used. Nurses must be active participants in the design of automated documentation to ensure that information is recorded appropriately and in a format that can be accessed and useful to all health care providers. Nurses also have a responsibility to safeguard the security and privacy of client information via education, policy, and technical means.

In 1994, Harsanyi, Lehmkuhl, Hott, Myers, and McGeehan argued that understanding current and evolving technology for the management and processing of nursing information helps the nursing profession assume a leadership position in health reform. That argument remains true now. If nurses understand the power of informatics, they can play an active role in evaluating and improving the quality of care, cost containment, and other consumer benefits. For example, nurses who are able to understand and use an information system that analyzes trends in client outcomes and cost can initiate appropriate changes in care. Nurses empowered by IT may also design computer applications that enhance client education, such as individualized discharge instructions, medication instructions and information, and information about diagnostic procedures. In these and other ways, nurses can integrate IT into nursing practice and administration as a means to manage client care, document observations, and monitor client outcomes for ongoing improvement of quality.

Nurses also handle information in the roles of educator and researcher. For example, educators must track information about students' classroom and clinical performance. Computers facilitate this process and allow educators to compare individuals with group norms. Nursing education must also prepare students to handle data. This is accomplished in several steps: teaching basic computer and information literacy, using nursing information systems, realizing the significance of automated data collection for quality assurance purposes, and recognizing the benefits of using computers to manage clinical data for research.

Researchers use computers to expedite the collection and analysis of data. One possible project, for example, uses data obtained from nursing documentation systems to study the relationship between frequent turning and positioning and the client's skin integrity. Nursing information systems are rich in data to support this type of research, and the growing prevalence of information systems increases research opportunities. As a result, nurses can expand the scientific base of their profession.

THE NURSE AS KNOWLEDGE WORKER

Health care professionals need to know more today to perform their daily jobs than at any previous point in history. Health care delivery systems are knowledge-intensive settings with nurses as the largest group of knowledge workers within those systems (Pittman 2000; Robert Wood Johnson Foundation 1996; Snyder-Halpern, Corcoran-Perry, and Narayan 2001). Advancements in knowledge, skills, interventions, and drugs are growing at an exponential rate. This makes it impossible for any one individual to keep up with all the knowledge needed to practice nursing or any of the other health care disciplines without making use of available resources and continuing education. The present health care delivery system fails to consistently translate new knowledge into practice and to apply new technologies safely and appropriately (Healthcare Information and Management Systems Society [HIMSS] 2002; IOM 2001). Several years typically elapse before new knowledge and advancements make it into the clinical setting. At the same time, the acuity level of clients continues to rise, making the work of the health care workers more difficult.

The nurse assumes several roles during the course of client care (Snyder-Halpern et al. 2001). Each role requires a different level of decision making and a different type of decision support. These roles include:

- *Data gatherer.* In this role the nurse collects clinical data such as vital signs.

- *Information user.* The nurse interprets and structures clinical data, such as a client's report of experienced pain, into information that can then be used to aid clinical decision making and patient monitoring over time. Quality assurance and infection control activities exemplify other ways in which nurses use information to detect patterns.

- *Knowledge user.* This role is seen when individual patient data are compared with existing nursing knowledge.

- *Knowledge builder.* Nurses display this role when they aggregate clinical data and show patterns across patients that serve to create new knowledge or can be interpreted within the context of existing nursing knowledge.

IT can support the nurse in each of these roles. Computerized assessment and documentation forms facilitate data collection by including prompts to help nurses to remember questions that they should ask and facts that should be recorded. These same tools strengthen the quality of clinical databases. The data gatherer role is also facilitated when input from monitoring devices is put directly into clinical documentation systems. The information user role is supported when computer capability quickly discerns patterns that help translate data into information. This saves time and labor for the nurse and provides useful information in a timely fashion.

Applications to support the knowledge user have yet to be prevalent in clinical settings; examples include making resources available at the point of care. These might include clinical practice guidelines, expert systems to support decision making, or research that supports evidence-based care and/or online drug databases. Although clinical information systems have the capability to aggregate data, currently that capability is not routinely available at the bedside. Knowledge builders examine aggregate data for relationships among variables and interventions. According to Davenport, Thomas, and Cantrell (2002), managers of knowledge workers have the responsibility to optimize the work process through improvements in design of the workplace as well as the application of technology. The unfortunate reality to date is that resource allocation for technology has been limited and the current health care environment fails to use technology well to streamline paperwork, transform data into information and knowledge, and eliminate redundancy for nurses (HIMSS 2002).

THE SIGNIFICANCE OF GOOD INFORMATION MANAGEMENT

Good information management ensures access to the right information at the right time to the people who need it. Vast amounts of information are produced daily. This information may or may not be readily available when it is needed. Its volume exceeds the processing capacity of any single human being. Part of good information management ensures that care providers have the resources that they need to provide safe, efficient, quality care. Some examples of these resources include clinical guidelines, standards of practice, policy and procedure manuals, research findings, drug databases, and information on community resources. IT can help to ensure access to the most recent versions of these types of resources. This solution eliminates the uncertainties of whether reference books are available in all clinical areas of any given facility and whether all areas have the correct version. Good information management also eliminates redundant data collection. Redundant data collection wastes time and irritates clients (HIMSS 2002).

THE DEFINITION AND EVOLUTION OF INFORMATICS

Informatics is the science and art of turning data into information. The term can be traced to a Russian document published in 1968 (Bemmel and Musen 1997). It is an adaptation of the French term *informatique*, which refers to "the computer milieu" (Saba 2001). More recently, informatics has been defined as "the study of the application of computer and statistical techniques to the management of information" (Academic Medical Publishing & CancerWEB 1997). The term has been applied to various disciplines. **Medical informatics** refers to the application of informatics to all of the health care disciplines as well as to the practice of medicine. Informatics has subsequently emerged as an area of specialization within the various health

Table 1–3	Informatics Definitions

Informatics. The science and art of turning data into information.

Medical informatics. May be used to refer to the application of information science and technology to acquire, process, organize, interpret, store, use, and communicate medical data in all of its forms in medical education, practice and research, patient care and health management or more broadly to the application of informatics to all of the health care disciplines as well as the practice of medicine.

Nursing informatics. Specialty "that integrates nursing science, computer science, and information science to manage and communicate data, information, and knowledge in nursing practice. Nursing informatics facilitates the integration of data, information and knowledge to support patients, nurses, and other providers in their decision-making in all roles and settings. This support is accomplished through the use of information structures, information processes, and information technology" (American Nurses Association [ANA] 2001, p. 17).

Health informatics. The application of computer and information science in all basic and applied biomedical sciences to facilitate the acquisition, processing, interpretation, optimal use, and communication of health related data. The focus is the patient and the process of care, and the goal is to enhance the quality and efficiency of care provided.

Bioinformatics. The application of computer and information technology to the management of biological information including the development of databases and algorithms to facilitate research.

Biomedical informatics. The science underlying the acquisition, maintenance, retrieval, and application of biomedical knowledge and information to improve patient care, medical education, and health sciences research.

Consumer health informatics. Branch of medical informatics that analyzes consumer needs for information and methods for making information accessible and implements those methods modeling consumer preferences into medical information systems (Eysenbach 2000).

Dental informatics. Application of computer and information sciences to improve dental practice, research, education, and management (Schleyer and Spallek 2001).

Clinical informatics. Multidisciplinary field that focuses upon the enhancement of clinical information management at the point of health care through improvement of information processes, implementation of clinical information systems, and the use and evaluation of clinical decision support (CDS) tools as a means to improve the effectiveness, quality, and value of the services rendered.

Public health informatics. Application of information and computer science and technology to public health practice, research, and learning.

SOURCES: Amercian Nurses Association (2001). Scope and Standards of Nursing Informatics Practice. Washington DC: Amercian Nurses Publishing. G. Eysenbach (June 24, 2000). Consumer health informatics. *British Medical Journal, 320,* 1713–6; and T. Schleyer and H. Spallek (2001). Dental informatics. A cornerstone of dental practice. *Journal of the American Dental Association, 132*(5), 605–13.

care disciplines and is one of the fastest growing career fields in health care (Abbott and Lee 2001). Table 1–3 displays some informatics terms and definitions; many are similar, but not all can be used interchangeably.

Nursing informatics may be broadly defined as the use of information and computer technology to support all aspects of nursing practice, including direct delivery of care, administration, education, and research. The definition of nursing informatics is evolving as advances occur in nursing practice and technology; there have been many different definitions throughout the years as the discipline has evolved. According to the American Nurses Association (ANA) (2001) and Staggers and Thompson (2002), these may be broken down into the following categories: 1) definitions with an information technology focus, 2) conceptually oriented definitions, and 3) definitions that focus on roles. Early definitions emphasized the role of technology. This may be seen in the statement by Scholes and Barber (1980) that nursing informatics is the "application of computer technology to all fields of nursing." Ball and Hannah (1984) later used a definition of medical informatics to define nursing informatics as the "collected informational technologies which concern themselves with the client care decision-making process performed by health care practitioners" (p. 3). In 1985 Hannah added the role of the nurse within nursing informatics to the definition that she and Ball developed. It retained its technical focus. The emphasis on technology remained evident in several later definitions as well. Critics note that many definitions emphasize technology and downplay the role of the informatics nurse in processing information that can be done without the aide of a computer. Staggers and Thompson (2002) also note that when clients are mentioned, it is usually in the role of passive recipients of care rather than as active participants in the care process.

The conceptually driven definitions started to appear in the mid-1980s as models and relationships were added to definitions (ANA 2001; Staggers and Thompson 2002). Schwirian (1986) used Hannah's 1985 definition but added a model that depicted users, information, goals, and computer hardware and software connected by bidirectional arrows. Schwirian called for a solid foundation of nursing informatics knowledge built on research that was model driven and proactive rather than problem driven. Graves and Corcoran (1989, p. 227) built on Hannah's definition to include "a combination of computer science, information science and nursing science designed to assist in the management and processing of nursing data, information and knowledge to support the practice of nursing and the delivery of nursing care." This definition addressed the purpose of technology and provided a link between information and knowledge. It built on an earlier model developed by Graves and Corcoran. In 1996 Turley introduced his model, which shows nursing informatics using theory from cognitive science, computer science, and information science on a base of nursing science with information present at the point that all areas overlap. Figure 1–1 displays the model proposed by Turley.

Role-oriented definitions began to appear at the same time that nursing informatics gained acceptance as an area of specialty practice. In 1992 the ANA's Council on Computer Applications in Nursing incorporated the role of the informatics nurse specialist into a definition derived from work by Graves and Corcoran. According to this definition, the purpose of nursing informatics was "to analyze information requirements; design, implement and evaluate information systems and data structures that support

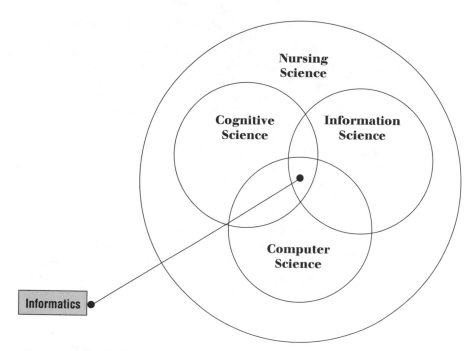

FIGURE 1–1 • Nursing informatics model (Turley 1996; reprinted by permission of Sigma Theta Tau International)

nursing; and identify and apply computer technologies for nursing." The ANA revised its definition again in 1994 to "legitimize the specialty and to guide efforts to create a certification examination" (ANA 2001, p. 16). The 1994 definition follows.

> Nursing informatics is the speciality that integrates nursing science, computer science, and information science in identifying, collecting, processing, and managing data and information to support nursing practice, administration, education, research, and expansion of nursing knowledge. Nursing informatics supports the practice of all nursing specialities in all sites and settings whether at the basic or advanced level. The practice includes the development of applications, tools, processes, and structures that assist nurses with the management of data in taking care of patients or in supporting their practice of nursing. (p. 3)

The ANA revised its definition of nursing informatics again in 2001, noting the need to address the core elements of "nurse, patient, health environment, decision making and nursing data, information knowledge, information structures, and information technology" (p. 17). The ANA prepared its definition for North America. This newer definition attempts to recognize the more active role of the patient in his or her own care and to more clearly articulate the role of the informatics nurse in today's health care environment. This definition is as follows:

Nursing informatics is a specialty that integrates nursing science, computer science, and information science to manage and communicate data, information, and knowledge in nursing practice. Nursing informatics facilitates the integration of data, information and knowledge to support patients, nurses, and other providers in their decision making in all roles and settings. This support is accomplished through the use of information structures, information processes, and information technology. (ANA, 2001, p. 17)

Groups and individuals in other parts of the world are working on definitions for nursing informatics as well. The Nursing Informatics Special Interest Group of the International Medical Informatics Association (2003) amended their definition of *nursing informatics* in 1998 to read that nursing informatics "is the integration of nursing, its information, and information management with information processing and communication technology, to support the health of people worldwide." At approximately the same time, a National Steering Committee in Canada solicited feedback via the National Nursing Informatics Project (Hebert 1999) from nursing organizations, edcuational institutions, and employers to arrive at the following definition for Canada.

Nursing Informatics (NI) is the application of computer science and information science to nursing. NI promotes the generation, management and processing of relevant data in order to use information and develop knowledge that supports nursing in all practice domains. (p. 5)

Despite national differences, agreement exists on the need for a definition to shape the specialty, obtain funding for studies, design educational programs, and help other disciplines define informatics practice within their own areas and to set expectations for employers (Hebert 1999; Staggers and Thompson 2002). There is also agreement that the goal of nursing informatics is to ensure that data collected and housed within automated record systems are available as information that can be used by health care professionals at the bedside as well as by those in administrative and research positions (Newbold 2002).

INFORMATICS COMPETENCIES FOR NURSES

Nursing informatics affects all nurses in some way because all nurses deal with data information and knowledge. The move toward electronic records and use of the Internet change the way that health care information is accessed. Informatics offers advantages to nurses in project management, consultation, and marketing, as well as in clinical practice, administration, education, and research. For these reasons, all nurses need to establish at least a minimal level of awareness and competence in informatics (ANA 2001; Heller, Oros, and Durney-Crowley 2003). This expectation also reflects employer and consumer expectations (Graveley, Lust, and Fullerton 1999; Petro-Nustas, Mikhail, and Baker 2002; Yee 2002). The terms *computer literacy* and *information literacy* are not synonymous. *Computer literacy* is a popular term used to refer to a familiarity with the use of personal computers, including the use of software tools such as word processing, spreadsheets, databases, presentation graphics, and e-mail. In recognition of these expectations, the American Association of Colleges of Nursing (AACN 1998) identifies information management as a skill needed by baccalaureate nursing graduates. More specifically, the AACN wants graduates to be able to use in practice existing and evolving methods of discovering, retrieving, and using information. This requires computer literacy but is broader in scope. Nursing programs now offer courses in basic computer skills as a gateway to information management skills. This provides a foundation for learning how to manage patient information using hospital and nursing information systems.

Information literacy is an important aspect of information management. Information literacy is defined as the ability to recognize when information is needed as well as the skills to find, evaluate, and use needed information effectively (Association of College and Research Libraries [ACRL] 2002). Information literacy is particularly important in today's environment of rapid technological change and knowledge growth, with information available from many sources and in different formats, including text, graphics, and audio. It is important to all disciplines because it forms the basis for ongoing learning. Nursing informatics education has moved from a focus on computer literacy skills to a model of information processing, computer science, and cognitive science (McNeil and Odom 2000).

Until recently there has been little consensus on the skills that comprise informatics competency. This situation made it difficult for educators and employers to ensure that all nurses possessed these skills. Hobbs' (2002) review of previous studies of informatics competencies found conceptual, methodology, and measurement problems that made it difficult to make generalizations across the research, although there was agreement that nurses should have skills in basic word processing and the ability to use databases, spreadsheets, document care, and e-mail. Yee (2002) found that employers want graduates to have these skills as well as Internet search skills and the ability to use statistical software, clinical information systems, and scheduling systems. Arnold (1996) also noted the need for familiarity with presentation graphics, data analysis, and decision support for administrators and educators. More recently, Heller, Oros, and Durney-Crowley (2003) note that the technology explosion brings the additional use of telehealth and electronic records as well as the need to quickly access several different views of data. They also note that nurses need to be adept at these uses of computer technology.

Computers are prevalent throughout the workplace. They are used for office applications such as word processing and spreadsheets, communication via e-mail, and the collection and storage of patient data via hospital and nursing information systems. Increasingly, nurses must interact with both patients and computer technology. Therefore they need to have basic competencies in both patient care and information management. Computer skills and information management competencies differ according to the level of nursing practice (Bickford 2002). Staggers, Gassert, and Curran (2001) identify four levels of informatics competencies for nurses.

The Beginning Nurse

- Has fundamental information management skills
- Can use information systems

The Experienced Nurse

- Is proficient in his or her area of specialization and highly skilled in the use of IT and computers to support that area of practice
- Sees the relationship between data elements and makes judgments based on observed trends and patterns
- Uses information systems and works with the informatics specialist to enact improvements in information systems

The Informatics Nurse Specialist

- Has advanced preparation in information management
- Focuses on informatics applications to support all areas of nursing practice
- Uses skills in critical thinking, data management and processing, decision making, and system development and computer skills

The Innovator Nurse

- Is educationally prepared to conduct informatics research and generate informatics theory
- Holds the vision of what is possible and has the ability to make things happen
- Is creative in developing solutions, possessing a sophisticated level of understanding and skills in information management and computer technology

Required competencies are further delineated in the Scope and Standards of Nursing Informatics Practice (ANA 2001). In this statement the beginning nurse must be able to identify, collect, and record data relevant to patient care, to analyze and interpret information as part of planning care, to use informatics applications designed for nursing practice, and to implement policies relevant to information. At the next level of practice, the experienced nurse is proficient in information management and one or more areas of practice. This expertise includes the ability to serve as a content expert in system design; to see relationships among data elements, execute judgments based on observed data patterns, to safeguard access to quality of information, and active involvement in efforts to improve information management and communication. The reality lay somewhere in between. Although younger nurses may enter nursing with well-developed computer and information management skills, there are many practicing nurses who identify IT training as a major need (Richards 2001; Werrett, Holm, and Carnwell 2001).

The informatics specialist has all of the competencies expected for the beginning and experienced nurse (ANA 2001; Curtin and Simpson 2001). The standards of practice are organized around a problem-solving framework that resembles the nursing process. This framework supports all aspects of informatics practice. The nursing informatics specialist is able to assess current work processes; design, select, implement, and evaluate data structures and technological solutions intended to improve productivity; and facilitate creation of nursing knowledge.

APPLICATIONS OF NURSING INFORMATICS

Informatics offers many solutions to support the work of the health care professional and health care consumer as they seek self-help and care (Brennan 2000). Some examples of how informatics and computers support the various areas of nursing and consumer health follow.

Nursing Practice

- Worklists to remind staff of planned nursing interventions
- Computer-generated client documentation including discharge instructions and medication information
- Monitoring devices that record vital signs and other measurements directly into the client record
- Computer-generated nursing care plans and critical pathways
- Automatic billing for supplies or procedures with nursing documentation
- Reminders and prompts that appear during documentation to ensure comprehensive charting
- Quick access to computer-archived patient data from previous encounters
- Online drug information

Nursing Administration

- Automated staff scheduling
- Online bidding for unfilled shifts
- Electronic mail for improved communication
- Cost analysis and finding trends for budget purposes
- Quality assurance and outcomes analysis
- Patient tracking and placement for case management

Nursing Education

- Online course registration and scheduling
- Computerized student tracking, and grade management
- Computer-assisted instruction
- Course delivery and support for Web-based education
- Remote access to library and Internet resources
- Teleconferencing and Webcast capability
- Presentation software for preparing slides and handouts
- Online test administration
- Communication with students

Nursing Research

- Computerized literature searching
- The adoption of standardized language related to nursing terms
- The ability to find trends in aggregate data, which is data derived from large population groups
- Use of the Internet for obtaining data collection tools and conducting research
- Collaborate with other nurse researchers

These examples demonstrate the importance of information sharing. Nursing informatics, through the use of computers, can facilitate and speed information sharing in all practice areas. For this to be most effective, nurses must have a basic understanding of informatics.

Consumers turn to the Internet for health information and services as well. A recent survey (Eaton 2002) found that nearly one third of Europeans and slightly more than one third of Americans used the Internet to obtain health information during the last year. Additional consumer applications may include:

- Communication with health care providers via e-mail and instant messaging
- Remote monitoring and other telehealth services
- Support groups
- Online scheduling

THE CURRENT STATUS OF HEALTH CARE DELIVERY

The health care delivery system is driven by several factors. These include patient safety and medication errors; the nursing shortage; consumer demands for cost-efficient, quality care based on best practices, managed care, economic survival, and pressure to implement IT solutions that include computerized physician order entry with decision support, bar code medication administration, electronic or computerized patient records, and e-prescribing (Baldwin 2002; Morrissey 2002).

Patient Safety

The issue of patient safety is primarily related to the prevention of medication errors and adverse events. According to the IOM (1999), at least 44,000 to 98,000 deaths per year in U.S. hospitals are due to medication errors. The IOM is a division of the National Academy of Sciences that was created by the United States government to advise in scientific and technical matters. Its Committee on the Quality of Health Care in America was formed in 1998 with the charge to develop a strategy that would substantially improve the quality of health care over a 10-year period. The committee subsequently published the landmark reports *To Err Is Human: Building a Safer Health System* and *Crossing the Quality Chasm: A New Health System for the 21st Century.* Despite recent attention to this area and recommendations for the use of IT to prevent adverse drug interactions, inappropriate doses, and potential side effects, recent reports indicate that little has been done as yet to introduce this technology on a widespread scale (Boodman 2002a, 2002b; Forster 2002).

Several professional organizations and accrediting bodies are looking at patient safety issues as well (Ball and Douglas 2002; Centers for Disease Control and Prevention [CDC] 2001; Detecting Medical Errors 2003; Health and Human Services 2003, Levine 2003; Patient Safety Task Force Fact Sheet 2001; Zurlinden 2003). These include:

- Joint Commission for Accreditation of Healthcare Organizations (JCAHO)
- Healthcare Information and Management System Society (HIMMS)
- American Hospital Association (AHA)
- Leapfrog Group
- National Advisory Council on Nurse Education and Practice (NACNEP)
- Council on Graduate Medical Education (COGME)
- National Committee for Quality Assurance (NCQA)
- National Patient Safety Foundation
- Patient Safety Task Force of the U.S. Department of Health and Human Services
- Institute for Healthcare Improvement
- Institute for Safe Medication Practice
- Centers for Disease Control (CDC)
- U.S. Food and Drug Administration (FDA)
- Agency for Healthcare Research and Quality (AHRQ)

In the United States, concerns over patient safety initiated a flurry of legislative activity (Beu 2002; Federal Safe Staffing 2003; Library of Congress 2002). Fifty bills were introduced before the 107th Congress. The 108th Congress will see a similar number. Recent legislation proposes protection for voluntary reporting of safety problems, the creation of national databases to study regional variations in care, grant and loan monies for the application of technology to improve health care, the creation of an advisory board to determine the best practices in medical technology, standards for staffing, and standards for information technology and security.

The Nursing Shortage

The nursing shortage has the attention of the public and health care providers because studies have shown that there is a relationship between the number of patients assigned to a nurse and clinical outcome (Grady 2002; Needleman, Buerhaus, Mattke, Stewart, and Zelevinsky 2002). This shortage comes at a time when the overall population is aging, placing greater demands on the health care system. The number of unfilled positions has caused hospitals to close units and curtail services.

The causes of the nursing shortage are numerous. Technology cannot solve problems that result from staffing shortages, but it can help prevent errors by giving busy nurses a system of double checks (Baldwin 2002). The IOM (2001) identified 10 domains or areas of concerns demanding action to bring about positive changes for nursing and the health care systems. Technology is an important aspect of each of these domains and can support and enhance the work of the nurse in these times of shortage. The 10 domains identified by the IOM are:

- Leadership and planning
- Economic value
- Delivery systems
- Work environment
- Legislation/regulation/policy
- Public relations/communication
- Professional/nursing culture
- Education
- Recruitment/retention
- Diversity

Pressure to Implement Information Technology

Hospitals and health care providers have been slow to adopt IT that is commonly found in the business sector. Advocates for its use claim that IT can support the work of health care professionals and benefit consumers.

The desire to reduce or eliminate medication errors focuses attention on **computerized physician order entry (CPOE),** bar code medication administration, and e-prescribing.

CPOE is the process by which the physician directly enters orders for client care into a hospital information system that provides clinical decision support to help the physician avoid adverse drug reactions (Ball and Douglas 2002; Eisenberg and Barbell 2002; Morrissey 2002). This support integrates client information from separate systems such as the hospital information, pharmacy, and laboratory systems with drug databases to warn physicians of potential problems with dosages, potential drug interactions, allergies and contraindications to use such as pregnancy, or other health conditions. CPOE is a major strategy to improve patient safety and reduce medication errors. The Leapfrog Group and Institute for Safe Medication Practices have placed demands on the health care delivery system to enact changes to provide safer, more effective care. The Leapfrog Group is a coalition of large corporations that have mobilized their purchasing power to promote changes in the health care delivery system by channeling patients to facilities that meet specified safety standards that include CPOE (Ferren 2002).

Bar code medication administration (BCMA) has been advocated as a means to reduce errors and streamline work processes (Bates et al. 2001; Meadows 2002; Sublett 2002). Bar coding was previously used in inventory control and for automatic capture of charges. With BCMA patients receive a unique bar code that is affixed to their wristband and record. Once a treatment or medication has been ordered, the bar code is scanned with an optical scanner and client details are automatically entered into the hospital information system. This eliminates the need for redundant data entry as well as the opportunity for transcription errors. It also allows staff at the bedside to verify a match between client identity and ordered medications before administration, reducing stress over potential errors and streamlining work flow. BCMA can also eliminate communication delays that occur when medication orders are changed.

E-prescribing refers to the electronic transmission of drug prescriptions generally from a computer at or near the location of the client (Bard 2002; Kuznar 2001). Its advantages include fewer errors, improved communication, lower costs, and less time to fill prescriptions. Errors are reduced because problems with illegible handwriting are eliminated and the system incorporates lists of patient allergies and other medications. Information may also be available that suggests the best drug for a particular problem and even on insurance co-payment.

Consumer Demands for Quality and Cost-Effective Care

The current health care delivery system does not make the best use of its resources, including IT (Kavanagh 2002). It is highly fragmented and often wasteful, creating unnecessary duplication of services as well as long periods of waiting and delays for treatment (IOM 2001). Consumers are asked to repeatedly provide the same information, but that information is not conveyed to all providers. As a consequence, providers are often forced to act without complete information from prior treatment episodes, often with the result of an increased incidence of treatment errors. Consumers also want options in their care that the current system does not typically provide. The IOM states that safety and quality problems occur largely because of an ongoing reliance on outmoded work systems that set up the workforces to fail despite their best efforts. Correction of this situation requires redesign of work processes.

Research

One aspect of the demands for quality and cost-effective care is that treatment should be based on research or evidence-based practice. **Evidence-based practice** is the process by which nurses and other health care practitioners use the best available research evidence, clinical expertise, and patient preferences to make clinical decisions (DiCenso, Cullum, and Ciliska 1998). Evidence-based practice represents the ideal. At this time there is still great variability in practice and a serious lack of research utilization. The domain of reliable data that nursing can rely on for informed decision making is limited. Therefore, evidence-based practice is in its infancy. Evidence-based practice is gaining ground in disease management. The Disease Management Association of America (1999) defines **disease management** as a "multidisciplinary, continuum-based approach to care that proactively identifies populations with, or at risk for, established medical conditions that:

- Supports the physician/patient relationship and plan of care
- Emphasizes prevention of exacerbations and complications using cost-effective evidence-based practice guidelines and patient empowerment strategies such as self-management education
- Continuously evaluates clinical, humanistic, and economic outcomes with the goal of improving overall health" (p. 1)

A significant number of the population have chronic diseases and use a disproportionate amount of health care dollars. Careful management of individuals with these chronic conditions can minimize complications and health care costs. Technology provides a tool to help nurses individualize care based on patient health status and evidence-based guidelines.

Managed Care

Limits to what providers can charge and capitated reimbursement plans that provide coverage for a particular diagnosis at a set rate force institutions to increase efficiency to maintain profitability. Downsizing, acquisitions, and mergers represent attempts to increase efficiency. Other methods include automation and cross-training personnel. Simply put, downsizing means that fewer people do more work. Unfortunately, the clinician also faces higher client acuity levels in many managed care scenarios. Acquisitions and mergers also allow providers to extend their reach by offering a more comprehensive set of services and encouraging clients to stay within the health care network. Smaller providers form alliances for the same purposes.

Alliances such as these encourage the sharing of information. The advantages of acquisitions and mergers may be minimized by the problem of having different computer systems from different organizations begin to work together. In an attempt to operate more efficiently, administrators are turning to IT as a tool. The following represent current and emerging technological tools: client server computing; thin client technology; wireless systems; document imaging for the storage of records on optical disks; optical scanning; digital picture archiving of diagnostic images; bar coding for demographic, insurance, and prescription information; handheld computers for material management; and telemedicine, voice recognition, and the use of Internet technologies.

BENEFITS OF NURSING INFORMATICS FOR OTHER HEALTH CARE PROFESSIONALS

Nursing informatics benefits other health care providers. For example, other providers can use data collected and documented by nurses using automated systems. In addition, multidisciplinary critical pathways are used by nurses and providers to plan and document care for a client. The aggregate critical pathway data may be analyzed for trends related to overall effectiveness of client care.

Other health care disciplines may have information systems that use data collected by nursing systems. For example, pharmacy information systems make use of data collected by nursing information systems, such as current medications, allergies, client demographic information, and diagnosis. This feature eliminates redundant data collection by different professionals, saving them time. Laboratory information systems may also connect to nursing systems. When a laboratory test is ordered and entered into the computer on the hospital unit, the information is transferred to the laboratory computer system. This replaces handwritten paper requisitions, saving time and improving communication. Similarly, other hospital departments may receive requests for consults.

Other uses of automation within health care may also improve communication and increase profitability. One example is inventory control. Health care product suppliers use technology to decrease administrative costs and to attract customers with improved inventory control. Specifically, suppliers can more quickly fill orders, check hospital inventory, and allow customers to receive prices, place orders, and confirm orders through information systems. Some suppliers provide the inventory system for customer use. Customers get a more accurate inventory, automatic replacement of supplies as they are used, and the ability to maintain a smaller inventory to reduce costs. This process is known as Web-based purchasing or e-procurement (Sandrick 2001; Schierhorn 2002). Thus, client care and consumer demands drive the health care delivery system toward working smarter, which is often best accomplished through automation.

Many of the benefits of automation in health care are seen with the development of the electronic medical record, which is an electronic version of the client data found in the traditional paper record (Budnick, Miley, Molfetas, and Pion 2002; Pifer, Smith, and Keever 2001; Rogoski 2002; Stammer 2001; Waegemann 2001; Zolot 1999). Some specific benefits of electronic medical records include the following:

- *Improved access to information.* The electronic medical record can be accessed from several different locations simultaneously, as well as by different levels of providers.
- *Error reduction and improved communication.* Automation eliminates problems associated with illegible handwriting and provides a series of checks and balances.
- *Decreased redundancy of data entry.* For example, allergies and vital signs need be entered only once.
- *Convenience.* Diagnostic images are a part of the record and can be viewed from various locations.
- *Decreased time spent in medication administration and documentation.* Automation facilitates the automation of medication administration and allows direct entry from monitoring equipment, as well as point-of-care data entry.
- *Increased time for client care.* More time is available for client care because less time is required for documentation and transcription of physician orders.
- *Facilitation of data collection for research.* Electronically stored client records provide quick access to clinical data for a large number of clients.
- *Improved quality of documentation.* Prompts help to ensure that key information is noted.
- *Improved compliance with regulatory requirements.* Automated systems can require information needed for regulatory bodies, ensuring that it is included in documentation.
- *Improved record security.* Access to the health record is limited to individuals with computer access.
- *Improved quality of care and patient satisfaction.* Built-in tools remind nurses to provide interventions appropriate for certain patient problems.
- *Decreased administrative costs for location and maintenance of client records.*
- *Creation of a lifetime clinical record facilitated by information systems.*

Other benefits of automation are related to decision-support software, computer programs that organize information to aid in decision making for client care or administrative issues. Some of the benefits that can be realized with these systems include the following (Waegemann 2001):

- Decision-support tools as well as alerts and reminders notify the clinician of possible concerns or omissions. For example, the client states an allergy to penicillin, and this is documented in the computer system. The physician orders an antibiotic that is a variation of penicillin, and this order is entered into the computer system. An alert informs the clinician that a potential allergic reaction may result and asks for verification of the order.

- With access to reference databases, nurses can easily review information on medications, diseases, and treatments as part of the automated system.

- Effective data management and trend-finding include the ability to provide historical or current data reports.

- Extensive financial information can be collected and analyzed for trends. Information related to cost by diagnosis and treatment can be more easily tracked using computer systems. For example, one can determine the least expensive drug that is effective for a particular diagnosis.

- Data related to treatment such as inpatient length of stay and the lowest level of care provider required could be used to decrease costs.

NURSING INFORMATICS AS A SPECIALTY AREA OF PRACTICE

Nursing informatics was first recognized as a specialty by the ANA in 1992. Informatics nurses are knowledgeable about patient care and technology; for that reason, they provide a valuable communication link between health care and technology professionals (Abbott 2002). Informatics nurses work in hospitals and other health care settings, in educational facilities, in research, as consultants, and with vendors.

The Scope and Standards of Nursing Informatics Practice (ANA 2001) notes that nursing informatics displays 5 of the 12 defining characteristics that must be present for a nursing specialty. These attributes were derived from earlier work by Styles (1989) and later modified by Panniers and Gassert (1996) and include the following:

- *A differentiated practice.* Nursing informatics differs from other specialties within nursing because it focuses on data, information, and knowledge; the structure and use of the same; and efforts to guarantee that nursing information is represented in efforts to automate health information. It shares an interest in the client, the environment, health, and the nurse with other areas of specialty practice.

- *Defined research priorities.* Target areas for research were identified and published in the early 1990s. These centered primarily on the development of a standard language for use within nursing, which would allow nurses, from different regions of a country or the world, to establish that they were describing the same phenomenon as well as conduct studies that could be replicated. In more recent years, survey results identified additional areas deemed critical for research, although the development of a standard nursing language remains crucial. The development of databases for clinical information is another priority area.

- *Representation by one or more organization(s).* This criterion is met because nursing informatics interests are represented by work groups within the American Medical Informatics Association (AMIA) and the International Medical Informatics Association, in a number of regional groups within the United States, and in national groups abroad. Table 1–4 displays some of these groups, and Table 1–5 lists official publications for informatics groups as well as other journals and resources.

- *Formal educational programs.* Early leaders in nursing informatics obtained their expertise through experience as well as classes in related areas such as computer science and information science. Grant monies from the Division of Nursing, Health Resources and Services Administration (National Advisory Council on Nurse Education and Practice 1997) were used to establish the first two graduate programs in nursing informatics at the University of Maryland in 1988 and at the University of Utah in 1990. There are now several graduate programs as well as certificate programs and doctoral education in this area. Some nurses still elect to enter programs in health care informatics and medical informatics as a means to pursue their interests.

- *A credentialing process.* The American Nurses Credentialing Center (ANCC 2001) used the foundation provided by the ANA in its 1994 definition of nursing informatics and scope and standards of practice. Applicants for the credentialing examination are required to meet the following criteria:

  a) Have a baccalaureate or higher degree in nursing or a baccalaureate in a relevant field such as science, one of the professional disciplines, or liberal arts

  b) Current licensure as a professional nurse

  c) A minimum of 2 years of professional practice as a nurse and a minimum of 2,000 hours of practice in informatics in the past 3 years or a minimum of 12 semester hours of graduate credits in informatics courses with at least 1,000 hours of practice in informatics nursing within the previous 3 years or completion of a

Table 1–4	A Partial Listing of Nursing Informatics Organizations and Groups

United States

National

American Medical Informatics Association (AMIA) Nursing Informatics Working Group

American Nurses Association Council for Nursing Services and Informatics

National League for Nursing (NLN) Nursing Education Research, Technology, and Information Management Advisory Council

American Medical Informatics Association (AMIA) Nursing Informatics Working Group Informatics Special Interest Group

Regional

American Nursing Informatics Association (ANIA)—California

Boston Area Nursing Informatics Consortium (BANIC)—Greater Boston Area

Capitol Area Roundtable on Informatics in Nursing (CARING)—Washington, DC

Informatics Nurses from Ohio (INFO)

Michigan Nursing Informatics Network (MNIN)

Midwest Alliance for Nursing Informatics (MANI)

Midwest Nursing Research Society (MNRS)

Nursing Informatics Research Section

Minnesota Nursing Informatics Group (MINING)

New Jersey State Nurses Association (NJSNA) Computer Forum on Nursing Informatics

Nursing Informatics Council—Kansas City

Nursing Information Systems Council of New England (NISCNE)

Puget Sound Nursing Informatics Group— Northwest Washington State

South Carolina Informatics Nursing Network

South West Michigan Informatics

Utah Nursing Informatics Network (UNIN)

International

IMIA Nursing Informatics Special Interest Group

Australian Nursing Informatics Council (ANIC)

Brazilian Nursing Association Nursing Informatics Group

British Columbia Computer Nurse Group

Canadian Organisation for Advancement of Computers in Health (COACH) Nursing Informatics Special Interest Group

British Computer Society Nursing Specialist Group

Nova Scotia Nursing Informatics Group

NURSINFO (Hong Kong)

Nursing Informatics Special Interest Group of the GMDS (The German Association of Medical informatics, Biometry and Epidemiology)

Ontario Nursing Informatics Group (ONIG)

ONIG-NCAN—Nursing Computers Application Network

Spanish Society of Nursing Informatics and Internet (SEEI)

Swiss Special Interest Group Nursing Informatics (SIG-NI)

graduate program in nursing informatics that includes at least 200 hours of clinical practicum

d) Thirty contact hours of continuing education applicable to nursing informatics within the past 3 years (waived for candidates who completed a graduate nursing informatics program with at least 200 hours of clinical practicum)

Table 1–5   Health Care Informatics Journals

ADVANCE for Health Information Executives Online

Artificial Intelligence in Medicine

Bioinformatics (formerly: Computer Applications in the Biosciences)

BioSystems

British Journal of Healthcare Computing & Information Management

Computerized Medical Imaging and Graphics

Computer Methods and Programs in Biomedicine

Computers in Biology and Medicine

Computers, Informatics, Nursing (formerly Computers in Nursing)

European Journal of Information Systems

Health & Medical Informatics Digest (H&MID)

Health Data Management

Health Informatics Europe

Health Informatics Journal

International Journal of Medical Informatics (formerly International Journal of Bio-Medical Computing)

Health Information & Libraries Journal (formerly Health Libraries Review)

Healthcare Information Management and Communications Canada

Health Management Technology Online

Healthcare Informatics Online

Information Technology in Nursing (ITIN)

Informatics in Primary Care

Informatics Review

International Journal of Medical Informatics (formerly International Journal of Bio-Medical Computing)

International Journal of Technology Assessment in Health Care

Journal of Biomedical Informatics (formerly Computers and Biomedical Research)

Journal of AHIMA

Journal of Clinical Monitoring and Computing

Journal of Healthcare Information Management (HIMSS publication)

Journal of Medical Internet Research

Journal of the American Medical Informatics Association (JAMIA)

Journal of the Medical Library Association (formerly Bulletin of the Medical Library Association)

Journal of Telemedicine and Telecare

LinuxMed News

Mathematical and Computer Modeling

MD Computing

Medical and Biological Engineering and Computing

Medical Computing Today

Medical Decision Making

Medical Engineering & Physics

Medical Informatics and the Internet in Medicine

Medical Science Monitor

Methods of Information in Medicine

Micron

Neural Networks

Online Chronicle of Distance Education and Communication

Online Journal of Nursing Informatics Corporation (OJNIC)

RN Palm: The Journal of Mobile Informatics

SCAR News: Society for Computer Applications in Radiology

Telemedicine Today Magazine

The certification examination covers content on the theory, information management principles and database management, human factors, and the analysis, design, implementation, evaluation, and support of information systems as well as trends and issues (ANCC 2001).

In summary, although many basic programs lag behind in providing IT skills, nurses are well suited to this specialty area of practice because of their critical-thinking and problem-solving skills (Briggs 2003). Nurses are ideally positioned to participate in the design and development of clinical software to ensure that it meets their needs. Specialty preparation serves to enhance application of information technology.

THE ROLE OF THE INFORMATICS NURSE

The nursing informatics specialist is a nurse with formal education and practical experience with information management. This includes the use of computers and automation to support all facets of nursing practice. Although informatics nurses are sometimes removed from the bedside, they are still focused on client care as they work to improve clinical decision making and ultimately clinical outcomes (Abbott and Lee 2001; Newbold 2002). The nursing informatics specialist may include the following activities:

- *Theory development.* The nursing informatics specialist contributes to the evolving knowledge base related to nursing informatics.
- *Analysis of information needs.* This involves the identification of the information that nurses need to do their work, encompassing client care, education, administration, and research.
- *Selection of computer systems.* The nursing informatics specialist guides the user in making informed decisions related to the purchase of computer systems.
- *Design of computer systems and customizations.* The nursing informatics specialist collaborates with users and programmers to make decisions about how data will be displayed and accessed.
- *Testing of computer systems.* Systems must be checked for proper functioning before they are made available for use. For example, nursing documentation of vital signs must be tested to ensure that the nurse can enter and retrieve the values in the system.
- *Training users of computer systems.* Users must be taught how the system works, the importance of accurate data entry, and how the system may benefit them.
- *Education of users on information policies.* Regulations on the collection, use, transmission, and storage of information require the development of guidelines to help employees to handle information appropriately. The informatics nurse is in an excellent position to develop and enforce information policies.

- *Evaluation of the effectiveness of computer systems.* The nursing informatics specialist is in a unique position to conduct this process. The combined knowledge of computers and nursing provides the informatics nurse with specialized ability to evaluate systems.
- *Ongoing maintenance and enhancements.* This involves ensuring that the system continues to work properly. In addition, the nursing informatics specialist explores possible enhancements to the system that may better serve the needs of the users.
- *Identification of computer technologies that can benefit nursing.* The nursing informatics specialist must keep abreast of technology changes, including new hardware and software applications that may benefit nurses. This may occur within the context of consulting work.
- *Compliance with regulatory requirements for information handling.* The informatics nurse needs to be aware of regulatory requirements for information handling and to ensure compliance with regulations.
- *Project management.* Knowledge of nursing and the health care disciplines and informatics makes the informatics specialist a good candidate for project leadership.
- *Research.* Varied interests lead informatics practitioners into different areas. Knowledge gained through research adds to domain knowledge.

Informatics is helping to advance the field of nursing by bridging the gap from nursing as an art to nursing as a science (Saba 2001). The informatics nurse plays an instrumental role in the development of nursing but also collaborates with informatics specialists from other disciplines. Informatics is one of the fastest growing career fields in health care (Abbott and Lee 2001).

THE FUTURE OF NURSING INFORMATICS

As each day goes by, technology becomes more pervasive. This is evident in the gadgets and monitoring devices in our homes as well as in health care. This type of technology allows better monitoring of clients and better disease management while expanding options for health care delivery settings. The improved collection and use of aggregate data will add to nursing knowledge, adding to its scientific basis and improving overall care through the provision of evidence based practice. Richards (2001) predicts that the new generation of nurses will bring their familiarity with technology and information literacy to exert their power and influence in health care. The new generation of nurses will understand and exercise their power to transform research into practice. They will also exhibit their creativity, innovation, and practical know-how in the ways that they use IT.

Consumers will also demand more. These demands are likely to include improved quality and convenience of services and expectations for practitioners to demonstrate competencies in simulated situations before working with live persons. There is an entire branch of informatics that is designed to help empower consumers by making health information readily available (Eysenbach 2000). Consumers will continue to consult online resources for health information and as an alternative means of communications with health care providers. Online scheduling, consults, and insurance authorization for services will become common.

The nurse informatics specialist will play a greater part in the future of health care delivery as the industry incorporates present-day technology to improve patient safety, gain efficiencies, compete with other providers, and plan for the future. Informatics nurses will need to do more with cost-benefit analysis before the introduction of new innovations given that financial constraints will continue to plague the health care industry for some time.

CASE STUDY EXERCISE

A client arrives in the emergency department with shortness of breath and complaining of chest pain. Describe how informatics can help nurses and other health care providers to more efficiently and effectively care for this client.

 EXPLOREMediaLink

Multiple choice review questions, case studies, and other interactive resources for this chapter can be found on the Web site at *http://www.prenhall.com/hebda*. Click on "Chapter 1" to select the activities for this chapter.

SUMMARY

- Data are a collection of numbers, characters, or facts that are gathered according to some perceived need or analysis and possibly action at a later point in time.
- Data have little meaning alone, but a collection of data can be examined for patterns and structure that can be interpreted. At this point, data become information.
- Knowledge is the synthesis of information derived from several sources to produce a single concept or idea.

- Health care delivery systems are knowledge-intensive settings with nurses as the largest group of knowledge workers within those systems. Information technology offers several tools to support nurses and other health care workers in their knowledge work.

- Good information management ensures access to the right information at the right time to the people who need it. This is particularly important when the volume of information exceeds human processing capacity.

- Informatics is the application of computer and statistical techniques to the management of information.

- Nursing informatics is the use of information and computer technology as a tool to process information to support all areas of nursing, including practice, education, administration, and research. The definition of nursing informatics continues to evolve.

- A formal definition of nursing informatics serves to shape job descriptions and educational preparation for informatics practice.

- Nursing informatics is a necessity, not a luxury, in today's rapidly changing health care delivery system. All nurses need basic informatics skills.

- Computer technology facilitates the collection of data for analysis, which can be used to justify the efficacy of particular interventions and improve the quality of care.

- Other health care providers also benefit from nursing informatics.

- Nursing informatics allows nurses to have better control over data management.

- The nursing informatics specialist supports nurses in the design, development, use, and evaluation of computer technologies.

REFERENCES

Abbott, P. A. (2002). Introducing nursing informatics. *Nursing 2002, 32*(1), 14.

Abbott, P. A., and Lee, S. M. (2001). Informatics: A new dimension in nursing. *Imprint, 48*(3), 33, 51–52.

Academic Medical Publishing & CancerWEB. (1997). *On-line medical dictionary.* Available online at: http://cancerweb.ncl.ac.uk/cgi-bin/omd?query=informatics&action=Search+OMD. Accessed December 28, 2002.

American Association of Colleges of Nursing (AACN). (1998). *Essentials of baccalaureate education for professional nursing practice.* Washington, DC: AACN.

American Nurses Association, Council on Computer Applications in Nursing. (1992). *Report on the designation of nursing informatics as a nursing speciality.* Congress of Nursing Practice unpublished report. Washington, DC: American Nurses Association.

American Nurses Association. (2001). *Scope and standards of nursing informatics practice.* Washington, DC: American Nurses Publishing.

American Nurses Credentialing Center (ANCC). (2001). *Computer based testing for ANCC certification.* Available online at: http://www.nursingworld.org/ancc/certify/cert/catalogs/CBT.PDF. Accessed December 11, 2002.

Anderson, S. (1992). *Computer literacy for health care professionals.* New York: Delmar.

Arnold, J. M. (1996). Nursing informatics educational needs. *Computers in Nursing, 14*(6), 333–339.

Association of College and Research Libraries (ACRL). (2002). *Information literacy competency standards for higher education.* Available online at: http://www.ala.org/acrl/ilintro.html#ildef. Accessed November 18, 2002.

Ayer, A. J. (1966). *The problem of knowledge.* Baltimore, MD: Penguin.

Baldwin, F. D. (2002). Making do with less. *Healthcare Informatics, 19*(3), 37.

Ball, M. J., and Douglas, J. V. (2002). IT, patient safety and quality care. *Journal of Healthcare Information Management, 16*(1), 28–33.

Ball, M. J., and Hannah, K. J. (1984). *Using computers in nursing.* Reston, VA: Reston Publishing.

Bard, M. (2002). E-prescribing cuts costs and reduces medical errors. *Managed Healthcare Executive, 12*(5), 46.

Bates, D. W., Cohen, M., Leape, L. L., Overhage, J. M., Shabot, M. M., and Sheridan, T. (2001). Reducing the frequency of errors in medicine using information technology. *Journal of the American Medical Informatics Association, 8*(4), 299–307.

Bemmel, J. H., and Musen, M. A. (Eds.). (1997). *Handbook of Medical Informatics.* New York: Springer Verlag Publishing.

Beu, B. (2002). Current federal legislation on patient safety. *AORN Journal, 76*(3), 516.

Bickford, C. J. (2002). Informatics competencies for nurse managers and their staffs. *Seminars for Nurse Managers, 10*(3), 215.

Boodman, S. G. (December 3, 2002a). No end to errors, *The Washington Post.*

Boodman, S. G. (December 10, 2002b). Little progress made on reducing medical errors. *The Pittsburgh Post-Gazette,* E1–E2.

Brennan, P. F. (2000). Nursing informatics: Two foundational developments. *Health Informatics Journal, 6*(3), 127.

Briggs, B. (2003). Information technology fits nurses like a glove. *Health Data Management, 11*(2), 90–98.

Budnick, P., Miley, L., Molfetas, L., and Pion, D. (2002). Using a CPR for nursing. *ADVANCE for Health Information Executives, 6*(8), 51–54.

Centers for Disease Control and Prevention (CDC). (August 23, 2001). *CDC's seven healthcare safety challenges.* Available online at: http://www.cdc.gov/ncidod/hip/challenges.htm. Accessed May 25, 2003.

Curtin, L., and Simpson, R. L. (2001). Standards of practice for nursing informatics. *Health Management Technology, 22*(4), 52.

Davenport, T. H., Thomas, R. J., and Cantrell, S. (2002). The mysterious art and science of knowledge worker performance. *MIT Sloan Management Review, 44*(1), 23.

Detecting medical errors. (2003). *The American Nurse, 35*(3), 6.

DiCenso, A., Cullum, N., and Ciliska, D. (1998). Implementing evidence based nursing: Some misconceptions (editorial). *Evidence Based Nursing; 1,* 38–40.

Disease Management Association of America. (1999). *The Disease Management Association of America releases the first comprehensive definition of disease management.* Available online at: http://www.riskworld.com/pressrel/1999/PR99a146.htm. Accessed April 23, 2002.

Eaton, L. (November 2, 2002). A third of Europeans and almost half of Americans use Internet for health information. *British Medical Journal, 325,* 989.

Eisenberg, F., and Barbell, A. S. (2002). Computerized physician order entry: Eight steps to optimize physician workflow. *Journal of Healthcare Information Management, 16*(1), 16–18.

Engelhardt, H. T., Jr. (1980). Knowing and valuing: Looking for common roots. In H. T. Engelhardt and D. Callahan (Eds.), *Knowing and valuing: The search for common roots* (Vol. 4, pp. 1–17). New York: Hastings Center.

Eysenbach, G. (June 24, 2000). Consumer health informatics. *British Medical Journal.* Available online at: http://www.findarticles.com/cf_0/m0999/7251_320/63563322/p1/article.jhtml?term=%22consumer+health+informatics%22. Accessed January 7, 2003.

Federal safe staffing bill introduced. 2003 *The American Nurse, 35*(3), 1, 5.

Ferren, A. L. (2002). Gaining MD buy-in: Physician order entry. *Journal of Healthcare Information Management, 16*(2), 66–70.

Forster, S. (December 4, 2002). Drug dosing is major cause of hospital errors. *The Wall Street Journal,* D3.

Grady, D. (May 30, 2002) Fewer nurses, more deaths. *New York Times.* Available online at: www.crona.org/NJA 53002.HPML. accessed April 7, 2004.

Graveley, E. A., Lust, B. L., and Fullerton, J. T. (1999). Undergraduate computer literacy: Evaluation and intervention. *Computers in Nursing, 17*(4), 166–170.

Graves, J. R., and Corcoran, S. (1989). The study of nursing informatics. *Image: Journal of Nursing Scholarship, 21,* 227–231.

Hannah, K. (1985). Current trends in nursing informatics: Implications for curriculum planning. In K. Hannah, E. Guillemin, and D. Conklin (Eds.), *Nursing uses of computer and information science.* Proceedings of the IFIP-IMIA International Symposium on Nursing Uses of Computers and Information Science. Amsterdam: Elsevier Science.

Harsanyi, B. E., Lehmkuhl, D., Hott, R., Myers, S., and McGeehan, L. (1994). Nursing informatics: The key to managing and evaluating quality. In S. J. Grobe and E. S. P. Puyter-Wenting (Eds.), *Nursing informatics: An international overview for nursing in a technological era.* Proceedings of the Fifth IMIA International Conference on Nursing Use of Computers and Information Science, San Antonio, TX, pp. 655–659.

Healthcare Information and Management Systems Society (HIMSS). (2002). *Using innovative technology to enhance patient care delivery.* A report delivered by the Improving Operational Efficiency through Elimination of Waste and Redundancy Work group at the American Academy of Nursing Technology and Workforce Conference in Washington, DC. Available online at: http://www.himss.org/content/files/ AANNsgSummitHIMSSFINAL_18770.pdf. Accessed January 1, 2003.

Health and Human Services. (March 13, 2003). *Press release: Secretary Thompson announces steps to reduce medication errors.* Available online at: http://www.hhs.gov/news/press/2003pres/20030313.html. Accessed May 24, 2003.

Hebert, M. (1999). *National Nursing Informatics Project discussion paper.* Available online at: http://www.cna-nurses.ca/pages/resources/nni/ nni_discussion_paper.doc. Accessed June 24, 2003.

Heller, B. F., Oros, M. T., and Durney-Crowley, J. (June 24, 2003). The future of nursing education: Ten trends to watch. *NLN Journal.* Available online at: http://www.nln.org/nlnjournal/infotrends.htm. Accessed June 24, 2003.

Hobbs, S. D. (2002). Measuring nurses' computer competency: An analysis of published instruments. *Computers, Informatics, Nursing, 20*(2), 63–73.

Institute of Medicine (IOM). (1999). *To err is human: Building a safer health system.* Washington, DC: National Academy Press.

Institute of Medicine (IOM). (2001). *Crossing the quality chasm: A new health system for the 21st century.* Washington, DC: National Academy Press.

International Medical Informatics Association: (2003). The Special Interest Group on Nursing Informatics. Available online at: http://www.IMIA. org/NI/. Accessed April 7, 2004.

Kavanagh, J. (November 7, 2002). Healthcare IT sector is in disarray, warns BCS. *Computer Weekly,* 53.

Kuznar, W. (2001). E-prescribing aims to improve care, overcome prior authorization shortcomings. *Managed Healthcare Executive, 11*(3), 32.

Levine, R. (February 24, 2003). *Dailymed initiative enhancing patient safety through accessible medication information.* Available online at: http://www.fda.gov/cder/regulatory/ersr/2003_02_13_dailymed/. Accessed May 25, 2003.

Library of Congress. (2002). Thomas. Available online at: http://thomas.loc.gov/. Accessed December 31, 2002.

Meadows, G. (2002). Safeguarding patients against medication errors. *Nursing Economics, 20*(4), 192.

McNeil, B. J., and Odom, S. K. (2000). Nursing informatics education in the United States: Proposed undergraduate curriculum. *Health Informatics Journal, 6*(1), 32.

Morrissey, J. (April 22, 2002). Doctor's orders: Computerized decision-support system directs Vanderbilt physicians to the latest treatment data, helping to eliminate unnecessary costs. *Modern Healthcare, 32,* 32.

National Advisory Council on Nurse Education and Practice (NACNEP). (1997). *A national agenda for nursing education and practice.* Rockville, MD: US Department of Health and Human Services, Health Resources and Services Administration.

Needleman, J., Buerhaus, P., Mattke, S., Stewart, M., and Zelevinsky, K. (2002). Nurse-staffing levels and the quality of care in hospitals. *New England Journal of Medicine, 346*(22), 1715–1722.

Newbold, S. K. (2002). FAQs about nursing informatics. *Nursing2002, 32*(3), 20.

Nursing Informatics: Special Interest Group of the International Medical Informatics Association (IMIA-NI). (1998). Proceedings of the General Assembly Meeting, Seoul, Korea.

Pabst, M. K., Scherubel, J. C., and Minnick, A. F. (1996). The impact of computerized documentation on nurses' use of time. *Computers in Nursing, 14*(1), 25–30.

Panniers, T. L., and Gassert, C. A. (1996). Standards of practice and preparation for certification. In M. E. Mills, C. A. Romano, and B. R. Heller (Eds.), *Information management in nursing and health care*, pp. 280–297. Springhouse, PA: Springhouse Corporation.

Patient Safety Task Force Fact Sheet. (2001). Agency for Healthcare Research and Quality. Available online at: http://www.ahrq.gov/qual/taskforce/psfactst.htm. Accessed October 25, 2002.

Petro-Nustas, W., Mikhail, B. I., and Baker, O. G. (2002). Perceptions and expectations of baccalaureate-prepared nurses in Jordan: Community survey. *International Journal of Nursing Practice, 7*(5), 349–358.

Pifer, E. A., Smith, S., and Keever, G. W. (2001). EMR to the rescue. *Healthcare Informatics, 19*(2), 111–112, 114.

Pittman, L. (2000). Dealing with the knowledge explosion. *Australian Nursing Journal, 8*(5), 30.

Richards, J. A. (2001). Nursing in a digital age. *Dermatology Nursing, 13*(5), 365.

Robert Wood Johnson Foundation. (1996). *Chronic care in America: A 21st century challenge*. Princeton, NJ: The Robert Wood Johnson Foundation.

Rogoski, R. R. (2002). The ABCs of CPRs and EMRs: Definitions, semantics, product differences and the need for demonstrated results hinder wide-scale adoption. *Health Management Technology, 23*(5), 14–16, 19.

Romano, C. (October 1996). Nursing informatics. Paper presented at MISA/MISPA International Conference, Nashville, TN.

Saba, V., and McCormick, K. (1996). *Essentials of computers for nurses.* New York: McGraw-Hill.

Saba, V. K. (2001). Nursing informatics: Yesterday, today and tomorrow. *International Nursing Review, 48*(3), 177.

Sandrick, K. (2001). E-commerce is here. *Health Facilities Management, 14*(4), 16.

Schierhorn, C. (2002). What's taking so long? *Health Facilities Management, 15*(4), 22.

Scholes, M., and Barber, B. (1980). Towards nursing informatics. In D. A. Lindberg and S. Kaihari (Eds.), *Medinfo, 80* (pp. 70–73). London: North-Holland.

Schwirian, P. (1986). The NI pyramid—A model for research in nursing informatics. *Computers in Nursing, 4*(3), 134–136.

Snyder-Halpern, R., Corcoran-Perry, S., and Narayan, S. (2001). Developing clinical practice environments supporting the knowledge work of nurses. *Computers in Nursing, 19*(1), 17–23.

Staggers, N., Gassert, C. A., and Curran, C. (2001). Informatics competencies for nurses at four levels of practice. *The Journal of Nursing Education, 40*(7), 303–316.

Staggers, N., and Thompson, C. B. (2002). The evolution of definitions for nursing informatics: A critical analysis and revised definition. *Journal of the American Medical Informatics Association, 9*(3), 255–261.

Stammer, L. (2001). Chart pulling brought to its knees. *Healthcare Informatics, 18*(2), 107–108.

Styles, M. (1989). *On specialization in nursing: Toward a new empowerment.* Kansas City, MO: American Nurses Foundation.

Sublett, P. (2002). Technology's impact on reducing medication errors. *Health Management Technology, 23*(11), 24, 26.

Turley, J. P. (1996). Toward a model of nursing informatics. *Image: Journal of Nursing Scholarship, 28*(1), 309–313.

Waegemann, C. P. (2001). Leading edge: An electronic record for the real world. *Healthcare Informatics, 18*(5), 55–56, 58, 60.

Warman, A. R. (1993). *Computer security within organizations.* London: Macmillan.

Werrett, J. A., Holm, R. H., and Carnwell, R. (2001). The primary and secondary care interface: The educational needs of nursing staff for the provision of seamless care. *Journal of Advanced Nursing, 34*(5), 629, 10p.

Yee, C. C. (2002). Identifying information technology competencies needed in Singapore nursing education. *Computers, Informatics, Nursing, 20*(5), 209–214.

Zolot, J. S. (1999). Computer-based patient records. *AJN, 99*(12), 64, 66, 68–69.

Zurlinden, J. (2003). FDA bands importing certain high risk prescription drugs using the Internet. *Nursing Spectrum, 4*(2), 12.

Hardware, Software, and the Roles of Support Personnel

After completing this chapter, you should be able to:

- Explain what computers are and how they work.
- Describe the major hardware components of computers.
- Understand what networks are, and list the major types of network configurations.
- Explain some considerations for choosing and using a computer system.
- List the advantages and disadvantages of mainframe, client server, and thin client technology.

- Compare and contrast mobile and wireless devices, including personal digital assistants (PDAs), in terms of basic technology and implications for use.
- Understand the major types of software commonly used with computer systems.
- Discuss the roles and responsibilities of various computer support personnel.

 MEDIALINK

Additional resources for this content can be found on the Companion Website at *www.prenhall.com/hebda*. Click on "Chapter 2" to select the activities for this chapter.

Companion Website

- Glossary
- Multiple Choice
- Discussion Points
- Case Study: How Computers Work
- Case Study: Roles of Support Personnel
- Case Study: Infection Control
- MediaLink Application: Comparing PDAs
- Web Hunt: Emerging Technologies in Health Care
- Links to Resources
- Crossword Puzzle

A **computer** is an electronic device that collects, stores, processes, and retrieves data. Information output is provided under the direction of stored sequences of instructions known as computer programs. The physical parts of a computer are frequently referred to as **hardware,** and the instructions, or programs, are collectively known as **software.** A computer system consists of the following components:

- Hardware
- Software
- Data that will be transformed into information
- Procedures or rules for the use of the system
- Users

Rapid advances in technology reshape computer capabilities and user expectations. Many changes have occurred since the introduction of the first computers in the 1940s. In general, computers have become smaller but more powerful and increasingly affordable. This is particularly evident with current notebook, tablet, and PDA computers.

HARDWARE

Computer hardware is the physical part of the computer and its associated equipment. Computer hardware consists of many different parts, but the main elements are input devices, the central processing unit, primary and secondary storage devices, and output devices. These devices may be contained within one shell or may be separate but connected in some fashion. Figure 2–1 describes the relationship among these components.

Input Devices

Input devices allow the user to put data into the computer. Common input devices include the keyboard, mouse and trackball, touch screen,

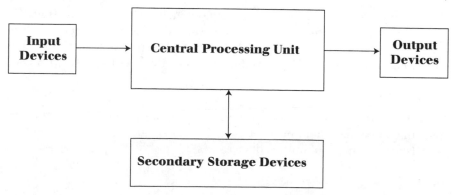

FIGURE 2–1 • Basic components of a computer

stylus, microphone, bar code reader, Fax modem card, joystick, scanner and digital camera, and Webcam.

Central Processing Unit

The **central processing unit (CPU)** is the "brain" of the computer. It has the electronic circuitry that actually executes computer instructions. The CPU can be divided into the following three components:

- The **arithmetic logic unit (ALU)** executes instructions for the manipulation of numeric symbols.
- **Memory** is the storage area in which programs reside during execution. Memory is subdivided into two categories: read-only memory and random access memory. **Read-only memory (ROM)** is permanent; it remains when the power is off. It typically cannot be changed by the user unless additional memory is installed. ROM contains start-up instructions that are executed each time the computer is turned on. **Random access memory (RAM)** is a temporary storage area that is active only while the computer is turned on. It provides storage for the program that is running, as well as for the data that are being processed.
- The **control unit** manages instructions to other parts of the computer, including input and output devices. It reads stored programs one instruction at a time and directs other computer parts to perform required tasks.

The CPU is located inside the system cabinet, which is the box that many people think of as "the computer." The cabinet contains other components as well. Figure 2–3 will show some items that may be inside a computer cabinet.

Secondary Storage

Secondary storage provides space to retain data in an area separate from the computer's memory after the computer is turned off. Common mechanisms for secondary storage include **hard disk drives, floppy diskettes, Zip drive disks, compact discs (CDs),** and **digital versatile** or **video discs (DVDs).**

Output Devices

Output devices allow the user to view and possibly hear processed data. Terminals or video monitor screens, printers, speakers, and Fax modem boards are examples of output devices.

COMPUTER CATEGORIES

Computers vary in size, purpose, capacity, and the number of users that can be accommodated simultaneously. The main categories of computers are:

- Supercomputers
- Mainframe computers
- Minicomputers
- Personal computers (also known as PCs or desktop computers)
- Laptop or notebook computers
- Tablet computers
- PDAs and other handheld devices

The PDA has become a very popular device that is revolutionizing information access in health care. Table 2–1 provides a brief description of the various types of computers and some advantages and disadvantages associated with each.

Supercomputers are the largest, most expensive type of computer. They are complex systems that can perform billions of instructions every second. Prohibitive cost limits use primarily to government and academic settings.

Mainframes, which are large computers capable of processing several million instructions per second, are used for quickly processing large amounts of data. Mainframe computers support organizational functions and therefore were the traditional equipment in hospital environments until recently. Software for mainframes supports many customized functions, and this level of specialization results in its high cost.

A **minicomputer** is a scaled-down version of a mainframe computer. Minicomputers are slightly less costly than mainframes but are still capable of supporting multiple users as well as the computing needs of small businesses. Because they have become more powerful, minicomputers may be used in hospitals.

Personal computers (PCs) are also known as desktop computers and were previously referred to as **microcomputers.** This computer category provides inexpensive processing power for an individual user. A PC may stand alone or be connected to other computer systems through a network, dial-up or wireless connection, or cable service. Improved reliability, availability, manageability, and processing capabilities allow PCs to assume responsibilities once associated with mainframe computers. Some variations of the microcomputer are the notebook or laptop, tablet PC, and handheld computers. These devices all offer portable computer capability away from the office or desktop. The **notebook** or **laptop** computer is a streamlined version of the personal computer, using batteries or regular electric current. These devices are more expensive than comparable desktop computers. The **tablet PC** can be carried in one hand like a clipboard and is smaller and lighter than a notebook computer but rivals notebook capability. It accepts handwritten input via a stylus but also incorporates a keyboard and supports Windows-based applications. The stylus can be used like a mouse. Devices may also be configured to accept dictation (MacVittie 2002; New products 2002). Handheld computers are special-use devices that offer portability and some of the features found in laptop and tablet

Table 2–1 Types of Computers

Type	Description	Advantages	Disadvantages
Supercomputer	Designed and used for complex scientific calculations	Performs complex calculations very quickly	Expensive Limited functionality
Mainframe	Used to support organizational information systems Multiple processors Varies in size	High-speed transactions Supports many terminals and users simultaneously Large storage capacity	Expensive Software expensive and inflexible
Minicomputer	Smaller version of a mainframe Designed for multiple users Supports corporate computing for smaller organizations	Less expensive than a mainframe Supports many terminals and users simultaneously	Relatively expensive
Personal computer (PC) or desktop computer	Usually a single-processor machine intended for one user	Inexpensive processing May be connected to other systems through a network, dial-up, or cable connection	High support costs Somewhat slower response with fewer capabilities than larger systems
Laptop or notebook computer	Streamlined, portable version of a PC or desktop system	Provides portable computer capability	Limited battery life More expensive than a comparably equipped PC Generally has a smaller keyboard than a PC
Tablet computers	Smaller than a notebook computer Weighs 2–3 pounds	Small size makes it easy to carry Generally accepts handwriting or keyboard input May receive and transmit data from and to other systems	Limited battery life Slightly more expensive than a desktop system May not be able to receive transmissions in some areas known as "deadzones"

(continued)

Table 2–1   **Types of Computers—*continued***

Type	Description	Advantages	Disadvantages
Handheld/personal digital assistant (PDA)	Small special-use device	Small, lightweight Inexpensive Quick learning curve Easily taken to the point of care Increases access to information Can improve productivity May accept handwriting, voice, or keyed input May download data from information systems and transmit data to other systems May incorporate the functionality of more than one device (i.e., PDA, e-mail terminal, cell phone)	Small screen size Offers less functionality than desktop and notebook computers Limited battery life Limited speed and processing ability May not hold up to rough use Synchrony with other computers may require special equipment E-mail connectivity/telephone service requires wireless service Small size makes it easy to steal Information security concerns related to theft May not be able to receive transmissions in some areas known as "deadzones"

PCs. Advances in technology add to the functionality of these devices. Some can accept handwriting and voice input as well as send and receive data. **PDAs** are a well-known type of handheld computer. These small devices were once used to keep appointment calendars, addresses, and telephone numbers. Advances in processing capability, memory, and design make PDAs attractive for a wide variety of functions, including many common software applications and data collection. PDAs can store extensive reference materials and have the ability to access patient information and transmit and receive information such as electronic prescriptions (Keplar and Urbanski 2003; Lewis and Sommers 2003; Schuerenberg 2003). Hybrids comprise another category of handheld devices. Hybrids may combine PDA capability with cell phones or other functions (Hochhauser 2002; Schuyler 2003).

PERIPHERAL HARDWARE ITEMS

Peripheral hardware or, more simply, a **peripheral,** is any piece of hardware connected to a computer. Examples of peripheral devices include:

- Monitors
- Keyboards
- Terminals
- Mouse and other pointing devices such as trackballs and touchpads
- Secondary storage devices such as tape, Zip, CD, and DVD drives
- Backup systems
- External modems
- Printers
- Scanners
- Digital and Web cameras (Webcams)
- Multifunction devices that combine functions such as printers that also scan, copy, and Fax

The **monitor** is the screen that displays text and graphic images generated by the computer. Many PC monitors use television technology to generate colors by combining amounts of red, green, and blue. **Refresh rate** and **resolution** are terms that refer to monitor characteristics. The refresh rate is the speed with which the screen is repainted from top to bottom. Early monitors had a slow refresh rate that caused the screen to flicker. Higher refresh rates eliminate flicker. **Resolution** is the number of pixels, or dots, that appear horizontally and vertically on the screen, making up the image. Resolution is expressed as the number of horizontal pixels by vertical pixels. Higher resolution numbers provide a better screen image. Most laptops and flat monitors use **LCD (liquid crystal display)** technology. LCD technology uses two sheets of polarizing material with a liquid crystal solution between them. An electric current sent through the liquid causes the crystals to align so that light cannot pass through them. Each crystal acts like a shutter, either allowing light to pass through or blocking the light. LCD displays may be monochrome or color. Monitors that accept handwriting via a stylus use an electromagnetic field under or over an LCD to capture the movement on the screen. The monitor may be housed separately from the CPU or contained within the same box. Touch screens offer another variation in monitor technology. Touch screens are sensitive to contact; this allows users to enter data and make selections by touching the screen.

    Keyboards are input devices with keys that resemble those of a typewriter. Keyboards allow the user to type information and instructions into a computer.

    A **terminal** consists of a monitor screen and a keyboard. It is used to input data and receive output from a mainframe computer. Unlike a personal computer, the terminal itself does not process information, thus giving rise to the expression "dumb terminal."

The **mouse** is a device that fits in the user's hand and can be moved around on the desktop to direct a pointer on the screen. It is often used to select and move items by pressing and releasing a button. A mouse pad optimizes function by providing a surface area with the proper amount of friction while minimizing the amount of dirt that enters the mouse.

Some other examples of pointing devices include joysticks, touchpads, and trackballs. A **joystick** allows the user to control the movement of objects on the screen and is primarily used with games. A **touchpad** is a pressure- and motion-sensitive surface. When a user moves a finger across the touchpad, the on-screen pointer moves in the same direction. A **trackball** contains a ball that the user rolls to move the on-screen pointer. Touchpads and trackballs work well when available space is limited, as with laptop computers.

Secondary storage devices are generally provided via the hard disk drive, floppy diskette drive, as well as magnetic disk or tape, Zip, CD and DVD drives. Some of these devices are no longer offered with new computers but remain in use with older computers and large mainframe computers. The hard disk drive allows the user to *retrieve*, or read, data as well as *save*, or write, new data. Data are stored in the hard drive magnetically on a stack of rotating disks known as *platters*. The amount of information that can be stored on disk is known as its *capacity*. Capacity is measured in bytes. Hard disk drives generally offer a larger capacity than do secondary storage devices. Home and office PCs offer hard disk drives with a capacity that is measured in gigabytes. One gigabyte is equivalent to 1,073,741,824 characters.

DVD drives offer more flexibility than CD drives. DVD drives can read or play CDs as well as DVDs but access data more quickly. DVD-ROM drives only read, not write, data. Some DVD drives can also write data. DVDs can store up to seven times more data than a CD. Another features is that a DVD (digital versatile or video disc) is similar to a CD (compact disc) and is commonly used to store multimedia or full-length movies. The traditional CD-ROM drive allows the user to read, but not change, information stored on CDs. Some CD drives can write data and, in some cases, rewrite data many times. A CD is the same type of disc on which music is recorded, but it usually stores more forms of data than just sound. The CD provides improved storage capacity and access rate over traditional magnetic floppy diskettes, or disks, which are the storage medium used by the floppy disk drive. A *floppy disk* is a thin plastic platter within a plastic cover. Earlier diskettes were larger in size and had a flexible cover. Currently, the most common diskettes have a 3.5-inch-square plastic outer cover. Most hard drives, CD-ROM drives, and floppy disk drives are located internally within the system cabinet, but they may also be located externally and connected using cables.

Additional secondary storage can be provided through the use of other devices internal or external to the cabinet. These may include Zip drives, optical disk drives, magnetic disk or tape drives, and RAID. A **Zip drive** is a high-capacity floppy disk drive. Zip disks are slightly larger than 3.5 inch floppy diskettes in both capacity and thickness. Zip disks are a relatively inexpensive device that were popular when hard disk space was expensive and limited.

A **tape drive** copies files from the computer to magnetic tape for storage or transfer to another machine. A **file** is a collection of related data stored and handled as a single entity by the computer. The tape drive uses tiny electromagnets to write data to a magnetic media by altering the surface. **Optical disk drives** rely on laser technology to write data to a recording surface media and read it later. The advantage of this technology is its large storage capacity.

A **redundant array of inexpensive or independent disks** (**RAID**) is precisely what the name indicates: duplicate disks with mirror copies of data. Using RAID may be less costly than using one large disk drive. In the event that an individual disk fails, the remaining RAID would permit the computer to continue working uninterrupted.

Backup systems are devices that create copies of system and data files. These systems use secondary storage device technology. The copies are generally kept at a location separate from the computer. A backup system is an important measure for protection against computer failure or data loss.

A **modem** is a communication device that allows computers to transmit information over telephone or cable lines. Faster modems transfer information more quickly. This, in turn, saves time and telephone charges. Modem speed is measured by the number of bits that can be transferred in 1 second of time, or **bits per second (bps).** A **bit** is the smallest unit of data that can be handled by the computer. In actuality, transfer occurs in thousands of bits per second, or **kilobits (kbps).** Many PCs include modem and Fax capabilities via a Fax modem board. A **Fax modem** board allows computers to transmit images of letters and drawings over telephone lines. **Wireless modems** allow users to send and receive information via access points provided with a subscription to wireless service.

A **printer** produces a paper copy of computer-generated documents. Several types of printers are available. Laser printers offer the highest quality print by transferring toner, a powdered ink, onto paper like a photocopier does. Ink-jet printers heat ink and spray it onto paper to provide a high-quality output. Dot matrix printers create letters and graphics through the use of a series of metal pins that strike a ribbon against paper. Color is an option with all three printer types. Prices vary according to quality and capability with prices starting under $100 and ranging upward. Dot matrix and ink-jet printers are relatively inexpensive to operate. Before the development of these three printer types, printers resembled typewriters. Some printers perform multiple functions and may be used as a printer, a scanner, a copier, and a Fax machine. Users should base their selection on need. Laser printers are the office standard because they are quiet and provide a high-quality print. Ink-jet printers are suitable for interoffice communication but are slow, and their ink may smear when exposed to moisture. Dot matrix printers are noisy and may provide a poor-quality print.

The **scanner** is an input device that converts printed pages or graphic images into a file. The file can then be stored and revised using the computer. For example, a printed report can be scanned, stored in the computer, and sent electronically to another output device. **Digital cameras** offer a means to capture and input still images without film. Digital images may be downloaded to a computer, manpulated, and printed. A **Webcam** is a small camera used by a computer to send images over the Internet. **Multiple function devices** combine functions such as printers that also scan, copy, and Fax.

NETWORKS

A **network** is a combination of hardware and software that allows communication and electronic transfer of information between computers. Hardware may be connected permanently by wire or cable, or temporarily through modems, telephone lines, or radio signals. This arrangement allows sharing of resources, data, and software. For example, it may not be practical to have a printer for every PC in the house or office. Instead, several PCs are connected to one printer through a network. Common use of hardware requires consideration of overall needs, convenience of location, priority by user and job, and amount of use. Figure 2–2 depicts a network.

Networks range in size from **local area networks (LANs),** with a handful of computers, printers, and other devices, to systems that link many small and large computers over a large geographic area. For example, some LANs provide support for **client/server** technology. In client/server technology, files are stored on a central computer known as the

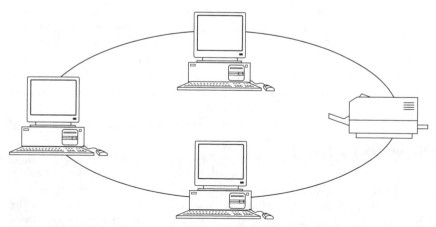

FIGURE 2–2 • Schematic representation of a network

server. Any type of computer may act as a server, including mainframes, minicomputers, and PCs. **Client** computers can access information stored on the server. One major advantage of a LAN is that only one copy of a software program is needed for all users since it can be stored on the server. The client computers then access the server to use the software. This contrasts with the need to supply a separate copy of a software program for each PC user. The primary disadvantage to client/server technology is vulnerability. If the server fails, the network fails. Multiple servers circumvent this problem. Larger, more expansive systems are known as **wide area networks (WANs).**

Thin client technology, also known as **server-based computing,** represents another networking model that relies on highly efficient servers (Mitchell 2002; Rand, Witt, Hunger, and Gulle 2002; Seltzer 2002). All system processing occurs on the server, rather than on the client or local PC, as seen in traditional client/server technology. The thin client is primarily a display, keyboard, and mouse or other pointing device. It sends keystrokes and mouse movements to the server over the network and the server sends back changes in the display. Any PC can serve as a thin client. The minimal hardware requirements for this model give rise to the name "thin client" as opposed to "fat client," as seen in traditional client/server technology. This model helps to reduce hardware costs; older equipment can be used longer and new thin clients cost less than traditional PCs because no local drives or storage devices are required. The absence of local drives and storage also reduces maintenance and administrative costs and facilitates software upgrades. Software resides on the server requiring one upgrade at the server rather than a physical visit to each PC or client. Security is enhanced because users cannot run foreign disks locally that may contain a virus.

The largest and best known network in the world is the **Internet,** also known as the **Net.** The Internet actually consists of thousands of interconnected networks. The Internet was once limited to individuals affiliated with educational institutions and government agencies, but access is now available to the public. Variations of Internet technology are available via intranets and extranets. Both intranets and extranets use software and programming languages designed for the Internet. **Intranets** are private company networks that are protected from outside access. **Extranets,** on the other hand, apply Internet technology to create a network outside of the company system for use by customers or suppliers.

HOW COMPUTERS WORK

Computers receive, process, and store data. They use binary code to represent **alphanumeric** characters, which are numbers and alphabetic characters. **Binary code** is a series of 1s and 0s. All 1s are stored on the disk as magnetized areas and 0s are stored as areas that have not been magnetized. Each 1 or 0 is called a **bit.** Eight bits make up one **byte.** The

Box 2–1   Binary Representation of an Arabic Number

The arabic number 13 is represented using the binary system as 00001101. Each bit (0 or 1) represents a particular power of 2, depending on its position. If the position is taken by a 0, then it has no value. If a position is taken by a 1, it has the value of the associated power of 2. The arabic number represented is the total of the powers of 2 represented by the 0s and 1s.

Binary represention of 13:	0	0	0	0	1	1	0	1
Powers of 2 by bit location:	2^7	2^6	2^5	2^4	2^3	2^2	2^1	2^0
Arabic value of position:	128	64	32	16	8	4	2	1
Actual value of bit:	0 +	0 +	0 +	0 +	8 +	4 +	0 +	1 = 13

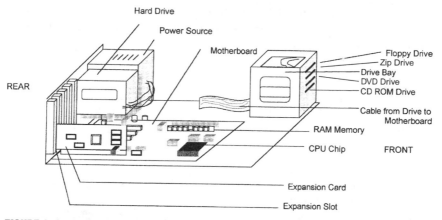

FIGURE 2–3 • Internal view of a PC

unique code for each character is eight bits long. In the code for numeric characters, each position corresponds to a specific power of 2. Box 2–1 provides a binary representation of the number 13.

Computer programs, or software, use binary code to provide the instructions that direct the work computers do. PCs, notebooks, and PDAs differ slightly from supercomputers, mainframe computers, and minicomputers in the structure of their CPU. The CPU in larger computers is generally composed of one or more circuit boards, while smaller computers rely on a **microprocessor chip,** which contains the electronic circuits of the CPU etched on a silicon chip, mounted on a board, otherwise known as the **motherboard.** All electrical components, including the main memory, connect to this board. Figure 2–3 depicts the internal components of a PC. The motherboard also provides slots for network interface cards and peripheral device interface cards. The **network interface card** physically connects a computer to a network, controlling the flow of information between the two.

Likewise, **peripheral device interface cards** connect equipment such as printers to the computer and control the exchange of information. The slot arrangement on motherboard allows users to change or add computer system components easily. Portable or laptop computers can be connected to networks or peripheral devices through the use of a **PCMCIA (Personal Computer Memory Card International Association) card.** These cards can be inserted into a slot, in the case of the laptop computer, to add increased functionality such as additional memory or network connections.

Processor speed is measured in **megahertz** or **gigahertz.** One megahertz (MHz) represents 1 million signal voltage cycles per second. A gigahertz (GHz) represents 1 billion cycles per second. The processor speed determines how rapidly instructions are handled. In general, each new PC model offers a faster CPU speed.

Whenever the power to a PC is turned on, the computer performs a start-up process. The program code for this test is stored in permanent memory and is known as **BIOS (basic input/output system).** The BIOS confirms that information about component parts is present and that this information coincides with existing hardware.

SELECTION CRITERIA

Equipment selection should be based on needs and expectations. When selecting a computer system and related hardware, it is important to consider the following:

- *The types of applications required.* For example, some people use primarily word processing programs, while others need applications to perform numeric calculations.

- *The program execution time and computer capacity needed to process jobs.* Complex jobs require higher processor speed and more memory for timely execution.

- *The number of workers who need computer access at any one time.* Single-user access demands can be met by a PC. Multiple demands for access may be better served by a network.

- *Storage capacity.* Storage needs are determined by the amount of information that must be kept and the length of time that it must be retained.

- *Backup options.* When information stored and processed on computers is critical to conduct daily business, another copy should be available to restore normal services after a crash.

- *Budget considerations.* The cost of hardware and software for various options should be considered in relation to the benefits and limitations associated with each.

- *Maintenance considerations.* There are several issues related to maintenance. These include durability, battery life and time required for recharging batteries, and the ability to easily disinfect or clean equipment to minimize the chances of spreading infection. Infection control may be accomplished via placement of computer equipment in areas away from splatter, the use of handwashing and antimicrobial hand cleaners, keyboard skins, and designated cleaning procedures with periodic cultures of equipment (Devine, Cooke, and Wright 2001; Neely and Sittig 2002).

These factors will help to determine which type of computer or network is the best option, as well as the required hardware features. Advance planning ensures that current and future computer needs are well served.

User Needs

Human factors should be considered in every work environment. Human factors, otherwise known as **ergonomics,** involves the study and design of a work environment that maximizes productivity by reducing operator fatigue and discomfort (The American Heritage Dictionary 2000). Ergonomics considers physical stresses placed on joints, muscles, nerves, and tendons as well as environmental factors that can affect hearing and vision. Poor placement of computer equipment can lead to a number of somatic complaints, including headaches, eye strain, irritation, stress, fatigue, and neck and back pain. **Repetitive stress injuries (RSIs), or repetitive motion injuries,** have also been reported. Repetitive motion injuries result from using the same muscle groups over and over again without rest (Black and Matassarin-Jacobs 1997). One well-known example of a repetitive motion injury is **carpal tunnel syndrome.** Carpal tunnel syndrome occurs when the median nerve is compressed as it passes through the wrist along the pathway to the hand. This compression results in sensory and motor changes to the thumb, index finger, third finger, and radial aspect of the ring finger. Other repetitive motion injuries may involve the neck and shoulders. Good ergonomics can save money by avoiding Workers' Compensation claims and keeping employees productive. Box 2–2 provides a checklist to ensure good ergonomic design when designing and working at computer workstations. Another aspect of ergonomics addresses worker concerns about alleged health risks associated with computer use. The list of alleged health risks includes, but is not limited, to the following: cataracts, conception problems, miscarriage, and/or birth defects. Research has not established any clear links between computer use and these risks. Table 2–2 lists several examples of commercially available ergonomic devices. Controversy exists regarding the degree to which these devices benefit the user and prevent injury.

Physical Constraints

Space is a chronic problem in health care settings. For this reason, workstation planning is less a function of good ergonomics and more a function of finding a place to put the equipment. Ergonomics rarely receives high

Box 2–2	Measures to Ensure Good Ergonomics When Using a Computer-Work Station

Determine how a workstation will be used. Choose optimal settings for the chair, desk, keyboard, and monitor for the person who will use the area or that can easily be adjusted for each user. Adjustments are appropriate when wrists are flat and elbow angle is 90 degrees or more to prevent nerve compression.

Determine the length of time the user will be at the workstation. Individual adjustments are less critical if use is occasional or for very brief periods.

Configure work areas for specific types of equipment. Most workstation desks are designed for PCs rather than notebooks. Use a docking station if needed to ensure proper monitor and keyboard height.

Select sturdy surfaces or furniture with sufficient workspace. Desks should have room to write and use a mouse.

Provide chairs with good lumbar support. Relaxed sitting requires chairs that allow a reclined posture of 100 to 110 degrees.

Educate all workers on the need for good body mechanics when working with computers. Good posture is essential to reduce physical strain whether the individual works from a standing or sitting position.

Position monitors just below eye level approximately one arm's length away. This will help to prevent neck strain, especially for bifocal wearers.

Adjust screen resolution and font size as needed. Sharp screen images help to reduce eye strain.

Periodically look away from the monitor to distant objects. This helps to avoid eye-focusing problems.

Minimize screen glare. Purchase nonglare monitors or place monitors at right angles to windows. Provide blinds or draperies, or adjust area lighting as needed.

Take frequent breaks. Intersperse computer work with other activities to avoid repetitive stress injuries.

Avoid noisy locations. Noise is distracting and stressful.

Place the workstation in a well-ventilated area. Fresh air and a comfortable temperature enhance working conditions.

Use ergonomic devices with caution. Select items that have been researched. Do not continue use if it remains uncomfortable after a trial period. Just because an item carries the label "ergonomic" does not mean that it is beneficial.

---

priority in planning. Provisions should be made for adequate numbers of computers in the clinical setting, located in quiet areas such as conference rooms.

Another major constraint to the installation of computers and networks in any institution centers on wiring and cabling. Adding power lines and cables for network connections to a current work space may prove to be more expensive than building a new work area. This is one reason for the growing popularity of wireless systems.

Table 2–2   Examples of Ergonomic Devices

Device	Purpose
Glare filter	Reduces eyestrain related to glare or light reflected from a monitor and may help make images appear sharper and text easier to read
Negative tilt keyboard	Tilts away from the user with the keyboard below elbow height to allow the user to rest arms, shoulders, neck, and back during pauses in typing
Document holder	Keeps documents at the same height and distance from the user as the monitor, limiting head and neck movement and tension
Ergonomic mouse	Various designs which aim to reduce wrist and hand pain No consistent research findings to support its use
Lumbar support	Maintains the natural curves of the back, minimizing back pain
Wrist rests	May actually increase carpal tunnel pressure unless a broad, flat, firm surface provides a place to rest the palm, not the wrist
Support braces/gloves	May relieve carpal tunnel symptoms when worn at night There are no consistent research findings to support use while typing
Ergonomic keyboards	Split keyboard designed to improve posture Research fails to support the benefit of this device
Foot rest	Encourages proper posture and supports the lower back to keep the pelvis properly tilted

MOBILE AND WIRELESS COMPUTING

The terms **mobile** and **wireless** are often used interchangeably but are not the same. **Mobile computing** uses devices that can be carried or wheeled from place to place. These devices may not have the capability to transmit and receive information while mobile. The user must reestablish a connection periodically to receive updated information or to send collected information to a large computer on the network. This connection may be achieved by plugging into a network port, docking port, or, in the case of some handheld devices, the use of a special cable to communicate with a computer that is connected to the network. Mobile devices may include desktop, specialized workstations or notebook computers on carts as well as some PDAs (Huff 2002). **Wireless devices** are equipped with a special card enabling it to broadcast and receive radio or cellular signals that reach the network via access points (Gillespie 2001a). That network may be wireless or ultimately a traditional network connected by cable. Wireless devices are not tethered by a physical connection such as a cable or telephone line. Wireless devices can continually receive and transmit up-to-date information.

Both mobile and wireless computing have great appeal for several reasons (Briggs 2002; Coonan 2002; Gillespie 2001a); these include:

- *Both technologies bring computing to the bedside.* Bedside computer access allows health care providers and clients to access relevant information at the location that it is needed. Bedside access also eliminates the need to return to a hardwired workstation at the nurses' station, where there may be a wait for access.

- *Cost.* Mobile and wireless technology reduce the number of computers that are needed because the health care worker takes the device with him or her to where it will be used rather than require an administrator to provide a device at a fixed location. Mobile and wireless systems also reduce the costs associated with connecting a traditional network with cables. Installing cable is labor intensive, may disrupt care, and can be difficult to accomplish, particularly in older buildings.

- *Improved data collection.* Computers at the point of care facilitiates the collection of data. Care providers can collect and input data once rather than taking handwritten notes for later entry into a computer.

- *More efficient work processes.* Wireless technology and some redesign of work processes enable health care professionals to work more efficiently. A graphic example is seen with online prescription of drugs. The physician or nurse practitioner can quickly access allergy and drug interaction information and instantly send prescriptions to the hospital or patient's pharmacy without delay or problems with interpretation of handwriting.

- *Error reduction.* Wireless technology has been hailed as a means to prevent errors because it can deliver up-to-date information, provide decision support, and access to reference materials and even applications such as electronic prescriptions.

Until recently, wireless technology was plagued by a lack of interoperability. This obstacle was removed by the adoption of a standard for wireless data transmission, making it possible for all wireless devices manufactured after the adoption of the standard to communicate. Recent advances in processing capability make the PDA particularly attractive because it is small, lightweight, and easy to use.

The advantages associated with mobile and wireless technology also raise concerns (Bowman 2002; Coonan 2002; Gillespie 2001a; Koo 2001). Concerns include:

- *Theft and loss.* These devices are more subject to theft and easy to lose because they are mobile and small enough to carry away. This requires the implementation of safeguards to protect information contained on stolen devices.

- *Threats to data security.* The security of data may be compromised when devices are stolen. The technology used to protect data on wireless networks has been less secure than technology used to encrypt information on traditional, hardwired networks. Vendors have been working on this issue.

- *Battery life.* Battery life varies according to use patterns and processing demands. Around-the-clock use requires close attention to the use of charge units and/or spare batteries.

- *Data loss.* Mobile devices are used to collect and send information to another computer system. Damage to devices, theft, loss, or downtime related to dead batteries may lead to loss of data before it can be shared.

- *Memory limitations.* While advances continue to add to the capability of handheld devices, memory limitations remain an issue, particularly when users expect additional features and capabilities.

- *Limited ability to display and see information.* Small screen size limits the amount of information that can be viewed at one time.

- *Deadzones.* Wireless devices may not be able to transmit and receive information in certain locations.

- *Lack of a means to readily exchange data between hospital information systems and handheld devices.* Physicians typically want clinical information systems available to them on their PDAs. The ability to provide clinical data to handheld devices can be arduous and expensive to develop.

Another concern related to the use of PDAs is that organizations need to develop a comprehensive strategy for their use and support if they do not already have one in place (LaRochelle 2002). Many physicians and other health care providers are purchasing their own PDAs but cannot fully realize benefits associated with their use without organizational plans for PDA use and support. Purchase recommendations from Information Services (IS) staff can help to avert disappointment. Useful information related to PDA use and available applications and databases can be found through the publications and Web sites of professional organizations as well as *PDA Cortex*, an online journal for mobile computing for health care professionals.

SOFTWARE

Software is a set of instructions that tells the computer what to do. **Programs** and **applications** are forms of software. All software is written in **programming languages.** Each programming language provides a detailed set of rules for how to write instructions for the computer. Numerous programming languages exist. A few examples are listed here. COBOL (Common Business Oriented Language) remains popular for business applications. MUMPS (Massachusetts General Hospital Utility Multi-Programming System) is commonly used for health care applications. Ada is a high-level, general-purpose programming language orginally developed for the defense department. Ada supports real-time applications. C is a flexible language that is particularly popular for PCs because it is compact. C++ is a descendent of C. Unlike its predecessor it supports object-oriented programming, which allows reuse of some instructions. C++ is favored for graphical applications in the Windows and Macintosh environments. BASIC

(Beginners All-Purpose Symbolic Instruction Code) is widely found in home computing. Java is a popular language for the development of programs for use on the Internet. Visual Basic is a programming language used for the development of graphical user interfaces. Structured Query Language (SQL) is an example of a programming language that allows the user to query or search a database for specific information.

Several categories of software exist; each has a different purpose. Some major software categories include operating systems, application software, and utility programs.

Operating Systems

The most essential type of software is the **operating system.** The operating system is a collection of programs that manage all of the computer's activities, including the control of hardware, execution of software, and management of information. *Control of hardware* refers to the ability of different parts of the computer to work together. Operating systems allow users to manage information through the retrieval, copying, movement, storage, and deletion of files.

The operating system also provides a user interface. The **user interface** is the means by which the individual interacts with the computer. For many years PC users were required to enter specific text commands. The introduction of Microsoft Windows signaled a move to a **graphical user interface (GUI)** for PC users. A GUI provides a set of menus, windows, and other standard screen devices that are intended to make using a computer as intuitive as possible (Webopedia 2003). GUIs decrease the amount of time required to learn new programs and eliminate the need to memorize computer commands. Work is under way on natural interfaces. The most natural user interface is the voice. Natural user interfaces are expected to free the user from conventional constraints such as mechanical keyboards, pointing devices, and GUIs, thereby making computers easier to use. Significant progress has occurred in recent years. Wireless technology, a highly mobile lifestyle, and advances in interactive voice recognition contribute to the increased use of voice recognition in call centers and for dictation (Colvard and Charles 2002; Fass 2003; Reese 2001). Voice recognition will not replace keyed data for some time yet. There are still limits to the number of words that are recognized and it is necessary to create a model of the user's voice before use. There also is an issue with accuracy, which is less than 100 percent.

Operating systems exist for all categories of computers. MS-DOS (Microsoft Disk Operating System) and Windows represent two popular PC operating systems. Earlier versions of Windows required MS-DOS to operate and were not true operating systems. Windows 95, 98, 2000, Me, XP, and NT are actual operating systems. LINUX is another operating system. **Macintosh computers,** or **Macs,** have their own operating systems. Macs are commercial computers that offer a graphical interface and are available for home and office use. Macs are produced by Apple Computer

Incorporated. Fewer software programs are available for Macs, but adaptations are available that permit Macs to run PC software. UNIX is an operating environment developed in the 1970s that is frequently found on large, commercial mainframe computers.

Application Software

Application software is a set of programs designed to accomplish a particular task such as word processing, financial management, or drawing. Application software builds on the foundation provided by the operating system. Box 2–3 lists some common types of application software and their functions.

Another factor that facilitates computer use is the development of software tutorials and online help. Most software packages now offer tutorials for review before application use, making software much more accessible to first-time users. Help screens are available while the program is running.

Utility Programs

Utility programs help to manage the computer and its data. Early operating systems offered few utility options such as optimization of the hard disk, system backup, or virus checks. To fill this need, a separate category of software evolved. Many utility programs are now included as part of the

---

Box 2–3   **Common Types of PC Software Applications**

- *Word processing.* Allows the creation of documents, utilizing features such as spelling and grammar correction, thesaurus, and graphics or pictures.

- *Presentation graphics.* Supports the preparation of slides and handout materials.

- *Spreadsheet.* Performs calculations, analyzes data, and presents information in tabular format and graphical displays.

- *Database.* Helps to manage large collections of information, such as payroll information, phone directories, and product listing. Performs calculations and produces reports from the stored information. Allows the user to find specific information.

- *Desktop publishing.* Offers expanded features that may not be commonly found in word processing programs. Useful for the creation of newsletters and other publications.

- *Web design.* Allows the user to create or revise Web pages and content that can then be posted to a Web site.

- *Specialized software*
  Project management. Supports the management of projects with identification of tasks and time frames for completion, including PERT (program evaluation review technique) charts.

  Personal information managers. Enhance personal productivity with time management tools, including an appointment calendar, telephone directories, and reminder lists.

  Personnel scheduling. Automates the process of scheduling staff.

operating system. However, users may still choose to install and use utility programs that are independent of their operating systems.

ROLES OF SUPPORT PERSONNEL

Even though PCs have brought computers closer to users, many people remain blissfully ignorant of computer technology beyond what they absolutely need to know. As a result, support is extremely important to maintaining user productivity. For example, PC support costs for large organizations typically range in the thousands of dollars for each computer. Support costs may include time spent planning system upgrades, installation of upgrades for operating systems and various applications, troubleshooting, and user education. With help from support personnel, users can benefit from computers without knowing or understanding how they work.

In addition to personnel who support the computer user, other essential positions are needed by hospitals and health care organizations that use computers and information systems. A **healthcare information system (HIS)** consists of a computer, including associated hardware and software that is dedicated to the collection, storage, processing, retrieval, and communication of information relevant to patient care within a health care organization. Staff are needed to create and maintain networks, customize and maintain software, and provide administration and leadership related to the HIS.

Superuser

The **superuser** has additional computer experience over the average employee and serves as a local resource person. In the hospital setting, the superuser is generally someone who knows the clinical area well and is able to answer most questions from users about the hospital computer system. In some cases the superuser may be involved in user training.

Call Desk and Help Desk Personnel

The **call** or **help desk** is the first line of user support within an organization (Wilk and McCrary 2003). These individuals require good communication skills as well as technical knowledge. A formal process exists for users to contact the call or help desk, usually by telephone or pager. All problems are logged to ensure that proper follow-up and resolution have occurred. If the problem cannot be resolved via telephone, then someone is sent to assist the user.

Microcomputer or PC Specialist

The **PC specialist** provides users with PC information and training, enabling them to perform routine tasks. The PC specialist may also be called on to help users adapt to notebooks and PDAs including aspects of mobile computing. These specialists often have technical training or an associate or a baccalaureate degree in computer science or a related area. PC specialists provide valuable services, but their salaries tend to be lower than those of other support personnel.

Analyst

Health care information system analysts are responsible for a wide range of activities related to the successful automation of information management. They may be clinicians who became involved in system selection and training. Many learned their role on the job and furthered their education by taking computer or information science classes. Analysts interview staff, determine user needs, write specifications for software performance, participate in some computer programming and debugging, implement new automated functions, and document program specifications and changes. Analysts who lack a clinical background may not be paid well initially, but with experience and additional preparation, their earning potential increases.

Clinical Liaison

Clinical liaisons are clinicians who represent the interests and needs of the users and work with the information system team to address these issues during system design and implementation. They may or may not have formal computer or information system training. Liaisons sometimes continue their clinical role while fulfilling this responsibility.

Programmer

Programmers actually write the code, or instructions, that tell the computer what to do. They often lack a clinical background. For this reason, analysts are responsible for communicating user needs to programmers. In some institutions, one individual may serve as both analyst and programmer.

Network Administrator

Network administrators are responsible for the planning, management, and expansion of networks. Network administrators must decide whether to contract with outside agencies for network services and support or to educate in-house personnel for these functions. Unfortunately, many organizations lack a mechanism to coordinate equipment selection among different departments but expect the network manager to get the resulting hodgepodge of equipment linked together. This is particularly true as more users purchase their own devices and expect them to work seamlessly with an existing network. Organizations should involve network administrators in equipment decisions when the ultimate goal involves the creation or expansion of a network. It is possible to become a certified network engineer via special course work and an examination. Network administrators can access all data no matter who owns it. The salaries of network administrators typically exceed those of the personnel discussed thus far.

Trainer

Trainers are responsible for educating clinical users in one or more applications and may also be required to define and monitor user competencies. Trainers may or may not have a clinical background but have knowledge of the specific computer application that they are teaching. This role may be filled as a permanent position or may be done by other information systems or clinical staff, as needed. Some organizations have a separate trainer for common office applications and PC use and another for information systems training.

Security Officer

Security officers are responsible for ensuring that measures exist to protect information privacy (Gillespie 2001b). This usually includes a process for assigning and monitoring system access identification codes and passwords as well as paper-based information. In some cases the security officer may be responsible for protecting the physical equipment and data stored there. Recent federal legislation and interest in data security make this an important role, although there are few full-time security officers at the present. Strategic planning, risk management, and the development of corporate wide policies and procedures are increasingly a part of the security office role. Security officers also need to educate administrators, physicians, and staff about security issues. The use of the Internet in health care means that the security officer must protect corporate information systems from outside threats in addition to protecting information found solely on desktop systems.

Chief Information Officer

The **chief information officer (CIO)** should have a broad view of the needs of the institution and the design, implementation, and evaluation of information systems. Responsibilities include strategic planning, policy development, budgeting, information security, recruitment and retention of information services staff, and overall management of the enterprise's information systems (Hagland 2001a; Kelly 2001). In some agencies the information services department is responsible for all computers and computer training. In recent years there has been a shift from chief technology officer to CIO as more CIOs play a greater role in developing their organization's strategies. The CIO is at the top of the compensation heap for computer-related positions. Preparation is usually at a master's or doctoral degree level.

Webmaster

The **Webmaster** is generally responsible for the design, maintenance, and security of materials placed on the Internet, intranet, and/or extranet. Growing concerns over information security, expanded use of Internet technology, and federal mandates require increased collaboration with other roles.

Chief Privacy Officer

Federal legislation mandates that each patient care organization name a **chief privacy officer (CPO)** to protect the personal health information of patients (Hagland 2001b). This includes paper and electronic information. At this time, there are uncertainties about the definition of the role, qualifications, its place within the organization, and compensation. The American Health Information Management Association (AHIMA) has published a sample job description and posted it on their Web site. AHIMA proposes that the health information management professional is uniquely qualified to serve as privacy officer through their professional preparation, experience, commitment to patient advocacy, and professional code of ethics. Given staffing constraints, it is likely that this role will be added to other responsibilities for a medical records or information services manager.

Chief E-health Officer

The role of **chief e-health officer (CeO)** exists in organizations that are expanding their use of the Internet beyond Web sites that provide information to a strategy that includes interactive services (Goedert 2001). An understanding of what the Internet can do for an organization is a prerequisite. There have been some questions as to whether e-health and this role are more fads than an emerging trend given the fact that e-health has failed to meet projections for its success (Marhula 2003).

Compliance Officer

The role of **compliance officer** is emerging in many organizations as one person is designated to ensure that state and federal regulations and accrediting requirements are met both via paper and automated records and systems. It may or may not be assumed by a member of the information services department but the professional preparation and experience of information services professionals provides an advantage. Many information services personnel believe that compliance is more of an educational issue than a systems issue.

Disaster Planning and Recovery Officer

Disaster planning is an essential component of strategic planning that needs to extend beyond the walls of any one institution. To ensure that plans are up-to-date and that all contingencies have been covered, one person should be designated to coordinate and update plans for natural and man-made disasters, including acts of terrorism.

Interface Engineer

Any health care organization is typically composed of many different information systems. The majority of these systems were not specifically designed to work with other systems. The interface engineer ensures that information is exchanged between disparate systems and isolates and corrects problems behind the scenes invisible to the users of the individual systems.

CASE STUDY EXERCISES

You are appointed to the hospital's information technology committee as the representative for your nursing unit. The charges of the committee include the following:

- Identify PC software that is needed to accomplish unit work, such as word processing, spreadsheets, and databases.
- Determine criteria for the selection and placement of hardware on the units.

Discuss these issues and how they affect patient care and workflow.

• • •

Your committee is charged with setting up a computer system that will automate transcription of physician orders and reporting of results. Identify the support personnel that you need at this point and write job descriptions for each identified position.

• • •

The infection control nurse has traced the spread of a nosocomial infection to a computer keyboard on a hospital unit. It is located in a work area adjacent to four patient rooms. This computer is routinely used by staff for documentation, to check laboratory and radiology results, and to access reference materials. The infection control nurse has asked the unit director and staff to identify strategies to eliminate this problem. Identify measures that can help to eliminate this problem.

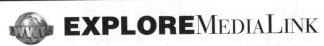

EXPLOREMEDIALINK

Multiple choice, review questions, case studies, and other interactive resources for this chapter can be found on the Web site at *http://www.prenhall.com/hebda*. Click on "Chapter 2" to select the activities for this chapter.

SUMMARY

- Computers are machines that process data under the direction of a program, or stored sequence of instructions.

- The major hardware components of computers are input devices, the CPU, secondary storage, and output devices.

- The major categories of computers are: supercomputers, mainframes, minicomputers, PCs or desktop systems, laptop or notebook computers, and tablet computers and handheld devices.

- Peripheral hardware items, such as the keyboard, mouse, monitor, modem, and printer, help the user put data into the computer, read output, and communicate with other users.

- Networks are linked systems of computers. LANs, WANs, and the Internet are all types of computer networks.

- Networks may use various technologies including cabling, radio signals, client/server, and thin client.

- In choosing a computer system, one must consider current and future information processing needs, budget, and human factors.

- Good ergonomics may reduce physical discomforts and injury associated with computer use.

- Mobile and handheld computer technology provide the promise of efficiency, improvements in the safety of care delivery, cost savings, and work redesign.

- Software is the set of instructions that make a computer run and control its resources. Operating systems, applications, utility programs, and programming languages are all types of software.

- Many institutions use support personnel to help people use computers effectively and to maintain and upgrade hardware and software.

REFERENCES

Black, J. M., and Matassarin-Jacobs, E. (1997). *Medical surgical nursing: Clinical management for continuity of care* (5th ed.). Philadelphia: Saunders.

Bowman, B. (2002). Health care's wireless expectations. *Advance for Health Information Executives, 6*(2), 46–48, 50.

Briggs, B. (2002). Is the future in the palm of your hand? *Health Data Management, 19*(1), 44–46, 50, 52, 54, 56, 60, 62.

Colvard, M., and Charles, S. (2002). Inching ahead with voice recognition. *Review of Ophthalmology, 9*(10). Available online at: http://www.revophth.com/index.asp?page=1_203.htm. Accessed January 18, 2003.

Coonan, G. M. (2002). Making the most of mobility. *Health Management Technology 23*(10), 32, 36–37.(10), 42.

Devine, J., Cooke, R. P., and Wright, E. P. (2001). Is methicillin-resistant Staphylococcus aureus (MRSA) contamination of ward-based computer terminals a surrogate marker for nosocomial MRSA transmission and hand-washing compliance? *The Journal of Hospital Infection*, *48*(1), 72–75.

Fass, A. (2003). Speak easy. *Forbes*, *171*(1), 135.

Gillespie, G. (2001a). Wireless catching up, catching on in health care. *Health Data Management*, *9*(8), 26–28, 30, 32, 34.

Gillespie, G. (2001b). Juggling skills a must for health care CSOs. *Health Data Management*, *9*(1), 50–52, 54, 56.

Goedert, J. (2001). Health care welcomes new CeOs. *Health Data Management*, *9*(2), 92–94, 96, 98.

Hagland, M. (2001a). Hire ups. *Healthcare Informatics*, *18*(3), 34–36, 38, 40.

Hagland, M. (2001b). The elusive CPO. *Healthcare Informatics*, *18*(7), 26–29.

Hochhauser, M. (March 18, 2002). It's a PDA! It's a phone! It's a data-enabled cell phone! *Network Computing*, *13*(6), 98.

Huff, J. W. (2002). Bringing in the COWS. *ADVANCE for Health Information Executives*, *6*(10), 47–48, 50.

Kelly, B. (2001). Retain staff is key to success. *Health Data Management*, *9*(1), 94, 96, 98.

Keplar, K. E., and Urbanski, C. J. (February 2003). Personal digital assistant applications for the healthcare provider. *The Annals of Pharmacotherapy*, *37*(2), 287–296.

Koo, C. (2001). Looking for the right fit. *ADVANCE for Health Information Executives*, *5*(5), 49–50, 52.

LaRochelle, B. (2002). Beyond vertical applications. *ADVANCE for Health Information Executives*, *6*(7), 66.

Lewis, J. A., and Sommers, C. O. (March–April 2003). Personal data assistants: Using new technology to enhance nursing practice. *MCN The American Journal of Maternal Child Nursing*. *28*(2), 66–71.

MacVittie, L. (February 18, 2002). Progear's an easy to swallow tablet. *Network Computing*, *13*(4), 61.

Marhula, D. C. (2003). Is e-health fact or fiction? *Healthcare Informatics*, *20*(1), 56–58.

Mitchell, R. L. (February 4, 2002). Thinfrastructure. *Computerworld*, *36*(6), 40.

Neely, A. N., and Sittig, D. F. (July 23, 2002). Basic microbiologic and infection control information to reduce the potential transmission of pathogens to patients via computer hardware. *Journal of the American Medical Informatics Association*, *9*, 500–508.

New products (November 2002). *District Administration*, *38*(11), 57.

Rand, D., Witt, C., Hunger, H., and Gulle, D. (September 2002). How thin will you go? *ADVANCE for Health Information Executives*, *6*(9), 20–21.

Reese, S. (July 19, 2001). Interactive voice response systems gaining importance. *New Straits Times-Management Times*.

Schuerenberg, B. (February 2003). When Goliath can't help, David does the job. *Health Data Management*, *11*(2), 72–80.

Schuyler, M. (March 2003). PDA Avoidance: They'll get you eventually! *Computers in Libraries, 23*(3), 32.

Seltzer, L. (January 15, 2002). Thin-client technology. *PC Magazine, 21*(1), 126.

The American Heritage Dictionary of the English Language (4th ed.). (2000). Boston: Houghton Mifflin Company. Available online at: http://dictionary.reference.com/search?q=ergonomics. Accessed January 8, 2003.

Webopedia. (2003). Graphical user interface. Jupitermedia Corporation. Available online at: http://webopaedia.com/TERM/G/Graphical_User_Interface_GUI.html. Accessed January 10, 2003.

Wilk, T., and McCrary, J. (2003). Getting serious about IT customers. *ADVANCE for Health Information Executives, 6*(10), 35–40.

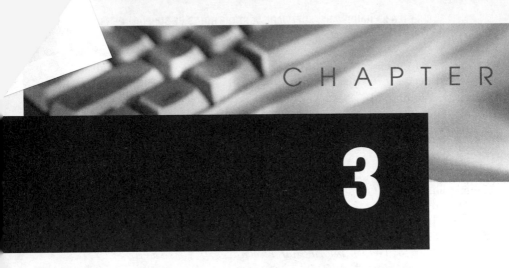

CHAPTER 3

Ensuring the Quality of Information

After completing this chapter, you should be able to:

- Define *data integrity* and its relevance for health care.
- Discuss the relevance of data management for data integrity.
- Identify strategies to ensure the accuracy of data.
- Differentiate between online and offline data storage.
- Explain how storage conditions can affect data integrity.
- Debate the relative benefits of outsourcing data storage.

- Discuss the factors that should be addressed when planning for data retrieval.
- Identify characteristics associated with quality information.
- Define *data mining* and discuss its use within health care.
- Discuss the significance of data cleansing for data warehousing and data mining.

 MEDIALINK

Additional resources for this content can be found on the Companion Website at *www. prenhall.com/hebda*. Click on "Chapter 3" to select the activities for this chapter.

Companion Website

- Glossary
- Multiple Choice
- Discussion Points
- Case Study: Accurate Data Entry
- Case Study: Correct Data Collection
- Case Study: Data Storage
- MediaLink Application: Outsourcing Data
- Web Hunt: Outsourcing
- Links to Resources
- Crossword Puzzle

D
ata provides the building blocks in the formation of knowledge. For this reason it is essential to understand the concepts of data integrity, principles of good data management, the characteristics of quality data, and the significance of data mining.

DATA INTEGRITY

Data integrity refers to the ability to collect, store, and retrieve correct, complete, and current data so it will be available to authorized users when needed. Data integrity is one of the most important issues related to computing and information handling in health care because treatment decisions are based on information derived from data. If the data are faulty or incomplete, the quality of derived information may be poor, resulting in decisions that may be inappropriate and possibly harmful to clients. For example, if the nurse interviewing a client collects data related to allergies but fails to document all reported allergies, the client may be given drugs that cause an allergic reaction. In this case, the data were collected but not stored properly.

Ensuring Correct Data Collection and Entry

Computer systems facilitate data collection but may increase the potential for entry of incorrect data through input errors. These errors may include hitting the wrong key on a computer keyboard, selecting the wrong item from a screen using touch or a mouse, or failing to enter all data collected. Several measures can be taken to decrease the likelihood of input errors, including educating personnel, conducting system checks, and verifying data.

Educating Personnel Staff who are proficient in the use of the input device and computer system are less likely to make data collection and entry errors (Wright and Bartram 2000). All personnel should attend classes that emphasize appropriate system access, input device use, potential harmful effects associated with incorrect data, data verification techniques, and error correction. On the completion of classes, all employees should demonstrate competence in system use. Even after staff have shown competence, continuing education should occur on a routine basis and as indicated by problems such as increases in data errors.

System Checks to Ensure Accurate Data Entry and Data Completeness Data entry systems should be easy to use and provide periodic checks to ascertain that data are correct and complete. A **system check** is a mechanism provided by the computer system to assist users by prompting them to complete a task, verify information, or prevent entry of inappropriate information. Computer systems facilitate data collection and verification in several ways. Examples of computer system safeguards and generated prompts include the following:

- *Data cleansing technology.* This software was originally developed to eliminate variations in name and address information for direct mail campaigns that led to multiple mailings for the same party (Faden 2000). When used at the point of data entry, it serves to prevent data input errors. This is best illustrated when the system asks the user to confirm whether there is a match already in the database for a patient, thereby eliminating duplicate entries with several variants in name or address.

- *Requesting information about a client's allergies when no entry has been made regarding allergies.* In the absence of an entry regarding allergies, the system may not accept medication and radiology orders.

- *Informing the user that an order already exists when the user attempts to enter a duplicate order.* The system requests verification before processing the duplicate order. This can prevent unintentional repetition of expensive diagnostic tests. For example, a physician previously ordered a complete blood count (CBC) to be drawn on the current day. Another physician has ordered a hemoglobin and hematocrit (H & H), also to be drawn on the current day. When the order for the H & H is entered into the computer, the system will alert the user that this is a duplicate order, because the H & H is part of the CBC.

- *Producing printouts alerting the nurse that a prescribed medication has not been documented as given.* This improves the quality of client care and documentation.

Data Verification Techniques Another means to ensure data accuracy is to have clients verify data that are collected during the admission and assessment processes (Brennan 1996). The active participation of the client in the data verification process remains a relatively new concept in relation to health care computer systems. This verification may be accomplished through one of the following methods:

- Verbal confirmation
- Asking clients to review data on selected screens
- Asking clients to review printouts of entered data

Each of these methods has potential problems. For example, with verbal confirmation clients may answer "yes" without actually hearing or understanding what was said to them. Screen review is difficult for the visually impaired or may be done too quickly for the client to scan all information. Finally, reading printouts is impractical for the visually impaired or illiterate. It also creates the additional problem of papers that must be disposed of with consideration for their confidential nature. All methods may be problematic for the individual who does not speak English.

Although the initial data collection and entry process provides an excellent opportunity to verify data accuracy and completeness, it should not be the only time that this is done. Health care consumers should be able to review their records at any time and furnish additional information that they believe is important to their care or to dispute portions of their record with which they do not agree. Recent federal legislation ensures these rights (Hicks 2001).

How to Minimize Fraudulent Information   Another concern in the concept of data integrity is the entry of fraudulent information. Fraudulent information can lead to financial loss to the provider and third-party payer as well as sully the credit rating of an innocent victim whose identity and insurance information were used. It may also result in treatment errors. At present, admitting clerks and physician office staff ask for the client's insurance card at the time of treatment. This request should also include proof of identification, preferably photograph identification, as a means to decrease claims filed under another person's identity. Clients should be informed of the purpose of this request and sign a statement indicating that they are aware that insurance fraud is a criminal act and that use of another person's insurance data may result in bodily harm secondary to treatment decisions based on someone else's health record.

DATA MANAGEMENT

The changing health care delivery system provides the driving force for improved data management. **Data management** is the process of controlling the collection, storage, retrieval, and use of data to optimize accuracy and utility while safeguarding integrity. Computers are an essential tool in this process. Good data management is essential for organizational decision making and is sometimes referred to as business intelligence (BI) (Kolar 2001). One important part of decision making is the distribution of information via reports. Good data management involves knowing who needs report information, what reports are generated and what they are called, and when reports are available (Liebmann 2000).

Several levels of personnel are involved in data management. Personnel at the point of data entry include employees and, in some cases, clients. System analysts help the users to specify the data that are to be collected and how this will be accomplished. Programmers create the computer instructions or program that will collect the required data. They also build the **database,** a file structure that supports the storage of data in an organized fashion and allows data retrieval as meaningful information. Some facilities may also employ a **database administrator (DBA),** who is responsible for overseeing all activities related to maintaining the database and optimizing its use.

A **relational database** is designed using data that are represented as tables. This type of database is easily updated and can provide specific information to answer a query. Additional types of databases may be used as well. A **data warehouse** provides an even more powerful method of managing and analyzing data. A data warehouse is a repository for storing data from several different databases so that it can be combined and manipulated to provide answers to complex analytic questions (Benander and Benander 2000).

Costs and benefits are additional considerations in the management of data. Storage and management of paper and film records are labor intensive and expensive. Retrieval of paper and film records must be done manually, and information may not be available when and where it is needed. Physical records are also subject to loss. One current solution is **document imaging,** which involves scanning paper records onto computer disks or other media to facilitate electronic storage and handling (Bizzell 2002; Documented Savings 2001). Converting paper records to other storage media may facilitate management, but a better solution is to move away from paper, with data entered directly to automated records. Although automated solutions may also be costly, they provide increased efficiency and improved access.

Automation of health care records creates new issues related to data storage and retrieval. Recent estimates project that PC, network, and mainframe storage requirements will grow 50% per year. Along with an increase in volume and types of materials for storage, data storage and retrieval require special conditions to ensure data integrity.

Data Storage

There are two basic types of data storage: online and offline. **Online storage** provides access to current data. Online storage is rapid, using high-speed hard disk drives or storage space allocated on the network. **Offline storage** is used for data that are needed less frequently, or for long-term data storage, as may occur with old client records. Offline storage can be done on any secondary storage device. Access to data stored offline is slower than with online storage. Immediacy of need for particular data is a key factor in determining whether it is stored online or offline. Table 3–1 describes various types of storage media, along with their advantages and disadvantages.

To protect computerized information, organizations need a storage strategy that addresses the following issues (Digital Preservation Coalition 2002):

- *Environmental conditions and physical hazards.* These include temperature, humidity, shock, dust control, and protection from damage by fire, water, or electromagnetic fields. Some media are more sensitive to environmental factors than others. Strict environmental controls protect the storage media and the data it contains. In general, temperatures in the 10°C range in conjunction with ideal environmental conditions help to maximize the shelf life for media.

Table 3–1 Storage Media

Type	Description	Advantages	Disadvantages
Optical media	A laser is used to alter the recording surface, which is then read as data	High data capacities Two major types: WORM (write once read many) and rewritable WORM: Does not use previously written sectors Difficult to alter Provides good data protection Identification is stamped into disks at production Sets aside corrupt data sectors May be accessed repeatedly over 30-year shelf life	Readable only in specific drives Disc swaps may be time-consuming Use of high-capacity discs decrease number of swaps and increases retrieval performance Limited expectations for future use as the price and perfor- mance for other media continue to improve Media subject to damage through poor handling or storage
Removable/portable hard drives	Easily removable from computer "docking bays"	Quick	Requires plug-and-play
Compact disc recordable (CD-R)	Inexpensive optical variant	Fairly large storage capacity	Slow
Compact disc read only memory (CD-ROM)	CD-R uses a light-sensitive dye layer as the data layer CD-ROM uses a series of pits and plateau in a metallic layer	Requires little storage space May have a shelf life of 3 months, and up to 75 years assuming ideal storage conditions and limited use	Not feasible for large-scale data storage CD-R technology less stable than CD-ROM
DVD	Inexpensive Can store up to 18 GB	Large storage capacity Requires little storage space Affords backward compatibility with CD-ROM discs Suitable for storage of data, images and sound May have a shelf life of 2 to 75 years contingent on storage conditions and use	Standardization in devices not reached

(continued)

Table 3–1	Storage Media—*continued*		
Type	**Description**	**Advantages**	**Disadvantages**
Redundant array of disks (RAID)	Uses two or more hard drives connected together to mirror data on duplicate drives	Very safe storage method Provides better performance at a better price than optical technology	Requires purchase of twice the needed storage
Magneto-optical	Uses a special alloy layer modified by a magnetic field later read by laser	Durable and transportable Rewritable Thirty-year shelf life	Slow search time
Magnetic tape or cartridges	The magnetic field on the media surface is altered using tiny electromagnets to "write" the data	Traditional mainframe storage media Inexpensive Available in several formats Can store large amounts of information Easy to duplicate and move to another location Reusable One to 75-year shelf life contingent on storage conditions and use	Slow May be difficult to use Backup requires verification Tape drives require maintenance Can be damaged by exposure to dust, electromagnetic fields, moisture Store under climate-controlled conditions, 20° to 22° C Minimize unnecessary handling to reduce wear

- *Control of equipment and media.* This refers to who may access computer equipment and data and is supported through a combination of physical and logical restrictions. Physical restrictions maintain a secure locked environment for the computer hardware and operations areas. Logical restrictions limit data access to only those staff who require this information. For example, admission clerks might be restricted from accessing clinical information such as test results but might be able to access demographic and insurance information.
- *Contingency planning.* A secondary or backup copy of the data is created as a safeguard in the event of loss or damage to the primary data. This backup copy should be stored at another location separate

from the computer, reducing the danger that a disaster will affect both the computer and the storage area.

- *Storage period for each record type.* The minimum length of time that client records must be stored is dictated by state laws. An organization may choose to retain records indefinitely, but cost and physical storage constraints must be considered.

- *Plans to transfer data to new media before degradation occurs.* For example, data stored on magnetic tape may degrade after 1 to 50 years, depending on storage conditions. If the organization intends to retain records indefinitely, the data must be transferred to other media.

- *Recognition that most electronic media will be threatened by the obsolescence of the hardware and software needed to access them.* Rapid advances in technology lead to the discontinuation of formats and media as more efficient storage modalities are introduced.

- *Maintenance of access devices.* Problems with access devices are one of the most common causes of damage to magnetic storage media. Consideration should be given to writing and reading archive copies from different devices as a means to protect against data loss from malfunctioning devices.

Outsourcing Data Management and Storage

Internal data storage is costly in terms of human resources and space that can be allocated for other purposes. Storage costs include the purchase price for devices and the costs of media, maintenance, and environmental control. These costs may consume a significant portion of the information services budget. Storage can be handled internally or outsourced. **Outsourcing** is the process by which an organization contracts with outside agencies for services. Outsourcing provides a means to cut costs that would otherwise be required for the physical space, special conditions, and support personnel needed to maintain storage media and data.

Outsourcing companies specialize in all aspects of data management for multiple customers, providing services at a lower cost than if the customers performed the tasks themselves. It is important to review the contract to ensure that the outsourcing company can meet all of the institution's requirements for data storage and retrieval.

Data Retrieval

Data retrieval is a process that allows the user to access previously collected and stored data. Data retrieval most commonly occurs as a function of a software application in conjunction with secondary storage media. Recent developments in technology have cut storage costs and improved access and capacity. In addition to new options in storage media, a variety of automated devices are available that provide access to stored data. Automated magnetic tape has been used to archive health care data for many years.

The significance of data retrieval may be seen in the development of an automated client record that covers the client's life span. Although these advances are critical to the development of a birth-to-death health record, many providers are still in the first phases of developing systems for each client visit and have limited archival access. Furthermore, present hospital data storage systems save data but often lack the ability to manipulate data to demonstrate patterns. For example, it should be possible to easily extract demographic data on the population served, individual and aggregate responses to specific treatment modalities, or abnormal laboratory values for a given client.

The following factors should be considered when planning for data retrieval:

- *Performance.* Performance refers to the ability of the system to respond to user requests for data retrieval. Some of the specific factors that define performance include acceptable retrieval response time and the ability to accommodate numerous simultaneous requests for data.

- *Capacity.* Capacity is the number and size of records that can be stored and retrieved.

- *Data security.* Data must be protected against unauthorized access and retrieval.

- *Cost.* The costs include hardware, software, and support personnel. Data storage and retrieval costs overlap in many cases.

Retrieval needs are frequently underestimated. For example, some systems sharply limit the amount of archival data available to users and may impede treatment. Determination of system performance requirements helps data management personnel and administrators choose storage and retrieval strategies for user needs. Generally, record demand is highest soon after data are collected, with the number of access requests and need for rapid retrieval diminishing with the passage of time.

Data Exchange

In the past, data retrieval was primarily performed for use within a single institution. Changes in the health care delivery system now mandate exchange of client information between institutions. For example, a client may have surgery at a major medical center but have follow-up appointments at a satellite location. The client's record must be accessible to clinicians at both sites. Several other factors contribute to the need to send client records in a timely fashion from one provider to another and to submit reimbursement claims in a timely fashion. These factors include, but are not limited to, a highly mobile population and consumer demands for efficiency. As the number of automated client record systems increases, so does the need to establish standard record structure and identifiers for individual data items to facilitate **electronic data interchange (EDI).** EDI is the communication of data in binary code from one computer to another.

Although EDI facilitates record exchange, there are problems associated with it. A major problem is that different computer systems use different formats for data. The data format from the sending system may not be understood by the receiving system. One solution to this problem is the development of a standard data format for EDI. At the present, no agreement exists among health care groups in the United States regarding a common EDI standard. Several groups are currently working toward a common standard. One proposed solution is **Health Level 7 (HL7)**. HL7 is both the name of the group and a standard for the exchange of clinical data. HL7 has an extensive set of rules that apply to all data sent.

CHARACTERISTICS OF QUALITY INFORMATION

If the recommended procedures for data collection, validation, storage, management, and retrieval are followed, then the end result is quality information. The significance of quality information is its potential impact on client care. High-quality information is needed by clinicians to make appropriate clinical decisions. In addition, quality information supports the ability of researchers to contribute to nursing science and the ability of health care administrators to perform outcomes analysis as a means to capture cost savings (Dakins 2001). The following characteristics describe quality information (Burke 1992; Kahn 1995; Tozor 1994; Zorkoczy and Heap 1995):

- *Timely.* Information is available when it is needed. The ability to access the client's insurance information at the time of an outpatient visit allows timely verification of coverage for specified procedures.

- *Precise.* Each detail is complete and clear. An example of a lack of precision is the client's report of previous "abdominal surgery." Precise data would be the identification of the specific surgical procedure, such as appendectomy.

- *Accurate.* Information is without error. An example of inaccurate data is documentation of the wrong leg in a below-the-knee amputation.

- *Numerically quantifiable.* The ability to measure data improves quality. An example is seen with the ability to measure and stage a decubitus ulcer, which aids the subsequent assessment of its status by other professionals.

- *Verifiable by independent means.* Two different people can make the same observation and report the same result. If two people listen to a client's apical heart rate simultaneously, they should both report the same rate.

- *Rapidly and easily available.* For example, the nurse can quickly retrieve a client's allergies from a past medical record stored by the computer system when a critically ill patient arrives in the emergency department.

- *Free from bias, or modification with the intent to influence recipients.* Data should be based on objective rather than subjective evaluation. Documenting that a client is depressed represents subjective interpretation. A better approach is to document observations about the client's activity level and interactions with others. These are quality data.
- *Comprehensive.* Required information is present. When a nurse asks a client for a list of current medications, it should include medication name, dosage, and frequency taken.
- *Appropriate to the user's needs.* Different users have different data needs. The appropriate data must be available for each user. For example, the nurse must be able to access data related to a client's previous diabetic teaching.
- *Clear.* Information is free from ambiguity, reducing the likelihood of treatment errors. An example is seen in the client's report of an allergy to eggs. On questioning, the nurse determines that the client only dislikes eggs and does not wish to be served them but has never had a truly allergic response.
- *Reliable regardless of who collects it.* There may be certain data that multiple professionals collect. Client allergies may be documented by the nurse, physician, and pharmacist. All documentation of allergies should agree.
- *Current.* All files should contain the most current information available to the health care team. For information to be kept current, a regular system for updating must be put in place. Having current information available on the computer will help avoid errors that could be harmful to clients. For example, data retrieved at an outpatient setting should include all recent inpatient data that is pertinent, not just the most recent outpatient data.
- *In a convenient form for interpretation, classification, storage, retrieval, and updates.* The user must be able to access and use the data without difficulty.

Quality is also an issue when large amounts of data on different computer types and using different formats must be extracted for storage or analysis (Faden 2000). Format variations can accentuate inaccuracies and erode data quality, particularly as the number of databases and the age of the stored data increase. For example, a client may have been registered and treated at one hospital a number of times, using a slightly different version of the client's name for each registration. One registration may have been created using a client's legal name, another using a nickname, and another omitting a middle initial. There also may have been a change in address during this period. It can be difficult in this instance to verify that all records belong to the same person; until recently, each record had to be examined individually for error. Software tools can now perform this task. The data source that

Box 3–1 | **Threats to Information Quality, Availability, and Confidentiality**

Threats to Information Quality

- *Alteration of files.* The accidental or intentional addition or change of data erodes the quality of the information. Accidental changes are known as data corruption. Intentional changes are viewed as forgery.

- *System alteration.* When systems are changed, the way that data are processed may be affected. For example, the addition of a new function may result in the loss of data due to planning or programming deficiencies.

- *Introduction of viruses, Trojans, or worms.* Viruses, Trojans, and worms are unwanted programs, created with malicious intent, that can damage, steal, or destroy data. These programs may be inadvertently introduced to a computer via infected disks or downloaded from another system or the Internet.

Threats to Information Availability

- *Destruction of hardware, software, and/or data.* This may occur through natural or manmade disasters or through lack of attention to environmental conditions and security.

- *Interruptions in power or radiofrequency disruption.* Interruptions in the processing of data may result in data loss.

- *Denial of service.* Malicious programs can overwhelm Web sites with the result that access to Internet-based health care information is impaired.

- *Sabotage.* Sabotage is the intentional destruction of hardware, software, or data. Potential sabotage should be considered in the design of security measures.

Threats to Confidentiality

- *Failure to adhere to information policies.* Misuse of computer access and inappropriate disclosure of information threaten confidentiality.

- *Eavesdropping.* Eavesdropping may involve unauthorized access to information, either looking at the system directly or reading confidential printouts. Security measures must limit computer access to authorized persons and provide appropriate guidelines for the handling and disposal of confidential printouts.

- *Unauthorized reception of wireless network technology transmissions.* The reception of radiofrequency transmission used in some wireless networks may provide another opportunity to eavesdrop. The use of technology safeguards, including coding data and changing frequencies, may minimize this threat.

---

is most likely to be correct is used for this purpose. Box 3–1 lists a summary of threats to quality, availability, and confidentiality of information.

DATA MINING

Data mining is a technique that uses software to look for hidden patterns and relationships in large groups of data. Data mining has been used in business to identify customer interests and marketing trends and has subsequently been embraced in the health care industry. Data mining is used in health care to identify successful standardized treatments for specific diseases, track performance, and chart quality improvement (Dakins 2001; Gillespie 2000; Kolar 2001). It does not look for specific answers to specific questions but allows users to sort and compare data in many different ways to discover relationships. One large advantage of data mining is that it can help to capture significant cost savings. Its power as a tool makes data mining a key component in business planning. Although data mining is now easier to use, the lack of standardized clinical language and work processes serve as roadblocks because both contribute to a lack of clean data needed for effective mining. TrendStar is an example of a data mining application used in health care. It is a product of the McKesson HBOC corporation, a major vendor of health information systems.

DATA CLEANSING

The first step in data cleansing is determining the extent of the problem. This can help users to decide where to focus their efforts for quality improvement for the input of new data as well as data that have already been collected. Manual review and correction of poor-quality data are extremely labor intensive. **Data cleansing** or **scrubbing** is a procedure that uses software to improve the quality of data to ensure that it is accurate enough for use in data mining and warehousing (Faden 2000). It uses technology to reconcile data inconsistencies that arise from different systems as well as duplicate entries in one system. These inconsistencies may include typographical errors, misspellings, and various abbreviations as well as address changes. According to Boyle and Cunningham (2002), data errors may be found in nearly one third of clinical records. The fact that abbreviations can have totally different meanings in different systems becomes a major problem with data warehousing. Another problem is the use of automatic defaults, which fill in blanks with information that is not accurate. One example is seen when the name of the ordering physician is "defaulted in" for the primary physician when it is not the same. Data cleansing is essential to data warehousing. Data inconsistencies that did not pose problems for daily operations do create a problem for data warehousing because it requires a higher quality data.

The use of the Internet technology for data entry by employees as well as clients serves to minimize some problems but accentuate others. This is because employees can be trained in data entry and can be called back for additional training if problems are noted. Clients have not had the benefit of system training to know what constitutes acceptable entries and may not have the incentive to correct errors in some cases. The use of data cleansing technology was once limited by its high costs and difficulties in implementation but improvements in the quality of data can improve safety and save money through elimination of duplication.

CASE STUDY EXERCISES

Agnes Gibbons was admitted through the hospital's emergency department in congestive heart failure. During her admission she was asked to verbally acknowledge whether her demographic data were correct. Ms. Gibbons did so. Extensive diagnostic tests were done, including radiology studies. It was later discovered that all of Ms. Gibbons' information had been entered into another client's file. How would you correct this situation? What departments, or other agencies, would need to be informed of this situation?

• • •

A non–English-speaking Vietnamese man was admitted through the emergency department with suspected tuberculosis (TB). The system carried information under his name. Mr. Nguyen nodded his head when the admitting clerk pointed to the demographic screen. Mr. Nguyen was tested and treated for TB. When the public health nurse went to Mr. Nguyen's address for follow-up, the man there was not the Mr. Nguyen who had been treated for TB. How would you address this problem? Explain your rationale.

• • •

You volunteered to serve on a committee to identify information from prior admissions that would be helpful to staff caring for current inpatients. What information, if any, would you select for ready access, and how long would you recommend that it remain active in the system? Remember that your system has limited capacity so that items must be carefully selected and prioritized. Identify the priority assigned to each item and provide your rationale for this priority.

 EXPLOREMEDIALINK

Multiple choice, review questions, case studies, and other interactive resources for this chapter can be found on the Web site at *http://www.prenhall.com/hebda*. Click on "Chapter 3" to select the activities for this chapter.

SUMMARY

- Data can be managed using a database application.
- A data warehouse is a collection of several databases that can be manipulated to provide complex data analysis.
- Information quality is ensured when measures to protect it are an integral part of its collection, use, storage, retrieval, and exchange.

- Data integrity strategies should provide safeguards against data manipulation or deletion, and entry of fraudulent facts.
- Data storage measures should provide safe, accessible storage to authorized persons through a plan that considers provider, client, and third-party payer needs; physical threats to information and media; performance requirements; pros and cons of on-site versus off-site storage; technological advancements; and future needs.
- Performance, capacity, data security, and cost should be considered when planning for data retrieval.
- Electronic data interchange standards provide timely access to providers at distant sites and computer systems.
- Quality information is essential to the delivery of appropriate client care.
- Data mining uses software to look for hidden patterns and relationships in large groups of data such as performance information and successful treatments for specific diseases. It allows users to sort and compare data in many different ways to discover relationships.
- Data cleansing uses software to improve the quality of data to ensure that it is suitable for all purposes including data mining and warehousing.

REFERENCES

Benander, A., and Benander, B. (2000). Data warehouse administration and management. *Information System Management. 17*(1), 71.

Bizzell, K. (2002). A giant step forward. *Health Management Technology, 23*(10), 56.

Boyle, D. I. R., and Cunningham, S. G. (2002). Resolving fundamental quality issues in linked datasets for clinical care. *Health Informatics Journal, 8*(1), 73.

Brennan, P. (1996). *Nursing informatics: Technology in the service of patient care.* Continuing education activity of West Virginia University Hospital, Morgantown, WV.

Burke, J. G. (1992). *System analysis, design, and implementation.* Boston: Boyd & Fraser.

Dakins, D. R. (2001). Center takes data tracking to heart. *Health Data Management, 9*(1), 32, 34, 36.

Digital Preservation Coalition. (2002). *Media and formats.* Available online at http://www.dpconline.org/graphics/medfor/media.html. Accessed February 9, 2003.

Documented savings.(October 2001). *Health Management Technology, 22*(10), 56.

Faden, M. (April 10, 2000). Data cleansing helps e-businesses run more efficiently. *Informationweek.com,* (781), 136, 138, 140, 144.

Gillespie, G. (2000). There's gold in them thar' databases. *Health Data Management, 8*(11), 40.

Hicks, G. T. (April 16, 2001). With privacy rule in effect, hospitals face two years of compliance actions. *AHA News, 37*(15), 1.

Kahn, M. G. (1995). The computer-based patient record and Robert Fulghum's 16 principles. *M.D. Computing, 12*(4), 253–258.

Kolar, H. R. (2001). Caring for healthcare, *22*(4), 46–47.

Liebmann, L. (April 10, 2000). ERP's second act: Online access. *Informationweek.com,* (781), 146.

Tozor, G. V. (1994). *Information quality management.* Cambridge, United Kingdom: Blackwell.

Wright, P., and Bartram, C. (2000). Text entry on handheld computers by older users. *Ergonomics, 43*(6), 702.

Zorkoczy, P., and Heap, N. (1995). *Information technology: An introduction,* (4th ed.). London: Pittman.

4

Electronic Communication and the Internet

After completing this chapter, you should be able to:

- Define *electronic communication*.
- Explain the Internet and the World Wide Web.
- Identify the process required to access both the Internet and the World Wide Web.
- Discuss services available on the Internet and the World Wide Web.
- Relate the advantages and disadvantages that the Internet and the World Wide Web have over traditional means of communicating information.
- Identify examples of Internet and World Wide Web resources that may be useful to nurses and other health care professionals and consumers.

- Compare and contrast a Web *page* and a Web *portal*.
- Discuss the terms *search index, search engine,* and *search unifier.*
- Evaluate the quality of a health information Web site.
- Compare and contrast the purpose and use of intranets and extranets to the purpose and use of the Internet.
- Discuss the advantages and disadvantages of the Internet as a platform for health care applications.
- Understand the concepts of *e-business* and *e-commerce* and their role in the health care arena.

 MEDIALINK

Additional resources for this content can be found on the Companion Website at *www. prenhall.com/hebda.* Click on "Chapter 4" to select the activities for this chapter.

Companion Website

- Glossary
- Multiple Choice
- Discussion Points
- Case Study: Advantages and Disadvantages of the Net
- Case Study: Access to Health Care Information
- Case Study: Consumer Education
- MediaLink Application: Evaluating Websites
- Web Hunt: Professionals Share Information and Data
- Links to Resources
- Crossword Puzzle

Computers can expedite the location and retrieval of information. This ability is particularly useful when material is difficult to obtain or quickly outdated. Electronic communication and Internet technology have the potential to support health care knowledge needs. **Electronic communication** is the ability to exchange information through the use of computer equipment and software. This is generally done through fixed network connections or the use of a **modem.** A modem is a communication device that transmits data over telephone or cable lines from one computer to another. This process allows individual users to communicate and share hardware, software, and information, and is otherwise known as **connectivity. Online** is a term that indicates a connection to various computer resources, such as the Internet and World Wide Web, that provide forums that encourage electronic communication and have revolutionized the way that information is shared.

The **Internet,** also called **the Net,** is a worldwide network that connects millions of computers. This technology first began as a United States government project to encourage researchers at different academic sites to share their findings. It now links government, universities, commercial institutions, and individual users. The Internet itself has been relatively free from the control of any government or single organization, although this situation is changing. Governments are looking at jurisdictional problems created by the Internet and ways to harmonize laws related to hacking, fraud, and child pornography. The Council of Europe drafted the Cybercrime Treaty in an attempt to provide common definitions of cybercrime (Stop Signs on the Web 2001).

On a different level, the nonprofit Internet Corporation for Assigned Names and Numbers (ICANN) allocates top-level domain names and settles domain name disputes. The U.S. government established the ICANN in 1998 (Geist 2003). It is the Internet Society that has the greatest overall influence on the Internet. The Internet Society is a nonprofit, professional organization that "provides leadership in addressing issues that confront the future of the Internet" and serves as a home for groups responsible for the promulgation of Internet infrastructure standards. These groups include the Internet Engineering Task Force (IETF) and the Internet Architecture Board (IAB). The Internet society serves as a global clearinghouse for information about the Internet and facilitates and coordinates Internet-related initiatives. The Society sponsors several events including the annual International Networking (INET) conference as well as training workshops, tutorials, research, publications, public policy, and trade activities for the benefit of people throughout the world (Internet Society 2003).

The Internet expands the range of available health care information through e-mail, discussion lists, file transfer protocol (FTP), Telnet, and World Wide Web resources. Many materials are no longer published on paper but are available only electronically. Some examples include research reports, journals, practice guidelines, educational materials, and conference proceedings.

The **World Wide Web** (Web or WWW) is an information service for access to Internet resources by content instead of file names. An easy-to-use graphical user interface (GUI) makes it simple to learn and use. The Web supports text, images, and sound as well as links to other documents. Users may search by specific words or move from one link to another. Links are displayed by highlighted keywords, text, or images. Selection of information in highlighted areas is accomplished through a click of the mouse button.

THE INTERNET

The Internet is the largest, best-known wide area network in the world. Its exact size is difficult to estimate because of its rapid growth, but its users number in the millions. One major factor in the growth of the Internet is the development of companies known as **Internet service providers** (**ISPs**) that furnish Internet access for a fee. Some well-known examples of ISPs include America Online (AOL), Microsoft Network (MSN), and EarthLink. Many other ISPs exist as well. ISPs opened the Internet to small business and home users. Internet access through an ISP requires computer access, a modem, and communication software. Several variations for connectivity exist, including the traditional access with telephone dial-up, or high-speed access such as digital subscriber line (DSL), cable, or satellite (Alsop 2003; Connect with High-Speed Internet 2003; Grimes 2002). The majority of users still rely on dial-up connections through existing telephone wires; however, high-speed access is gaining in popularity. DSL uses existing copper telephone wires but differs from the traditional dial-up connections in that it requires a special modem and is always "on." DSL service uses an individual line and is limited to customers who fall within a certain distance of the telephone switching station. Cable service uses the coaxial cable used to transmit cable television signals. Cable service also requires a special modem but is generally less expensive and provides a better level of performance. Satellite service has been plagued with a reputation of difficult and expensive installations, poor service, and suspect performance. For these reasons it has not been considered a viable option except in areas where neither DSL nor cable is available. Another option for connectivity that is in the pilot stage uses the existing electrical power grid to provide high-speed Internet service (Davidson 2003; Fox 2003; Markoff and Richtel 2003).

ISPs provide software and directions on how to access the Internet and a special **SLIP/PPP** account that provides Internet and World Wide Web access. SLIP/PPP refers to the serial line Internet protocol (SLIP) and point-to-point protocol (PPP). Both protocols allow passage of data through communication lines. Customers generally pay their ISP a monthly fee; in some cases there is an additional charge for access time. Most ISPs provide a local telephone number for customer use.

The Internet offers many types of services and resources, including the following:

- *Electronic mail or e-mail.* **E-mail** is the use of computers to transmit messages to one or more persons. Delivery can be almost instantaneous. Text messages may be accompanied by attachment files. E-mail may be sent anywhere in the world as long as the individual has an Internet address. Like street addresses, Internet addresses are specific to a location and type of institution or ISP.

- *File transfer.* This capability allows users to move files from one location to another. The benefit of file transfer is that users can capture, view, edit, or use work developed by others rather than starting anew.

- *Database searches.* This feature allows users to conduct comprehensive literature searches over a shorter period of time than could be accomplished via a manual approach. More than 200 universities and public libraries offer online databases for review. In this instance, "online" refers to databases that are available through Internet connections.

- *Remote log-on.* This feature allows use of computer facilities at other locations to access directories, files, and databases. This ability is accomplished through the Telnet protocol. Some systems such as the Virginia Henderson International Nursing Library require an account, identification, and a password for user access.

- *Discussion and news groups.* The Internet provides a place where specialty interest groups can address concerns, discuss solutions, and exchange information in a timely fashion.

- *Instant messaging.* This feature allows interactive discussions. At the present, most chats are typed. The Internet does have the capability to support voice, although both users must be online at the same time and have the same software to chat (Joyce 2002). Instant messaging was sometimes referred to as as *Internet relay chat (IRC)* in the past.

E-mail

E-mail is one of the most frequently used Internet applications. It is commonly found in private organizations, colleges, universities, corporations, and private homes. It is a powerful connectivity tool and often is the feature that first attracts users to the Internet. E-mail encourages networking among peers, yields helpful tips and shared resources, and saves time and money that would otherwise be spent on individual problem solving. E-mail is a convenient way to contact employees, colleagues, students, and recruiters. It allows users to participate in educational offerings and send announcements and resumes. Box 4–1 lists some advantages and disadvantages associated with e-mail. The next few paragraphs explain the composition and management of e-mail.

Box 4–1 **E-mail: Advantages and Disadvantages**

Advantages

- *Eliminates telephone tag.* Provides the ability to leave a written message.
- *Convenient.* Can be sent or retrieved from multiple locations, including work, home, or while traveling. Can be used on a 24-hour basis.
- *Easy to prepare and send.* Electronic mail requires less effort to prepare, address, and send than the traditional means of dictation and mailing.
- *Saves time and money.* Eliminates postage and paper expenses.
- *Delivery can be almost instantaneous.* Eliminates the time lag associated with traditional mail.
- *Messages are time- and date-stamped.* Provides documentation of the actual time of the mail transaction. Can also provide a log of when the message was received, read, and answered.

Disadvantages

- *Interpretation of messages without the benefit of voice inflection.* Unlike telephone conversations, e-mail eliminates the additional information that may be communicated through verbal cues.
- *High volume of messages sent and received.* E-mail's popularity and ease of use make it easy to generate large numbers of messages, including copies, forwarded messages, and "junk mail."
- *Viral contamination with e-mail attachments.* Attached files that contain a virus or worm may contaminate the recipient's computer.
- *Security concerns related to maintaining confidentiality.* E-mail is easily intercepted and forwarded, and may be read by unintended parties. Employers have the right to read e-mail transmitted using company resources. In addition, deleted messages may be retrieved during system backups.

Every e-mail message has a header and message text. The **header** lists who sent the message, when, to whom, and at what location and the address to which a reply should be directed if different from the sender's address. Message copies may also be directed to others. Messages can be composed online or in advance. In this case, "online" refers to the period that one computer is actively connected to another. Composing messages ahead of time may decrease costs for connection time and improve the organization of expressed thoughts. Mail received may be read while online or downloaded to the recipient's computer for later review.

An **e-mail application** is a computer program that assists the user to send, receive, and manage e-mail messages. Most have basic text editing and spell checking capability. Some popular commercial e-mail applications include Microsoft's Outlook Express, Lotus Notes, Eudora, and Send-Mail, which is used with Linux and UNIX operating systems. Individuals accustomed to working in an environment with large systems may still use a UNIX mail program or programs such as Elm or Pine, which are deemed to be friendlier alternatives to UNIX mail. Despite its popularity, health care workers have been among the last to receive e-mail accounts.

As e-mail popularity grows, so do concerns related to its use. These concerns include threats to data integrity and security, confidentiality, verification that messages emanate from the identified source, spam, and HIPAA (Health Insurance Portability and Accountability Act) compliance (Kelly and McKenzie 2002; Tabar 2002; Voelk and Geyer 2002). Data integrity may be threatened by **computer viruses.** Viruses are malicious programs that can disrupt or destroy data and sometimes overwhelm networks with traffic. Viruses are not transmitted via e-mail messages themselves but may be found as file attachments sent with messages or launched when infected Word or Excel files are opened. The threat of viruses can be minimized in several ways; one way is to not open e-mail and attachments from unknown sources. Obviously this option is not always practical. The next option is to avoid opening files with unrecognized file extensions. All remaining attachment files should be scanned before opening with the latest version of antivirus software. When content needs to be kept secure and confidential, **encryption** is recommended. Encryption uses mathematical formulas to code messages. Message recipients decode content with an encryption key. Encryption may be done at the desktop or at the server level. Encryption is available as a feature with many commercial e-mail packages. Encryption done at the desktop may protect the message but also prevents the e-mail system administrator from seeing viruses. Some organizations rely on an employee or small group of employees to encrypt messages and distribute decryption keys rather than use public keys. This situation invites violation of HIPAA's disclosure policies. Encryption of patient-related e-mail is one of HIPAA's mandates. Server-based encryption is a better alternative (Tabar 2002; Voelk and Geyer 2002). Many chief information officers are asking what to encrypt and who should do the encryption.

Methods to validate e-mail author identity include **public key infrastructure (PKI)** and digital credentialing. PKI provides a unique code for each user that is imbedded into a storage device. User information is stored in a database by the organization that created the code. Identity is confirmed when the storage device and a password or other form of ID match information stored in the database (Kelly and McKenzie 2002). A simpler alternative to PKI is the digital signature or credential. The digital signature is a unique identifier issued to the individual that can be verified against the sender's public key. Intel and the American Medical Association worked collaboratively to develop digital credentialing for physicians. Physician digital crendentials are routed through a firewall to the Intel Internet Authentication Service (ITAS) to validate user identity and create an audit trail. This same process is available for other health care workers. Although the digital credential does not require biometric measures to verify identity, there is increased interest in the use of biometric measures as a means to ensure that only authorized users access private health information.

Another issue that has been raised about the security of health information transmitted via e-mail is the security of the mail server, or the computer on which e-mail messages reside, both coming into an organization and leaving. Use of the health provider's e-mail for nonwork purposes can open up the server to viruses and hackers (Kelly and McKenzie 2002). Secure e-mail applications ensure that all information remains available to enterprise servers when it is needed. The use of a secure e-mail service provider is likened to using a private postal carrier, which helps to maintain data integrity as well as provide audit trails and proof of receipt. This arrangment usually requires that servers on both ends are registered, so it is best suited for organizations that communicate regularly. Yet another safeguard of confidentiality is the ability to screen outgoing messages for appropriate content and to block it if it is going to unknown or suspect addresses.

Other issues surrounding e-mail focus on its increasing volume; the time required to sift through e-mail messages; unwanted or "junk" e-mail, also known as **spam;** accurate interpretation of messages; and HIPAA compliance. The number of legitimate e-mail messages has grown exponentially, but so have the number of unwanted messages. Approximately one half of all e-mail traffic is now spam. Spam is a problem because thousands of messages may be sent at one time. Spam spreads advertisements and may be used to collect personal and credit card information. Unfortunately, the technical rules that govern how messages are transmitted allow spammers to forge return e-mail addresses and domain names, making it difficult to track and prosecute them when they engage in fraudulent claims and illegal activity (FTC Takes on Spam 2003). Efforts to block spam include lawsuits, state and federal legislation, industry initiatives, establishing separate e-mail accounts for different purposes, e-mail rules for incoming mail and filtering software, and challenge response tools (Gann 2003; Merline 2003; Schofield 2003; Woellert and Wildstrom 2003). Additional proposals for dealing with spam call for the establishment of a "do not e-mail" list, limiting the number of messages that can be sent out per day via free e-mail accounts, and a requirement that "ADV" appear in the spam header to indicate advertisement. Spam is costly in terms of user time to delete unwanted messages, costs for filtering and challenge software, and higher costs for ISP service.

Challenge response software works by asking the e-mail sender to answer a question or complete a task that requires human intervention. No mail is accepted unless its validity has been confirmed by a human being. Challenge response software is sometimes referred to as **Captohas,** which stands for "completely automatic public Turing test to tell computers and humans apart" (Vijayan 2003). Challenge response tools are effective in filtering out spam, but they create additional network traffic. Box 4–2 provides some informal rules to guide e-mail use.

Like other Internet services, e-mail is based on a client/server system. In client/server technology, files are stored on a central computer known as a **server.** In this case, the server receives mail from other Internet sites and stores it until it is read, answered, or deleted. The client computer requests

Box 4–2

Informal Rules for E-mail Use

- Change passwords for e-mail access immediately after they are first assigned, and frequently thereafter.
- Limit copies to the people who need the information. This keeps the number of messages manageable.
- Choose an accurate description for the subject line. This practice helps recipients to determine which messages should be read first.
- Give e-mail messages the same consideration given to business correspondence. E-mail may be seen by parties other than intended recipients. In an e-mail message, nothing should be written that one would not publicly post.
- Make messages clear, short, and to the point.
- Avoid the use of all capital letters. This is difficult to read, and may be perceived as shouting, according to e-mail etiquette.
- Limit abbreviations to those that are easily understood.
- Read mail, file messages in categories, and delete messages no longer needed on a regular basis. This frees storage space and helps to optimize system function, as well as making it easier to find and retrieve messages later.
- Consider using mechanisms to prevent unwanted mail.
- Do not reply to messages that do not require a reply unless adding relevant information.

mail access from the server and generates new mail that will be handled by the server.

File Transfer

File transfer is the ability to move files from one location to another across the Internet. Users may download archived files that they find interesting or give their files to others. Transferred files can include graphics, text, or shareware applications. One means to achieve the actual movement of data is through the **FTP.** FTP is a set of instructions that controls both the physical transfer of data across the network and its appearance on the receiving end (Webopedia 2003). The benefit of file transfer is that users can preview work developed by others rather than starting anew. FTP may be available with World Wide Web software. Internet etiquette traditionally calls for the transfer of large files after peak business hours to prevent slow response times. **Binary file transfer (BFT)** represents another standard for file transfer.

The World Wide Web

The World Wide Web is an information service that can access data by content and support a multimedia approach. It was first developed at the European Center for Particle Physics in Geneva for scientists to publish

| Box 4–3 | The World Wide Web: Advantages and Disadvantages |

Advantages

- Browser software is available for all types of computers, including mainframes and Mac- and IBM-compatible personal computers.

- Browser software is easy to use.

- Text, pictures, video, and sound are supported.

- The amount of information available on the Web is constantly expanding.

- Internet overload is decreased because it links to other documents instead of including them as attachments.

- The need to hold a line open while a document is read is eliminated because the document is transferred to the host computer and the connection is terminated.

- Document transfer is facilitated.

- Voice communications may be supported.

Disadvantages

- No one person or group controls the Web, just as no one controls the Internet.

- The quality of available information varies widely.

- Documents may not supply sufficient depth in content.

- Not all Web pages display a date of authorship.

- Web sites may change without a "forwarding address" being provided.

- The Web is vulnerable to hacker attacks.

- The large amount of available information may be overwhelming.

- Employers may be concerned over wasted company time and lost productivity as people explore the Web.

---

documents while linked via the Internet. The Web's GUI makes it the most user-friendly service on the Internet, as well as the fastest growing. The Web provides a forum for the exchange of ideas, free marketing, and public relations. It now serves as a platform for a growing number of businesses. Box 4–3 lists advantages and disadvantages associated with using the World Wide Web.

Figure 4–1 displays information uploaded to the Web by the American Nurses Association regarding its subsidiary and affiliate groups. Web pages frequently change as content is revised and new technologies are incorporated. This results in a different appearance for the page the next time the user accesses it. The use of new technology and software in Web page design may leave some users unable to access certain features or content. Periodic browser updates and the use of additional applications that can be downloaded from the Web or purchased in stores help to address this situation. It

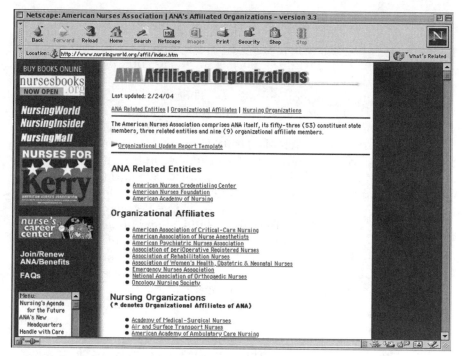

FIGURE 4–1 • "ANA Affilliated Organizations" (Reprinted from American Nurses Association web site http://nursingworld.org/affil/index.htm/ by permission of the American Nurses Association)

may also be necessary to evaluate, upgrade, and replace hardware and software to access and use desired Web features and applications.

One particularly popular Web feature is the **home page,** the first page seen at a particular Web location. The home page presents general information about a topic, a person, or an organization. Pages are written in hypertext markup language (HTML) or extensible markup language (XML). Markup languages include text as well as special instructions known as *tags* for the display of text and other media. HTML also includes highlighted references to other documents that the user may choose if additional information about that topic is desired. World Wide Web software interprets HTML tags for display. Tags specify formatting information such as the type of heading, font size, and alignment of type. Tags also indicate the location of other media such as graphics or even music. HTML can include links to other documents and may incorporate text, graphics or video, and sound files. Despite the fact that HTML is considered a standard, some variations exist to allow information to be displayed on personal digital assistants and other devices. XML was developed by the World Wide Web Consortium. The Consortium is a group of companies dedicated to the development of open standards to ensure the development of the Web.

Portal is a term that refers to some Web sites. Portal sites require registration and collect information from the user that can be used to personalize features for individual users. Services such as e-mail, news search capability, and online shopping may also be available. Portals organize data with different formats from multiple sources into a single, easy-to-use menu (Bland 2001). Portals started as entry points to the Web that added additional features to attract and maintain user interests. AOL and Yahoo represent general portal sites. There are also special interest or niche portals. Some examples of nursing portals include The Nursing Portal (*http://www.nursing-portal.com*) and The Virtual Nurse Web (*http://www.virtualnurse.com*). WebMD, HealthGate, OnHealth, and HealthCentral provide services for physicians, consumers, nurses, and office managers (Hussey 2000). CVS and other commerical pharmacies also have portal sites that provide information for consumers and allow prescriptions to be filled online. Portals are constantly evolving. Portals can also be used by health care organizations to enable technical and nontechnical staff to create and update information (Portal Technologies in Action, 2003). For example, a hospital portal may contain links to online continuing education such as safety and regulatory information. Employees can access this information independently at times convenient for them to complete required education. Other uses for portal technology include providing secure Web access to patient care systems or information contained within these systems. This includes making results available to physicians, as well as digital images and monitor strips, and the opportunity for electronic review and sign-off of medical records (Carlson 2003; New Portal Launched 2003). Basic portals furnish information in a static fashion. More sophisticated sites are interactive, allowing users to complete and submit forms online, complete health assessments, and perform other activities. There are variations on the portal theme. Active portals focus on a specific topic and use a customized search agent that automatically updates searches. Enterprise portals provide access to information quickly and easily, extending user access across departments and organizations (Hall 2002).

Links, also known as **hypertext,** are words or phrases distinguished from the remainder of the document through the use of highlighting or a different screen color. Links allow users to skip from point to point within or among documents, escaping conventional linear format. Clicking on links with the mouse establishes a TCP/IP connection between the client and server, which sends a request in the form of a hypertext transfer protocol (HTTP) command. TCP/IP (transmission control protocol/Internet protocol) are the most commonly used rules for exchanging information among the networks (Tabar 2000). The TCP/IP connection is closed after the information is sent, while the user is seamlessly transported to another area of the document or another Web site.

HTTP supports hypermedia information systems, including the Web. The initial portion of Web site addresses, "http," refers to this protocol. Links are maintained via a **uniform resource locator (URL),** a string of characters similar to a postal address. The URL identifies the document's Web location and the type of server on which it resides, such as HTTP or other Web server, FTP, or news server. Addresses that include an "s" (https) indicate secured sites, such as those that request entry and submission of credit card numbers.

Box 4–4 lists some steps required to create, post, and maintain a home page. Web sites may consist of a single page or hundreds of pages of information. They vary in complexity from simple text to sites with elaborate graphics, sound, and videos. The person responsible for putting a Web site together and maintaining it is known as the Webmaster. One popular type of Web site is the blog. **Blog** is an abbreviation for Web and log. The blog provides a forum for individuals to maintain an online journal on the Internet (Cox 2003; Ernst 2003; Everett 2003). Entries are time stamped. Simple blogs are regularly updated Web pages with the most recent entries appearing at the top of the page. Content varies widely from personal diaries, requests for contributions, and special interest blogs organized by topics. Blogging software and providers are available to help create and maintain blogs.

Nurses may use the World Wide Web to learn more about any of the following topics:

- *Undergraduate, graduate, and doctoral nursing programs.* Most schools have Web pages that provide information about their philosophy, curriculum, and application process. In some cases, potential candidates can complete an application online.

- *Professional associations.* Most groups, including the American Nurses Association, maintain Web sites that provide information about the purpose of the group and advantages of membership. This increases visibility for the group and serves as a recruitment strategy to attract new members.

- *Nursing informatics.* Announcements of upcoming meetings and calls for papers about nursing informatics can be found on the Web.

- *Online nursing journals.* Many traditional journals offer electronic versions of their publications in addition to the printed version. Some, however, may restrict general access to the electronic format, and require a subcription, which may have a fee. In addition, they may offer the option to purchase specific articles.

- *Continuing education offerings.* Program announcements and even entire courses may be found on the Web.

- *Disease-specific information and recommended treatment modalities.* This content may be directed to the health care consumer and/or the health care professional.

- *Consumer education.* The American Heart Association and the National Cancer Institute are among the growing list of groups that maintain Web sites.

A list of nursing Web sites and related sites of interest can be found on the Companion Website at www.prenhall.com/hebda.

Content and Design Considerations

- *Determine purpose, intended audience, and content.* A well-designed Web page starts with good planning.

- *Select a Web developer or an authoring tool.* A Web developer can help ensure the success of a site. A variety of tools can be used to create Web pages, including word processors, browsers, and dedicated Web-authoring tools. The complexity of design, user comfort, and experience are factors in tool selection. Basic knowledge of html markup commands is helpful but not essential.

- *Determine page layout.* Do not crowd pages with information and images. Limit introductory page information so that essential data are visible without scrolling. Review existing Web pages for pleasing appearance and useful features.

- *Readability.* Use high-contrast backgrounds for easy reading, such as black print on white. Dark backgrounds can cause fatigue. Use 12-point fonts or larger.

- *Choose links.* Links can make the site more interesting and useful. Organize links to help users find what they are looking for. Use specific link references rather than the phrase, "click here."

- *Include contact information.* Contact information, such as name, organization, credentials, an e-mail link, and a postal address, provide the appearance of credibility and a means to establish contact.

- *Update/revision information.* A date helps the user to determine whether posted information and links are current. Updates and revisions also maintain interest, giving users a reason to come back. Consider the addition of icons to identify new or recently revised materials.

- *Download time.* Lengthy download times can frustrate users, causing them to move to other sites.

- *Check the page for errors.* Spelling, grammar, and content errors reflect poorly on the author or site. Review all materials prior to posting.

- *Do not include a counter.* Visitors do not need to know how many people visited a site.

- *Consider including activities for users.* Users want more than just information.

- *Consider copyright issues.* Request permission prior to using work developed by others. Register original work with the U.S Copyright office and place a copyright notice with year next to protected material. Develop a written agreement that identifies copyright ownership when working with a Web developer.

Posting and Maintenance Considerations

- *Test the page before posting.* Ensure that it looks and performs as conceived. Use different browsers to view results. Pages that do not load properly or that have a sloppy appearance make a poor impression.

- *Gather information on Internet service providers and Web servers.* Compare service, cost, and support when selecting an ISP and home for Web pages.

- *Establish Internet access.* Internet access is essential for periodic review of Web materials and to receive mail generated by the site.

- *Find a Web server.* Many ISPs and Web sites offer space for home pages. Determine which service provider can best meet the requirements for the page being posted.

- *Obtain a Web or domain address.* An address provides a location to post pages. A domain name refers to one or more IP addresses. Domain names are used in URLs. Suffixes provide information about the type of affilliation. Memorable names help users to find and return to pages.

- *Review and revision procedures.* To remain timely, pages should include review or revision dates.

- *Security issues.* Use mechanisms to protect against unauthorized changes in posted materials.

Browsers

A **browser** is a retrieval program that allows access to hypertext and hypermedia documents on the Web by using HTTP. The computer, acting as server, interprets the client's HTTP request and sends back the requested document for display. Browsers can also use Telnet FTP protocols. Browsers may be obtained free from an ISP, as a download over the Internet or purchased. The National Center for Supercomputing Applications (NCSA) developed Mosaic, the first Web browser. Web use increased after the introduction of Mosaic. Examples of browsers include Netscape Navigator, Microsoft's Internet Explorer, AOL, RapidBrowser XP, Mozilla, and Opera. Netscape Navigator and Internet Explorer have dominated the market, but alternative browsers are expected to increase in popularity (Carroll et al. 2002; Hamilton 2003). Unlike Navigator and Explorer, which distribute advertisements, Opera and RapidBrowser XP are available advertisement free for a fee. Browsers use the URL to request a document from the server.

Browsers are available for many types of systems and frequently offer features that extend their utility. However, there are still many things that browsers do not do. **Helper programs** and **plug-in** programs evolved to fill this void. Helper and plug-in programs are computer applications that have been designed to perform tasks such as view graphics, construct Web pages, play sounds, or even remotely control another PC over the Internet. The main difference between helper and plug-in programs is that the first does not require the browser to be running to function, while the second does require the browser to be running. Both are typically available on the Web at no cost and are often written in **Java.** Java is a programming language that enables the display of moving text, animation, and musical excerpts on Web pages. Java is popular for the following reasons:

- Applications will run on any Java-enabled browser.
- Actual code can reside on the server until it is downloaded to the client computer as it is needed.
- Java reduces the need to purchase, install, and maintain on-site software.

Microsoft's ActiveX is an alternative to Java for the development of Internet-enabled tools and technologies.

Search Tools

The overwhelming amount of data available on the Web requires the use of tools to locate specific information. This is where **search tools** come in. Several types of search tools are available to help users find information on the Web. The distinction among the types of tools is sometimes blurred. Some sites, such as Yahoo, index links by broad subject categories. **Search**

indexes are appropriate when general information is requested. **Search engines** use automated programs that search the Web, compiling a list of links to sites relevant to keywords supplied by the user. The search may also include Usenet discussions. Search engines are indicated when it is necessary to find a specific topic. Google and AltaVista are examples of search engines. Each search tool maintains its own list of information on the Web and uses its own method to organize materials. Because of this variation in organization, searches conducted with different engines yield different results. Although subtle differences exist among each, all permit the user to enter a search word or phrase. Web sites that contain the search item are then displayed. The number of hits or Web sites that carry this word or phrase varies according to the search engine used and the time the search is done, since new sites are constantly being indexed. Search engines also weight the pages so that the most commonly useful links are displayed first (Carroll 2003). There are several ways to weight pages, but the best-known method is based on the popularity of each site as is represented by the number of other sites that link to it. Enclosing key phrases in quotation marks is recommended as a way to obtain better results with some, but not all, search tools; otherwise, all documents containing portions of the key phrase will be identified. Help pages are available to aid the user in conducting searches. The relevance of search results is also determined by whether the search engine is ad sponsored (Arnold 2003; McLaughlin 2002). Many results contain links that advertisers have paid the search engine to display. Paid links are not necessarily labeled as advertisements. Consumer groups have asked the Federal Trade Commission to look at this issue.

Despite the success of search engines, important information is frequently missed. This occurs for several reasons. Search engines have interfaces in the major languages but may miss results that are not in any of those languages. Another reason that information is missed is that it is password-protected or stored in formats that are not indexed (Clyde 2003). Yet another reason that information is missed is that the incorporation of multiple concepts makes indexing difficult (Hawkins 2003). Search tools are still evolving. Medical World Search (*http://www.mwsearch. com*) is a search tool for selected medical sites that requires a subscription fee. It uses indexing and a thesaurus of uniform health care terms, which users can view before conducting a search. There are also problems with filters designed to block pornography that also block access to health information sites.

Until recently, retrieval of comprehensive results meant repeating a search several times with a different search engine each time to identify all relevant sites. **Search engine unifiers** can shorten search time by using several engines at one time. There is some debate as to whether they actually yield better results than a good search engine. Some examples of search unifiers include Dogpile (*http://www.dogpile.com*), Search (*http:// www.search.com*), and MetaCrawler (*http://www.metacrawler.com/info.*

metac/dog/index.htm). Users should try several search tools to determine what provides the best results for their needs.

Listservs

A **Listserv** is actually an e-mail subscription list. A mailing list program copies and distributes all e-mail messages to subscribers. All mail goes through a central computer that acts as the server for the list. Some groups have a moderator who first screens messages for relevance. Listservs are sometimes referred to as *discussion groups, mailing lists,* or *electronic conferences* (Robinson 2001). Listservs provide information on thousands of topics. Subscription may be open to anyone with an e-mail addressed or restricted. A complete list of listservs may be obtained by visiting the Tile.net site (*http://www.tile.net*).

To subscribe to a listserv, individuals must send the e-mail message "sub" or "subscribe," followed by their first and last names. Exact commands may vary slightly. Most listservs provide help and instructions on request. Subscribers may participate in discussions or just monitor them. Listserv participants should read their mail frequently and skim messages for subjects of interest to keep up with discussions. Subscribers may terminate their participation at any time by sending an "unsubscribe" message.

News Groups

Usenet news groups are another available Internet feature. Usenet groups are similar to listservs in content and diversity (Morochove 2003). More than 100,000 discussion groups exist, each dedicated to a different topic. These groups provide a forum where any user can post messages for discussion and reply. Users do not subscribe to these groups, nor do they receive individual messages. Instead, they may participate at any time free of charge. ISPs do not carry every news group. ISP administrators decide which news groups will be available to their customers and how long messages will be stored. Only messages that are currently stored on the user's ISP computer may be read. Some ISPs restrict access to usernet groups or restrict the length of time that messages are saved. It may be necessary to subscribe to a usernet service to view older postings. Special broswer programs called **news reader software** are needed by the individual users to read messages posted on the news group. Many different news readers are available. News readers come bundled with Web browsers. A list of Usenet groups may also be found at the Tile.net site. Some examples of nursing Usenet groups are the following:

- *sci.med.nursing.* This is a general forum for the discussion of all types of nursing issues. A review of discussion topics reveals current concerns in the profession by country and practice area. Individual nurses may request assistance with particular problems and receive help from people across the globe.

- *alt.npractitioners.* Issues pertaining to nurse practitioners provide the focus for this group.
- *bit.listserv.snurse-l.* This is a group for international nursing students.

No single person is in charge of universal Usenet procedures, but informal rules and etiquette for participants have developed. The first rule is that all new users should read the **frequently asked questions (FAQ)** document before sending any messages of their own. The FAQ file serves to introduce the group, update new users on recent discussions, and eliminate repetition of questions. Additional Usenet guidelines call for:

- *Short postings.* This helps to maintain interest while preventing any individual or subgroup from monopolizing the group.
- *No sensationalism.* The intent of Usenet groups is the sharing of information, not gossip.
- *No outright sales.* Usenet originated in academia and relies on a cooperative environment. Advertising, by custom, is kept at a minimum.
- *Respect for the group focus.* Posting messages that are not relevant wastes time and resources.

News groups may be discovered through any of the following methods: searching the Web by topic, word of mouth from individuals with like interests, conferences, professional publications, or searching through lists of all available news groups. If no news group exists for a given topic, instructions on how to start one can be found on the Internet.

Bulletin Board Systems

Bulletin board systems (BBSs) started out as a computerized dial-in meeting and announcement system for users to make statements, share files, and conduct limited discussions. The original BBS did not require Internet access, just a computer and modem. Once very popular, BBSs have largely been replaced by Web sites. These sites may have a moderator who determines what messages will be posted.

Access to Health Care Information and Services

Internet and Web resources provide another means to increase access both to information for professionals and health care consumers and to select health care services. Much of this information is free. In this way, the Internet allows health care providers to share information with each other and consumers that is reliable, effective, and secure (Leary 2003). Federal agencies, health care institutions, physicians, nurses, psychologists, dentists, online journals, drug companies, equipment manufacturers, and discussion groups all offer information and advice. Information may be located by symptom, disease, drug interaction, nutrition, common injuries, or support group. Users can post inquiries, read documents of commonly asked questions and answers, or search by keyword or subject. Some services, such as consults and disease management, involve costs. Third-party payers may not pay for some Web-based services.

Professional Information Sharing

The Internet encourages timely sharing of information among professionals, health care organizations and alliances, vendors, federal agencies, schools, and students. It decreases geographic isolation and allows professionals in remote areas to keep informed of the latest discoveries, treatment modalities, regulations, trends, drugs, and adverse reactions or interactions. Nurses benefit from communication with experts, listservs and discussion groups, online literature searches, and access to Web sites. These resources offer tutorials, multimedia instruction, online journals, and continuing education. Electronic communication disseminates information quickly, allowing clinicians to learn about revisions in practice guidelines and new study findings. The Internet provides teleconferencing capability for distance learning and continuing education. Electronic communication facilitates networking among nurses, saves labor through the sharing of useful tips and policies, and facilitates collaborative research and writing.

Information for Consumers The rapid development and dissemination of new knowledge today means that the consumer may hear about discoveries and treatments before the professional does. Consumers may even consult the same source as their health care providers. Online resources can aid in diagnosis, present new treatment options, and help consumers locate support groups. The Web also presents another medium for health teaching. Despite the value of online resources, however, these materials cannot be considered as a replacement for actual health care. Most Web sites of health care providers guide users to follow-up care. Questions about professional liability for information found on the Web are unresolved at this time.

The number of client education materials and support groups is growing as more people access the Internet and Web. The Internet and Web offer a way to reach large numbers of people easily and inexpensively. In addition, materials can be updated easily and printed. Some examples of Web sites that furnish client education materials include the American Heart Association and American Cancer Society. Figure 4–2 shows a page from the American Heart Association Web site explaining heart attack. Some practitioners also provide information on the Web as a public service, although disclaimers are included stating that this advice does not replace a visit to a practitioner. Other sites, such as Your Family Doctor and VirtualDoctor.Net, offer individual consultations for a fee.

Evaluation of Online Information The Internet offers unprecedented access to health care information. Unfortunately, the accuracy, readability, depth, diversity, and presentation of this content vary greatly from site to site (Hebda, Czar, and Mascara 2003; Mack and Llewellyn 2003; Long 2003; RAND Health/California HealthCare Foundation 2001; WHO

Eval Criteria

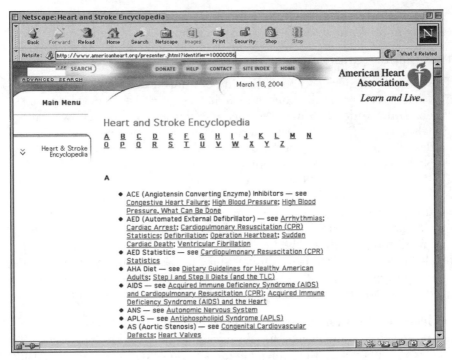

FIGURE 4–2 • http://www.americanheart.org/presenter.html?identifier=10000056.
(©2003, copyright American Heart Association. Reproduced with permission of Heart and Stroke Encyclopedia World Wide Web site.)

2003). Some online information can even be harmful. The lack of a controlling body over the Internet makes it impossible to regulate the quality of information before posting. For this reason, health care professionals and consumers must be wary. Online resources should be evaluated according to the following criteria:

- *Credentials of the source.* Large professional associations, such as hospitals, universities, government, and official health organizations, tend to have the most reliable sites. In some cases the source is not readily apparent. For example, it is important to consider whether the information provided mirrors the focus of professional education and expertise.

- *Ability to validate information.* Validation of information can be difficult unless the source can be traced back to a reputable university or other agency. Many messages and Web sites identify a person or persons to contact for further information. When facts and studies are cited, the original source should be stated so users can review it and draw their own conclusions. It should also be possible to corroborate information from independent sources.

- *Accuracy.* Because no single person controls information that is placed on the Internet, the mere existence of information does not indicate that it is accurate. Postings should identify contact persons or cite references that may be checked to allow evaluation of posted information.

- *Comprehensiveness of informaiton.* If the site professes to provide information about medications, it should discuss indications, contraindications, protocols, and dosages. If the user must go elsewhere to find relevant information, the site is not comprehensive. Sites with broad generalizations or poorly referenced research should be considered suspicious. The user should continue to use caution because the information could be biased.

- *Date of issue or revision.* One problem with the Internet and World Wide Web is that not all pages contain dates indicating when material was written, revised, or reviewed, making it difficult to determine whether information is current. Publication, review, and revision dates help the user to determine if material is current or outdated.

- *Bias or sponsorship.* Commercial uses of the Internet are growing daily. The consumer must consider whether information is biased in favor of a particular product or commercial service. One means to consider bias is to look for a funding and advertising policy.

- *Ease of navigation.* Content should be well organized with the appropriate use of hyperlinks. All links should be to current Web pages and download easily.

- *Intended purpose and audience.* Sites should indicate the intended audience and use terminology and a reading level appropriate to that population.

- *Disclaimers.* Sites that express individual opinions should contain a statement to that effect to help users distinguish between fact and opinion.

- *Site accreditaion.* Several groups have been working to ensure the quality of information found on health-related Web sites. As a consequence of these efforts, some sites display a "seal" that indicates that their sites meet a set of predetermined standards for the quality of information posted. Compliance is purely voluntary.

- *Privacy policies.* Sites that collect personal information need to identify how that information may be used so that visitors can determine whether they choose to disclose information.

A number of groups are looking at the quality of posted materials, including most professional organizations, the Health Internet Ethics (Hi-Ethics) Alliance, the Health on the Net Foundation (HON), HealthWeb, Healthfinder, the Healthcare Coalition, the American Accreditation Health Care Commission (URAC), the European Council, and the World Health

Organization. None of these groups impose mandatory controls over quality. Hi-Ethics published a set of 14 principles in 2000 that forms the basis for URAC accreditation. Sites that have URAC accreditation display a seal. The seal indiciates that the site meets more than 50 standards that include disclosure, site policies and structure, content currency and accuracy, linking, privacy, security, and accountability. The accreditation process is one way to quickly identify posted content that meets quality standards. It is also seen as a means to facilitate the growth of the health Internet by fostering trust (D'Andrea 2002). URAC recently approved HIPAA security accreditation standards (Kohn 2003).The European Union has also developed criteria for evaluation of Web content that largely mirror those already defined by URAC (Commission of the European Communities 2002).

Online Publications and Journals

Soaring costs for paper, layout, printing, distribution, and the time that it takes to get materials to press make traditional publication an expensive process (Barbour and Pini 2002; Birchard 2002; Dvivedi and Dvivedi 2003; Grech 2002; Savulescu and Boyd 2003). Although online publication does not eliminate the costs associated with the collection, writing, and editorial processes, it does offer several advantages over traditional approaches, including the following:

- *A shorter time frame between writing and publication.* This is particularly important when material is quickly outdated, as occurs in health care. Individuals can place information on the Internet as soon as it is written rather than wait until a formal article or manuscript is accepted for publication. Peer-reviewed publications expedite the publication process when reviews are done electronically. Timely articles can be published almost immediately rather than sit in a queue once accepted. This shortens the traditional period of 4 months or longer from the time that an article is submitted until it appears in print.

- *Lower printing and distribution costs.* Electronic publication eliminates the need for paper, postage, and handling costs. Instead, documents are transferred from computer to computer in binary code. This transfer process is known as **electronic document interchange (EDI).** EDI also lowers publication costs because information is typed only once. An example of EDI is seen when an author submits an article for publication via FTP. Lower printing and distribution costs encourage publication of diverse viewpoints and small studies. Electronic publication also eliminates the need to curtail article length.

- *Revisions can be made quickly and distributed instantly.* For example, recommended treatment modalities are often changed with the latest research findings. Texts, professional standards of practice, nursing procedure manuals, and advice for consumers must reflect current recommendations. The electronic format also eliminates the need to replace and discard large volumes of out-of-date print materials.

- *Facilitation of joint authorship.* Colleagues at any location can share ideas and revise manuscripts without actually meeting in one physical location or spending scarce resources for travel or telephone charges.
- *Rapid identification of knowledge deficits.* FAQ on the Internet may indicate areas where research is needed. Surveys can be conducted quickly via e-mail and other electronic means.
- *Multimedia capability.* The inclusion of sound, voice, still images, and video permits the inclusion of links and allows comprehensive simulation of clinical problems that can aid student learning.
- *Improved access to materials.* Persons can access materials at any time and from any location as long as they have online access. There is no need to wait until a library is open. As a consequence, users can view literature previously unavailable to them. Many publishers allow access by subscription only, whereas others permit purchase on an article-by-article basis.
- *Facilitates electronic document searches for keywords or phrases.* Users can locate relevant information more quickly.
- *Lower subscription and storage costs for libraries.* Electronic publications can save libraries monies otherwise spent on higher costs for hard copies and physical management and storage.

Several nursing and allied health journals are currently available online. Some are published in both print and electronic format, whereas others are available only electronically. The existence of online journals may be researched through many of the same methods discussed earlier to find discussion groups and Web sites.

Despite the many advantages of electronic publication, there are some disadvantages. Electronic documents lack the same type of portability provided by print media. Reading lengthy documents online can cause eye strain and take longer because of the time that it takes for documents to download. Plagiarism is easier to commit and more difficult to find as the volume of online materials soars. There are also unresolved issues about archiving electronic publications. Excessive use of links may confuse the reader. Consideration must also be given to the fact that there are still large numbers of persons who have no online access.

Marketing Services

Web sites are a cost-effective public relations tool in health care. This is particularly true for sites that attract return visitors through the incorporation of interactive features. The Internet and Web can provide a competitive edge in the health care delivery system in the following ways:

- *Job postings.* Both employers and persons who are job hunting can use the Web to advertise positions and find new opportunities. Several sites offer help in locating job opportunities. Nursing World is one site that offers job search capability. Several employment services make it possible to complete resumes online, and some employers incorporate employment applications into their Web sites for electronic completion.

- *Virtual tours of educational institutions.* Some schools use their Web sites to introduce their facility and key people as well as allow the potential student to view available resources and complete an application online.

- *Support groups.* Emotional support and information is available for professionals and health care consumers. For example, the listserv AANurses (*http://www.tktucker.net/nir/*) is a support group for nurses, and the newsgroup alt.support.arthritis is a support group for the lay population. The presence of these resources on the Internet makes them readily available to a large number of people 24 hours a day.

- *Advertisement of services and consumer education.* Many health care providers furnish information about their services, assist with finding a physician or dentist, and provide general health care information via Web sites.

- *Dissemination and revision of product information.* Pharmaceutical companies and hospital equipment suppliers may also maintain Web sites that provide additional information about their products.

- *On-line risk assessments.* Some health care providers post tools that users may complete to determine their risk for developing a particular health problem. Basic advice for follow-up care may be provided along with names of area providers.

- *Completion of forms.* The time spent in the health care delivery system can be shortened when online prescreening forms are completed at the same time that appointments are requested (Brakeman 2000).

- *Benchmarking information.* Many providers and educational facilities include information that notes how their services compare with like entities in recent surveys.

E-health

The Internet offers the potential to increase access to health care information, empower consumers, educate practitioners, and transmit information quickly and cheaply (Briggs 2002, 2003; Girzadas and Given 2003; Hagland 2001). It is already used for business transactions, electronic prescriptions, online hospital registration, consumer education via Web sites, continuing education, and communication among professionals. Numerous terms have been coined to describe these applications, including e-business, e-commerce, and e-health or e-healthcare. **E-business** and **e-commerce** are not specific to health care. Both of these terms refer to services, sales, and business conducted over the Internet. Benefits associated with e-business and e-commerce include real-time responses to inquiries, clinical alerts, and the ability to quickly submit claims. **E-health** brings information, products, and services online. It provides the opportunity for providers and insurers to provide new services as well as use their strengths and bargaining powers to lower costs and increase the efficiency of services delivered. **E-care** is a broader term used to refer to the automation of all parts of the care delivery process across administrative, clinical, and departmental boundaries. E-care can include online purchasing of supplies and client management. The Internet has even been proposed as the infrastructure to achieve the computerized client record by providing a network to link together all health care providers, as well as payers and clients. Examples of e-health include wellness tips found on Web sites, e-mail reminders of appointments, follow-up e-mail from health care practitioners to consumer questions, electronic prescriptions, centralized storage of health records on the Web, regional telemedicine networks on the Web, consults, and long-term management of chronically ill patients. Another major application is electronic submission of claims and payment. Electronic claims submission reduces time and costs for claims submission and results in fewer rejections.

The Internet provides easy access to health-related information, including medical literature, location of clinical trials, and support groups for persons with particular health problems. An increasing number of providers and third-party payors are taking advantage of the power of the Internet to market their services and to publish up-to-date patient education materials, wellness newsletters, and eligibility information in a cost-effective fashion. At the same time, the number of individuals seeking online health care information and services is growing. The result is an empowered consumer who demands services now found on other Web sites but have been slow to arrive in health care. These include personalized, service-oriented features, such as scheduling, reminders for care, physician messaging, personal Web pages for the storage of health care information, and remote monitoring. The majority of these feature streamline care, improve the quality of service, and improve client tracking.

Another service that ultimately benefits the consumer is the electronic prescription. Electronic prescriptions eliminate the problem of lost or unreadable prescriptions while providing access to Web-based personal health information, drug interaction warnings, formularies, and verifications that reduce the incidence of medication errors. Handheld prescribing devices facilitate the electronic prescription process. The use of the Web to store health care information makes it available from different locations and to practitioners with different computer systems. A number of current sites allow consumers to store information and modify it for access when it is needed. One Web-based application that holds great promise for improved patient outcomes and lower long-term costs is disease management (Morrison 2002; Walker 2002). Chronic illness now accounts for the majority of health care costs. Web-based management provides a way to monitor large numbers of clients efficiently on a daily basis. Client participation is stimulated through the development of health goals and recording improvements. A device may be used to measure overall health. In this case, readings are obtained and sent for review by a health care practitioner. Devices have been used for asthmatics and persons with congestive heart failure. Technology can warn practitioners of abnormal findings that require intervention. The simplicity of the Web allows the addition of features easily and relatively inexpensively.

E-health is changing the relationships between health care professionals and consumers as well as the way that the health care industry is conducted (Hagland 2001). Browsers and the Web provide a user-friendly environment that allows users to focus on their needs rather than the technology. The Web provides the framework to expedite the delivery of services and revolutionize the way that care is delivered. Web portals help to create virtual communities both for professionals and consumers. Educated consumers come for treatment armed with knowledge that empowers them and may lead them to question treatment modalities. Full realization of the benefits of e-health requires good strategic planning, financial commitment, redesign of processes, consideration of regulatory demands, physician acceptance, and adequate data protection (Briggs 2002, 2003; Hagland 2001). One cited reason for the slow development of e-health is the mismatch between consumer demand and services provided. Most major initiatives in health care have a Web component, and this must be considered in the planning and budgeting processes. The success of e-health also requires reimbursement for services.

Current trends in health care delivery include use of online services for purchasing, referrals, submission of claims, and storage of health information. There is a shift away from heavily modified information systems maintained by the individual organization toward Web-based applications supported by vendors for some functions. These are known as **application service providers (ASPs)**. ASPs are ready for immediate use and available at a lower initial cost (Briggs 2002; Extinction Thwarted 2002). Typically the vendor hosts both the application and the data warehouse. The software and data are accessed through an Internet or a dedicated connection. ASPs can facilitate administrative tasks such as billing and coding. ASPs can also support clinical functions, although issues related to patient information security and data ownership have slowed their use. Organizations can realize cost savings when ASPs are used because the initial capital expenditure is less and fewer support staff are needed.

CONCERNS RELATED TO THE USE OF THE INTERNET

The single largest concern related to Internet use in health care is the security of client data, followed by worries over slowdown, collapse, and the ability to transact business smoothly. Lesser concerns include viral contamination and a lack of adherence to Internet standards among some products.

Firewalls

The open design of the Internet invites security abuse, particularly for private networks with Internet access. Most organizations with an Internet connection are under continuous attack by human attackers and automated software applications (Karpinski 2003). Any of these attacks have the potential to pose a serious security breach or a launching pad for large-scale attacks on other computers. For this reason, private networks need a gateway to intercept and examine Internet messages before they are permitted to enter the private network. A **gateway** is a combination of hardware and software used to connect local area networks with larger networks. A **firewall** is a type of gateway designed to protect private network resources from outside hackers, network damage, and theft or misuse of information (Cain 2003). It consists of hardware and software that can use one of several mechanisms to protect data. A firewall should be transparent to users. A firewall does not preclude the need for a security plan or periodic security testing; outside intruders may still be able to penetrate firewall protection.

Not all threats to a network arise from outside sources; firewalls alone do not protect against internal attacks or prevent viral contamination. Strong security policies for employees can minimize these threats as long as users are aware of the policies, their responsibilities, and the implications for policy violations. Another key factor in network protection is knowledge. Network administrators must educate themselves about attacks on Internet sites and protective measures recommended by the federally funded Computer Emergency Response Team (CERT) Coordination Center and Usenet groups. Subsequent work by a coalition of federal and private organizations produced a set of security configurations entitled "Consensus Baseline Security Settings." This effort was geared toward the protection of government Windows-based workstations from external and internal attacks, but it is expected to help other systems administrators to protect their systems and provide guidance for the future development of network protocols and systems (FAQ—The Benchmarks 2003; Vasin 2002).

Web Security

Most organizations focus security efforts on their internal networks, for the obvious reason that any disruption in computer operation affects service. As a consequence of this action, Web sites receive less attention. This omission leaves Web sites vulnerable to attack because of their visibility and the fact that they have been easy targets. However, disruption of Web sites may affect business operation as well. For example, hacker changes to Web pages may prove embarrassing, endanger consumers who follow altered advice, and/or result in libel charges. This recognition brings with it a heightened awareness of the need to safeguard Web sites as well as internal networks. At the same time, Webmasters are being encouraged to put their organizations on the Web so the world can access them, but they must also protect the organization from intruders.

The following measures can protect Web sites and their information (Karpinski 2003):

- *Construct a separate firewall for the Web server.* Firewalls provide the same level of protection for Web servers as they do for private networks with Internet access. Some, if not all, hacker attacks can be prevented with a firewall for each Web server.

- *Limit access to Web page content or configuration.* The risk of internal attacks or accidental damage is directly related to the number of persons with authority to change Web information or setup.

- *Isolate Web servers.* Web servers should not have direct connections to other agency systems, nor should they be located at a site subject to attack. This action minimizes the chance of Web site damage.

- *Heed security advisories.* Updates on hacker attacks and warnings on new breach techniques are posted by several sites on the Web, including the WWW Security FAQ and commercial sites such as Symantec.com. Webmasters should anticipate attack and take proactive measures.

- *Keep antivirus systems up-to-date and install intrusion detection systems to hail attacks.* Webmasters or network administrators need to maintain up-to-date virus detection to avoid having their site(s) being brought down by the latest virus or worm. Alarms and tracking mechanisms alert administrators or Webmasters to attacks early so that action can be taken to mininize Web site damage.

Organizational Policy

All organizations with an Internet connection need policies that address the following areas (Corry and Nutz 2003; Mirchandani and Motwani 2003; Ruckman 2002):

- *E-mail privacy.* The organization has the legal right to read employee e-mail unless stated otherwise. Employees should be aware of their organization's e-mail policy. Some organizations may permit a limited amount of personal e-mail.

- *Encryption.* Potentially sensitive data should be coded or encrypted to prevent unauthorized people from reading it. Any client data are sensitive and should be encrypted for transmittal over the Internet.

- *Transmission of employee data or photographs.* Employers should obtain consent before the transmittal of employee pictures or personal data over the Internet.

- *Intellectual ownership.* Guidelines should establish how issues of intellectual ownership are determined for network postings and other communications. In other words, it is important to resolve who owns the information: the employee who developed it or the employer.

- *Free speech.* The organization's stance on ideas or images that it considers offensive or inappropriate should be plainly delineated. Pornographic or sexually explicit or otherwise offensive materials are not acceptable. This helps to protect the organization from liability for inappropriate statements made by employees.

- *Acceptable Internet uses in the workplace.* Permissible Internet uses must be identified and communicated to employees. Violations of accepted use may constitute grounds for dismissal. One example of unacceptable use is the downloading of pirated music or software. One means to enforce this policy is the inclusion of a section on acceptable Internet use in the employee's annual performance evaluation.

- *Citation of sources and verification of information downloaded from the Internet/Web.* Authors of materials on the Internet and Web deserve the same recognition as authors of any other media. Failure to cite sources is plagiarism. Guidelines for the citation of on-line resources can be found at the American Psychological Association and the Modern Language Association Web sites as well as at most college and university sites.

- *Monitoring policies.* Employess need to be aware that e-mail and Internet use may be monitored and that inappropriate use can be cause for dismissal.

- *Acknowledgment of receipt of Internet policies.* Employees should sign a statement that they have read and understand the organization's Internet policies at the time of hire and on yearly review.

Overload

The Internet consists of many interconnected networks. Actual collapse is improbable, although vendor and facility outages and problems will likely continue as the number of users increases. Many first-time providers are undercapitalized or have poorly trained staff, so periodic overload or slow service can be expected. These problems raise interesting questions about maintaining data availability and integrity for the health care institution that uses the Internet to transport health data.

The majority of overload and collapse problems result from technical problems such as traffic jams, transmission difficulties, attacks by worms and viruses, and poor Web site design. These problems may occur on the user's network or an outside network. The popularity of the Internet makes it difficult to accommodate the needs of all of the users. For this reason, work is in progress to launch another version of the Internet. Internet2 (About Internet2 2003) is a collaborative effort of universities, government, industry, and various research and educational groups. The purpose of the Internet2 effort is to build and operate a research network capable of enhancing delivery of education and other services, including health care. This includes the development and support of advanced applications and standards. Another project that is working on ways to improve Internet speed and efficiency is the Next Generation Internet launched by the Clinton Administration (Rapoza 2002). This program conducted research but did not actually build a secure, newer Internet.

Viral Contamination

Viruses may be spread when files are imported for use without subjecting them to a viral scan (Rachel 2003; Ruckman 2002). The danger of viral contamination cannot be eliminated, but it can be reduced through the following measures:

- *Strict policies on Internet use.* These policies should include scanning all files before use, including FTP files and deletion of files with unfamiliar file extensions. Viruses may be included in materials available for public consumption. Consider deleting all attachments with unfamiliar file extensions.
- *Using the latest version of antiviral software.* New viruses are created daily. Older releases of antiviral software cannot recognize new viruses; therefore, it is important to frequently update the virus files for antiviral software. This can usually be done using downloads from a Web site and may or may not require a fee.
- *Downloading and installing software security patches.* Security patches for operating systems and applications are available from the vendor once problems have been identified.
- *Install or enable a computer firewall.* Some operating systems come with a firewall. A firewall provides a barrier against outsiders infiltrating a computer or network.
- *Use security features that come with software.* Word and Excel documents may contain macros that open automically. This can be controlled by setting the security level to "high."

INTRANETS AND EXTRANETS

The terms *intranet* and *extranet* received considerable attention when they were introduced. The concepts remain viable but the terms themselves are used less frequently. Instead it is more common to speak of portals. **Intranets** are private computer networks that use Internet protocols and technologies, including Web browsers, servers, and languages, to facilitate collaborative data sharing (Kohn 2002; Ortman 2001; White 2003). They were first developed in response to concerns over slowdowns, security breaches, and fears of Internet collapse. Intranets sit behind firewalls or other barriers and may not normally be available to people outside of the organization. In some cases authorized users may be able to access content from remote sites.

Intranets allow integration of disparate information systems. Intranets can save money by providing an easy-to-use, familiar interface that is intuitive and therefore requires little training. Most organizations use the corporate intranet first for publication of internal documents. This cuts down on paper and distribution costs, makes materials available more quickly and widely, and helps to ensure version control. This type of intranet application may be used to distribute policy and procedure manuals or other reference materials. It also acclimates employees to using the intranet as the single source of information. Additional features may include the ability for employees to view and enroll in benefits, request vacation days, and apply for internal jobs. Intranets are also an effective tool for marketing and advertising. Intranets in health care enterprises may also be used for mail and messaging, conferencing, and access to clinical data once the infrastructure is in place to bring together clinical systems and authenticate authorized users. In some cases, clients may be able to view their own health information, schedule appointments, and register for the hospital online. The concerns associated with intranet use mirror those discussed earlier; these include data security, the need to develop and implement strong organizational policies on appropriate intranet use, and the development of the infrastructure to support an intranet. Remote access may present additional issues for users because intranet content is generally designed to take advantage of fast network connections.

Extranets represent another variation of Internet technology (Denison 2002; Poynder 2002; White 2002; Whiting 2002). **Extranets** are networks that sit outside the protected internal network of an organization and use Internet software and communication protocols for electronic commerce and use by outside suppliers or customers. Extranets are more private than a Web site that is open to the public but are more open than an intranet, which can be accessed only by employees. Many extranets offer information that is a byproduct of the organization's main business either gratis or for a fee. Customers benefit because information is available 24 hours a day. For example, a vendor may develop an extranet that customers can use to obtain prices and place orders for merchandise. Security measures can be used to restrict access and secure information, making extranets more private than the Internet. Extranets may be subject to viruses, worms, and hacker attacks. One example of an extranet in use is the initiative by the U.S. Navy Medical Information Management Center to share medical and benefit information, newsletters, and e-mails with more than 100,000 users worldwide (Simpkins 2003).

CASE STUDY EXERCISES

As the representative for your medical center's Better Care Initiative, a project with the purpose of identifying ways that services can be delivered in a more efficient manner, you have suggested that the Internet be made available to clinicians at the point of care. You must develop a report listing the potential uses of the Internet, as well as potential problems that might occur.

• • •

One of your clients has a rare genetic defect. The client is requesting additional information about this from you, but no reference books on the unit describe this condition. Discuss strategies for how you might obtain this information using the Internet and electronic communication.

• • •

The e-health committee at your facility is looking at ways to provide greater client involvement in accessing their own health information. What ramifications must be considered for this to occur in terms of security, interpretation of results, and training?

 EXPLOREMediaLink

Multiple choice review questions, case studies, and other interactive resources for this chapter can be found on the Web site at *http://www.prenhall.com/hebda*. Click on "Chapter 4" to select the activities for this chapter.

SUMMARY

- Electronic communication is the ability to exchange information through the use of computer equipment and software, using network connections or a modem.
- The Internet is a network of networks, connecting computers worldwide. It offers a wealth of information about many topics, and can be extremely useful for the exchange of health care information.
- The World Wide Web (Web or WWW), a popular Internet feature, allows users to find information more easily by conducting word searches using browser software or locating a specific Web site or address. It is characterized by a GUI that makes it easy to use.
- A popular Web feature is the home page, the first page seen at a particular Web location. The home page provides general information about a topic, a person, or an organization.

- Links are words, phrases, or pictures that are distinguished from other parts of a WWW home page, usually by color, and enable users to move directly to another Web location.

- Nurses, other clinicians, and consumers may use the Web to obtain information regarding clinical topics, diseases, treatments, and health care agencies.

- Electronic mail, or e-mail, is the use of computer technology to transmit messages from one person to another. Delivery can be almost instantaneous. The Internet allows e-mail to be sent anywhere in the world, as long as the recipient has an Internet address.

- File transfer is the ability to move files from one location to another across a network.

- Other forms of electronic communication include listservs (electronic mailing lists), usenet groups (message discussion groups), and instant messaging. These forums provide information and support.

- E-commerce, or e-business, uses Internet technology to provide health care organizations with mechanisms to safely and quickly exchange information with other business entities.

- E-health refers to online availability of health information, products, and services.

- E-care is a broad term used to refer to the automation of all parts of the care delivery process, including purchasing and patient management.

- Evaluation of online information entails consideration of the source of the information, validation, accuracy and depth, dates for publication or review and revision, possible bias or sponsorship, organization and linkage, intended audience, presence of disclaimers and privacy policies, and accreditation or sponsorship by reputable organizations.

- Security is a major concern surrounding the use of the Internet and electronic communication. Firewalls and encryption are two prevalent strategies for safeguarding information.

- Internet technology is used internally in an organization in systems known as intranets, or external to the organization in systems known as extranets. Increasingly, these applications are referred to as Web portals.

- ASPs represent an alternative to institutional purchase and customization of information systems and software applications. ASP advantages include lower initial expenses, reduced wait time, and easier upgrades.

REFERENCES

About Internet2. (2003). Available online at: http://www.internet2.edu/about/aboutinternet2.html. Accessed October 3, 2003.

Alsop, S. (2003). I covet my neighbor's broadband (it's about time!). *Fortune*, *147*(13), 132.

Arnold, S. (July/August 2003). The new Internet gold rush is search market-ing. *Information World Review, Issue 193,* 14.

Baldwin, G. (1999). New Internet technologies getting closer and closer. *Health Data Management,* 7(10), 14, 24.

Barbour, V., and Pini, P. (June 29, 2002). Early online publication. *Lancet, 359*(9325), 2216.

Behan, M. (1999). Internet security: Making your e-business a safe business. *Beyond Computing,* 8(5), 34–39.

Birchard, K. (September 27, 2002). Journal opts out of print and for the In-ternet. *Chronicle of Higher Education, 49*(5), A50.

Bland, V. (2001). Web portals. *NZ Business, 15*(5), 36.

Brakeman, L. (2000). Number of Internet users tops the 100 million mark. *Managed Healthcare, 10*(1), 48, 2p.

Briggs, B. (2002). E-health demand may finally catch up with supply. *Health Data Management, 10*(12), 40–46.

Briggs, B. (2002). The jury's still out on ASP's in health care. *Health Data Management, 10*(8), 52.

Briggs, B. (2003). E-health rises from the ashes. *Health Data Management, 11*(1), 40–52.

Cain, M. (2003). Cybertheft, network security, and the library without walls. *Journal of Academic Librarianship, 29*(4), 245.

Carlson, W. H. (2003). Making a splash with Web services. *ADVANCE for Health Information Executives,* 7(8), 45–48.

Carroll, S. (2003). How to find anything online. *PC Magazine, 22*(9), 80.

Carroll, S., Mendelson, E., Cohen, A., Ellison, C., Metz, C., Pike, S., and Sar-rel, M. D. (October 15, 2002). The bionic browser, *PC Magazine, 21*(18).

Clyde, L. A. (2003). Search engines are improving—But they still can't find everything. *Teacher Librarian, 30*(5), 44.

Commission of the European Communities. (2002). EEurope 2002: Quality criteria for health related Websites. *Journal of Medical Internet Re-search, 4*(3), e15.

Connect with high-speed Internet. (2003). *NEA Today, 21*(8), 34.

Corry, D. J., and Nutz, K. E. (2003). Employee e-mail and Internet use: Canadian legal issues. *Journal of Labor Research, 24*(2), p233.

Cox, L. (July/August 2003). "Blograising" begins. *Columbia Journalism Re-view, 42*(2), 9.

D'Andrea, G. (2002). Health Web site accreditation: Opportunities and chal-lenges. *Journal of Healthcare Information Management, 16*(3), 9–11.

Davidson, P. (April 14, 2003). High-speed net service: Coming to a plug near you? *USA Today.*

Denison, D. C. (May 6, 2002). Corporate extranets enable new forms of col-laboration with partners, customers. *The Boston Globe.*

Desai, V. (1997). Web-based management: Welcome to your next nightmare. *Internetwork,* 8(1), 40–42.

Dvivedi. J., and Dvivedi, S. (May 2003). Online medical publication and the medical student. *Asian Student Medical Journal.* Available online at: http://asmj.netfirms.com/article0103.html. Accessed September 17, 2003.

Dyer, K. A. (1999). Cybermedicine enters the new millennium. *MDComputing*, *16*(6), 49–50.

Ernst, W. (June 30, 2003). Building blogs. *PC Magazine*, *22*(11), 60.

Everett, J. (July 2003). All the science news that's fit to print (and some that's not). *Popular Science*, *263*(1), 98.

Extinction thwarted. (June 10, 2002). *eWeek*.

FAQ—The benchmarks. (May 2003). The Center for Internet Security. Available online at: http://www.cisecurity.org/. Accessed September 24, 2003.

Fox, S. (July 2003) Fast net access from your power outlet. *PC World*, *21* (7), 37.

FTC takes on spam. (June 30, 2003). *eWeek*.

Gann, R. (April 2003). Get rid of all that spam! Use Outlook Express rules to deal with unwanted email messages. *Internet Magazine*, 34.

Geist, M. (March 3, 2003). Governments hold reins in those national domains. *Toronto Star*.

Grech V. (2002). The legitimacy and advantages of electronic publication. *Images in Pediatric Cardiology*, *10*, 1–3.

Girzadas, J., and Given, R. (2003). Distinguish yourself with e-health. *Healthcare Informatics*, *20*(3), 39–40.

Grimes, B. (2002). Ditch your dial-up. *PC World*, *20*(2), 68.

Hagland, M. (2001). Finding the e in healthcare. *Healthcare Informatics*, *18*(11), 21–22, 24, 26.

Hall, M. (2002). Web services open portal doors. *Computerworld*, *36*(26), 28.

Hamilton, D. (2003). Mozilla. *Searcher*, *11*(1).

Hawkins, D. T. (2003). The eighth search engine meeting. *Information Today*, *20*(6), 1.

Hebda, T., Czar, P., and Mascara, C. (2003). Information technology. In Haynes, L. C., Butcher, H. K., and Boese, T. (2003). *Nursing in contemporary society: Issues, trends and transition to practice*. Upper Saddle River, NJ: Prentice-Hall.

Hussey, J. S. (2000). Healthcare on-line. *Healthcare Informatics*, *17*(2), 100.

Internet Society. (August 11, 2003). *All about the Internet Society*. Available online at: http://www.isoc.org/isoc/. Accessed August 23, 2003.

Joyce, J. (September 2002). Instant messaging. *Scientific Computing & Instrumentation*, *19*(10), h12, 61.

Karpinski, R. (2003). Web site security. *B to B*, *88*(6), 15.

Kelly, G., and McKenzie, B. (2002). Security, privacy, and confidentiality issues on the Internet. *Journal of Medical Internet Research*, *4*(2), e12. Available online at: http://www.jmir.org/2002/2/212/. Accessed August 24, 2003.

Kohn, C. (June 2, 2003). URAC board approves HIPAA security accreditation standards. *Managed Care Weekly*, 25.

Kohn, D. (2002). E-health initiatives for today's information systems. *ADVANCE for Health Information Executives*, *6*(12), 17–22, 96.

Leary, B. (2003). The quest for administrative simplification and cost reduction. *ADVANCE for Health Information Executives*, *7*(7), 37–42.

Long, C. (August 2003). Evaluating Web sites. *Nursing2003, 33*(8), 82.

Markoff, J., and Richtel, M. (April 10, 2003). Internet via the power grid: New interest in obvious idea. *New York Times,* 7.

Mack, J. and Llewellyn, P. (2003). Internet Healthcare Coalition and Polling Pharma launch new survey: Quality of Pharma-sponsored health information on the internet. Available online at: http://www.ihealthcoalition. org/about/ihcc_pr18.html. Accessed May 9, 2004.

McLaughlin, L. (2002). The straight story on search engines. *PC World, 20*(7), 115.

Merline, J. (2003). Can e-mail be saved from 'spam'? *Consumers' Research Magazine, 86*(7), 10.

Mirchandani, D. and Motwan, J. (2003). Reducing internet abuse in the work place. *SAM Advanced Management Journal, 68*(1), 22.

Morita, R. (1997). Taking management to the Web. *Internetwork, 8*(1), 8.

Morochove, R. (August 4, 2003). It's not flashy but Usenet still vital to Net. *Toronto Star.*

Morrison, M. H. (2002). e-Healthcare: A new service for older consumers. *Nursing Homes Long Term Care Management, 51*(2), 48.

Nash, K. S. (1996). Policing the net. *Computerworld, 30*(27), 1, 89.

New portal launched to serve 2000 clinicians, 46,800 patients. (June 16, 2003). *Managed Care Weekly Digest,* 29.

Ortman, N. (2001). Healthcare Intranets are healthy investments that pay for themselves. *Managed Healthcare Executive, 11*(8), 42–44.

Poynder, R. (February 2002). Paying the price for security. *Information Today, 19*(2), p1.

Portal technologies in action. (2003). *ADVANCE for Health Information Executives, 17*(1), 75–90.

Rachel, R. (August 14, 2003). Latest virus new breed of computer parasite. *Toronto Star.*

RAND Health and California HealthCare Coalition (2002). Proceed with caution: A report on the quality of health information on the internet. Available at: http://www.chcf.org/documents/consumer/ ProceedWithCautionCompleteStudy.pdf. Accessed May 9, 2004.

Rapoza, J. (July 15, 2002). It's time for next Internet. *EWeek, 19*(28), 58.

Robinson, D. (2001). Listservs 101: What they are and how to make the best use of them. *Feliciter, 47*(6), 292.

Ruckman, S. (2002). Helping protect computer networks from the inside: Education as a security tool. *Techniques, 77*(5), 42.

Saunders, J. (1999). Corporate portal opens data door. *Computing Canada, 25*(43), 23.

Savulescu, J., and Boyd, K. M. (February 2003). Institute of Medical Ethics prize for the most innovative Web publication. *Journal of Medical Ethics, 29*(1), 1.

Schofield, J. (August 19, 2003). Challenge-response systems could beat spam. *Computer Weekly,* p. 2001.

Semeria, C. (1996). Internet firewalls and security. *Enterprise Systems Journal*, *11*(7), 32, 34, 36–38.

Simpkins, A. (February 2003). Navy secures healthcare network. *Communications News*, *40*(2), 20.

Spanbauer, S., and McDonald, A. B. (September 2002). IE alternatives: Three new contenders. *PC World*, *20*(9).

Stammer, L. (February 2000). ASPs will transform healthcare into a truly Internet-friendly business. *Healthcare Informatics*, *17*(2), 46, 48.

Stop signs on the web. (January 1, 2001). *Economist*, *358*(8204), 21.

Tabar, P. (2000). The latest word. *Healthcare Informatics*, *17*(3), 75–132.

Tabar, P. (2002). You've got mail. Plus problems? *Healthcare Informatics*, *19*(1), 13–14, 18.

Vasin, R. (July 22, 2002). Feds endorse guide for Windows security. *Federal Computer Week*. Available online at: http://www.fcw.com/fcw/articles/2002/0722/pol-win-07–22–02.asp. Accessed September 24, 2003.

Vijayan, J. (2003). Captohas eat spam: Ingenious computer tests may also advance machine vision and AI. *Computerworld*, *37*(24), 32.

Voelk, R., and Geyer, A. (2002). Got a grip on email security. *Healthcare Informatics*, *19*(4), 50.

Walker, T. (2002). Successful e-DM initiatives rely on the connectivity of patient, provider, insurer. *Managed Healthcare Executive*, *12*(7), 34.

Webopedia. (July 24, 2003). FTP. Available online at: http://webopaedia.com/TERM/F/FTP.html. Accessed August 27, 2003.

White, M. (June 2002). Intranets and extranets: Playing the numbers. *EContent*, *25*(6), p 40(2p).

White, M. (April 2003). Passing through. *EContent*, *26*(4).

Whiting, R. (May 20, 2002). Extranets go the extra mile. *InformationWeek* Issue 889, p 72 (3p).

Woellert, L. and Wildstrom, S. H. (August 11, 2003). Out, out, damned spam: Junk e-mail accounts for roughly half of all network traffic. Here are five ways to beat it back. *Business Week, issue* 3845, p. 54(3).

World Health Organization (WHO). (2003). Medical products and the Internet: A guide to finding reliable information Available online at: http://www.who.int/medicines/library/qsm/who-edm-qsm-99–4/medicines-on-internet-guide.html. Downloaded September 14, 2003.

Two

Health Care Information Systems

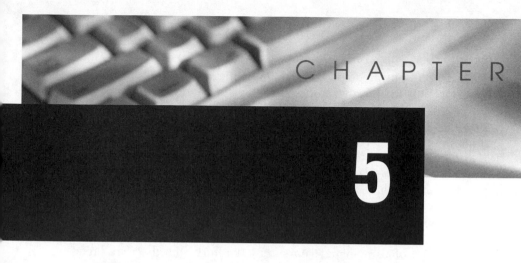

Health Care Information Systems

After completing this chapter, you should be able to:

- Identify the various types of information systems used within health care institutions.

- Define the terms *health care information system, hospital information system, clinical information system, nursing information system, physician practice management system,* and *administrative information system.*

- Explain the functions of a nursing information system.

- Differentiate between the nursing process and critical pathways/protocol approaches to the design of a nursing system.

- Review the key features and impacts on nursing and other health care professionals associated with order entry, laboratory, radiology, and pharmacy information systems.

- Describe the functions of client registration and scheduling, and coding systems.

- Explain the purpose of decision support and expert systems.

- Identify ways that mobile devices such as personal digital assistants and tablet personal computers can improve the utility of health care information systems.

MEDIALINK

Additional resources for this content can be found on the Companion Website at *www. prenhall.com/hebda*. Click on "Chapter 5" to select the activities for this chapter.

Companion Website

- Glossary
- Multiple Choice
- Discussion Points
- Case Study: Medication Documentation System
- Case Study: Implementation of CPOE
- Case Study: Radiology System
- MediaLink Application: Clinical Information Systems
- Web Hunt: Health Care Advocacy Groups
- Links to Resources
- Crossword Puzzle

An **information system** can be defined as the use of computer hardware and software to process data into information to solve a problem. The terms **healthcare information system** and **hospital information system (HIS)** both refer to a group of systems used within a hospital or enterprise that support and enhance health care. The HIS comprises two major types of information systems: clinical information systems and administrative information systems. **Clinical information systems (CISs)** are large, computerized database management systems that support several types of activities that may include physician order entry, result retrieval, documentation, and decision support (Clinical Information Systems 2002). Clinicians use these systems to access client data that are used to plan, implement, and evaluate care. CISs may also be referred to as *client care information systems.* Some examples of CISs include nursing, laboratory, pharmacy, radiology, medical information systems, and physician practice management systems. **Administrative information systems** support client care by managing financial and demographic information and providing reporting capabilities. This category includes client management, financial, payroll, and human resources, and quality assurance systems. Coding systems use clinical information to generate charges for care . Figure 5–1 shows the relationships between various components of a hospital information system.

Clinical and administrative information systems may be designed to meet the needs of one or more departments or functions within the organization. These can be implemented as stand-alone systems, or they may work with other systems to provide information sharing and seamless functionality for the users. Any one health care enterprise may use one or several of the clinical and administrative systems but probably will not use all of them. Increasingly, organizations are looking at the need to improve productivity, increase the quality of care, and reduce costs across the enterprise. Information technology is seen as the means to achieve these ends through improved work flow and better management of resources (Lavelle 2002).

CLINICAL INFORMATION SYSTEMS

Although many CISs are designed for use within one hospital department, clinicians and researchers from several areas use the data collected by each system. For example, the nurse documents client allergies in the initial assessment. The physician, the pharmacist, the dietician, and the radiologist can then use these data during the client's hospital stay. The goal of CISs is to allow clinicians to quickly and safely access information, order appropriate medications and treatments, and implement care while avoiding duplicate services (Lavelle 2002; Morrissey 2001). The following descriptions of CISs address those that are most frequently seen in the hospital setting.

Nursing Information Systems

A **nursing information system** supports the use and documentation of nursing processes, activities, and provides tools for managing the delivery

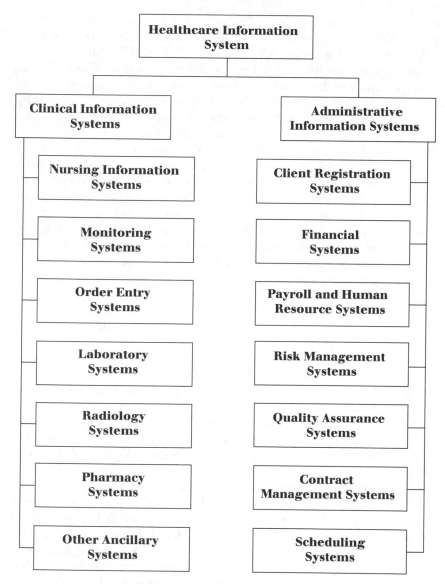

FIGURE 5–1 • Relationship of the healthcare information system components

of nursing care (Hendrickson 1993). An effective nursing information system must accomplish two goals. The first goal is that the system should support the way that nurses function, allowing them the flexibility to use the system to view data and collect necessary information, provide quality client care, and document the client's condition and the care that was given. Necessary information includes past health medical history, allergies, test results, and progress notes, among other things. The second goal of an effective nursing information system is that it should support and enhance nursing practice through improved access to information and tools. These include online literature searches such as the Cumulative Index of Nursing and Allied Health Literature (CINAHL) and MEDLINE, and automated drug information and hospital policy/procedure guidelines. Consideration of these two goals in the selection and implementation of a nursing system will ensure that it benefits nursing. The challenge for nursing is to identify and implement technology and information systems solutions that provide more breadth, depth, flexibility, and standardization (Hughes 1997).

In general, there are two approaches to nursing care and documentation using automated information systems. These are the *traditional nursing process* approach and the *critical pathway*, or *protocols*, approach. The traditional nursing process approach allows documentation of nursing care using well-established formats such as admission assessments, problem lists, and care plans. A more organized version of this approach incorporates **standardized nursing languages (SNLs)** accepted by the American Nurses Association (Prophet, Dorr, Gibbs, and Porcella 1997). These include nursing diagnoses defined by the North American Nursing Diagnosis Association (NANDA), Nursing Interventions Classification (NIC), and Nursing Outcomes Classification (NOC). SNLs provide a common language across the discipline of nursing that allows all nurses to describe nursing problems, treatments, and outcomes in a manner that is understood by all nurses. SNLs facilitate data collection and research that can be replicated and shared across all of nursing (Powelson, McGahan, and Wilkinson 2000). The University of Iowa Hospitals and Clinics have been working for 20 years on the development of a clinical database to support patient care planning and documentation via their INFORMM NIS (Information Network for Online Retrieval & Medical Management Nursing Information System) (Prophet 2000). The recent adoption of the first international standard for nursing, *The Integration of a Reference Terminology Model for Nursing*, at the International Organization of Standardization Technical Committee for Health Informatics represents an important step in representing nursing diagnosis and other key concepts in a manner suitable for computer processing (Health Informatics Standards 2003). Despite this progress in representing nursing language in automated systems, the use of interdisciplinary pathways remains popular. These protocols suggest specific treatments related to the client's diagnosis and outline the anticipated outcomes. The advantages of using a nursing information system are listed in Box 5–1.

Nursing Process Approach The nursing process approach to automated documentation is based on the paper forms traditionally used by nurses. The nursing diagnosis often serves as the organizational framework. Many current information systems follow this format.

- *Documentation of nursing admission assessment and discharge instructions.* A menu-driven approach to the admission assessment ensures capture of essential information. A **menu** lists related

Box 5–1

Advantages of a Nursing Information System

- Increased time to spend with clients
- Better access to information
- Enhanced quality of documentation
- Improved quality of client care
- Increased nursing productivity
- Improved communications
- Reduced errors of omissions
- Reduced medication errors
- Reduced hospital costs
- Increased nurse job satisfaction
- Compliance with JCAHO regulations
- Development of a common clinical database
- Improved client perception of care
- Enhanced ability to track client's record
- Enhanced ability to recruit/retain staff
- Improved hospital image

SOURCE: Saba, V., and McCormick, K. (1998). *Essentials of computers for nurses,* 2nd ed. New York: McGraw-Hill. Used with permission from The McGraw-Hill Companies.© 1996

commands that can be selected from a computer screen to accomplish a task. For example, the menu may include selections such as past medical history, advanced directives, organ donation status, psychosocial history, medications, and review of body systems. This approach can also be used to ensure that all necessary information is covered in the client's discharge instructions, including follow-up appointments and diagnostic studies; diet and activity restrictions; wound care; and medication information such as drug names, instructions for administration, and common side effects that the client should report. The system should generate printed copies of these instructions for clients to review on discharge and for their use at home, as well as for use by the Home Health staff.

- *Generation of a nursing worklist that indicates routine scheduled activities related to the care of each client.* These activities can be grouped according to scheduled time or skill level.

- *Documentation of discrete data or activities such as vital signs, weight, and intake and output measurements.* The automation of this type of data promotes accuracy and allows the data to be readily available to all care providers at any time.

- *Documentation of routine aspects of client care, such as bathing, positioning, blood glucose measurements, notation of dietary intake, and/or wound care in a flowsheet format.*
- *Standardized care plans that the nurse can individualize for clients as needed.* This feature saves time yet allows flexibility to address the client's needs while promoting quality care.
- *Documentation of nursing care in a progress note format.* The nurse may accomplish this through narrative charting, charting by exception, or flowsheet charting. Regardless of the method, automated documentation can improve the overall quality of charting by prompting the nurse with predefined selections. Box 5–2 describes three of these traditional formats and some typical automation approaches.
- *Documentation of medication administration.* This complex procedure may require several steps, described below.
    1. The system can generate a medication list, indicating which medications are scheduled for administration during the nurse's shift. This list may also include unscheduled or PRN medications for each client, as well as instructions related to administration. For example, the list might include a reminder to check the client's pulse before giving digoxin and to hold the medication if the pulse falls below a standard rate or the physician's ordered parameter. The nurse may use this list to write notes and check off medications as they are given if a portable device is not available for direct documentation into the system.

Box 5–2 **Automation of Traditional Nursing Documentation Methods**

Many forms of nursing documentation have been automated by various nursing information systems. Some of these formats are listed below.

- *Narrative charting.* Traditionally, nurses complete charts using narrative text. In a nursing information system, this may be accomplished using free text entry or menu selections.
- *Charting by exception.* Client-specific documentation addresses only the client's exceptions to normal conditions or ranges. Automated documentation should provide all normal standards and allow the nurse to easily document any exception observed. This may involve menu selections or free text entry.
- *Flowsheet charting.* Routine aspects of care are documented in tabular form. This format is most effective when presented in a personal computer–based graphical user interface. A pointing device such as a mouse is used to make menu selections or text entries. One form of flowsheet charting is the automation of medication administration records.
- *Standardized nursing languages.* This approach uses NANDA nursing diagnosis as well as the Nursing Interventions Classification and Nursing Outcomes Classification languages. It removes the ambiguity of meaning found in other documentation systems.

2. The nurse can then access the medication administration record (MAR) in the information system to document medications that were given or held. An automated MAR helps the nurse document administration of medications in a manner that satisfies regulatory and nursing policy requirements.

3. The system prompts the nurse to enter other related information, such as injection site, pulse, or pain scale value. If a medication is not given, the system prompts the nurse to enter the reason.

4. The system can generate a report indicating medications that were not charted as a reminder to the nurse.

5. The system can issue a warning when medications are charted as given two or more times for the same time slot and then request verification or correction of the same.

6. Some systems allow automatic patient billing for medications and related supplies such as intravenous (IV) tubing and IV dressing changes based on documented care.

Recent initiatives to improve patient safety and decrease medication errors call for the use of barcode medication administration systems (Baldwin 2002; Gryskevich 2002). While these are not considered to be a part of a nursing documentation system, bar code systems are designed to prevent common medication administration errors at the bedside, document medication administration, and capture charges. These systems require the nurse to scan the bar codes found on his or her identification, the patient's identification bracelet, and on all prescription medications during the medication administration process. These systems are designed to help the busy nurse to ensure that the right medication is given in the correct dosage and form at the correct time for the right patient. Bar coding systems often include warnings for high-risk drugs, for medications with sound-alike names, and for maximum dosages.

Critical Pathway or Protocols The critical pathway or protocol approach to nursing documentation is another approach used in automated nursing information systems, particularly with the onset of managed care. This approach is often used in a multidisciplinary manner, with many types of care providers accessing the system for information and to document care. Nurses, nursing or patient care assistants, dietitians, social workers, respiratory therapists, physical and occupational therapists, case managers, and physicians all use these systems for documentation. Critical pathway systems include the following features:

• *The nurse, or other care provider, can select one or more appropriate critical pathways for the client.* If more than one path is selected, the system should merge the paths to create one "master" path or protocol.

- *Interaction with physician orders.* Standard physician order sets can be included with each critical pathway and may be automatically processed by the system.
- *Tracking of protocol variances.* The system should identify variances to the anticipated outcomes as they are charted and provide aggregate variance data for analysis by the providers. This information can be used to fine tune and improve the critical pathways, thereby contributing to improved client outcomes.

Clinician Information Systems

CISs are information systems that may be used by any clinician. These users can include nurses, physicians, pharmacists, social workers, respiratory therapists, dieticians, physical therapists, and any other clinician requiring access to the client record. CISs may allow the user to document client condition and response to treatment, or they may limit the user to viewing client information without the capability of entering data. Rapid developments in technology are revolutionizing CISs. Mobile and wireless technology are used with CISs to allow information entry and retrieval at the point of care or wherever it is needed by the health care professional. Most often this is at the bedside, but it may be in another hospital department. This is best illustrated by the health care professional who can view client lab results while walking. This type of access enhances worker productivity because they do not need to walk back to a central location to view test results, and it improves client service because treatments can be ordered and initiated in a more timely fashion. Internet technology is also changing the way that users interact with CISs. This capability allows a physician to view client test results from the comfort of his or her home or office or even while on the golf course or at the mall. Despite the fact that the technology exists to permit this type of access, not all facilities can provide it at this time.

Monitoring Systems

Monitoring systems are devices that automatically monitor biometric measurements in critical care and specialty areas, such as cardiology and obstetrics. These devices may send information to the nursing documentation system. For example, a monitoring system would directly enter measurements such as blood pressures, eliminating the need for the nurse to enter these data manually. Another example may be seen with blood glucose monitors that send client readings to the laboratory system for display with other laboratory tests. Box 5–3 describes some additional features of monitoring systems.

Order Entry Systems

With **order entry systems,** physician orders for medications and treatments are entered into the computer and directly transmitted to the appro-

Box 5–3	Some Common Features of Monitoring

- *Alarms alerting the nurse of significant abnormal findings.* Sophisticated systems provide different alarms indicating various abnormalities. For example, the nurse may be able to hear a specific alarm sound that indicates which cardiac arrhythmia the client is experiencing.
- *Portable monitoring systems.* These allow easy transportation of the client throughout the facility without loss of data or functionality.
- *Records of past abnormal findings.* The system maintains a record of all past abnormal findings during this monitoring episode. The system allows the user to find trends in data using graphical displays and to focus on specific details.
- *Download capabilities.* The system may be able to transfer patient data to a separate system in another facility to provide a continuous patient record.

priate areas whether that is the pharmacy, the laboratory, the radiology department, or social service. The preferred method is direct entry of orders by the physician because this eliminates issues related to illegible handwriting and transcription errors, speeds the implementation of ordered diagnostic tests and treatment modalities, and can enhance staff productivity and save money (Dorenfest 2003; Marshalek and Cassey 2003; May 2003; Stablein and Drazen 2003). This process is known as **computerized physician order entry (CPOE).** CPOE represents a major initiative on the part of the Institute of Medicine and Leapfrog Group to improve the quality of care and reduce medication errors. While most CPOE is found in inpatient settings, its use in outpatient and ambulatory settings is under exploration for all of the same reasons that it is advocated in primary care settings. CPOE systems are also made safer through the incorporation of built-in reminders and alerts that help the physician to select the most appropriate diagnostic test or medication for a particular patient as well as the appropriate dose and form. Implementation of CPOE has been slowed by such factors as difficult system sign-on, limited system access or response time, funding constraints, inadequate access to clinical data to support the expert decision-making features of CPOE, and the perception by many physicians that CPOE affords them few advantages. In some settings, transcription of physician orders into the clinical information system is still done by a nurse or by ancillary personnel. When entries are made by ancillary personnel, nurses are responsible for ensuring that entries are correct.

Entry of an order into a clinical information or order entry system *alerts all departments* to carry out physician orders. For example, when a physician orders a barium enema, the order entry system can automatically notify the dietary department to hold the client's breakfast, the pharmacy to send the appropriate medications, and the radiology department to schedule the test. These systems prompt the clinician to provide the information necessary for carrying out the order.

Another feature of an order entry system is *duplicate checking*. When an order is entered, the system checks to see if a similar order has been placed within a specified time frame. If this is the case, the system can alert the user with a message, or automatically combine the two orders, permitting only one execution of the order.

The order entry system can reflect the *current status* of each order. For example, the status may be listed as pending, complete, or canceled. This allows the user to see a comprehensive list of the client's orders at any point in time. It can also afford a mechanism for the entry of charges for a procedure once it has been completed.

One mechanism that is used in some order entry systems uses rules-based or knowledge-based programming. Rules provide guidelines to assist physicians to select the preferred and most cost-effective medication along with the best route and dose for a particular patient problem. Rules can also provide prompts for when patients should be seen next and diagnostic tests that should be performed. These automated reminders help to improve the quality of care (Calabrisi, Czarnecki, and Blank 2002).

Laboratory Systems

Laboratory information systems (LISs) can provide many benefits, including a shorter turnaround time for results, prevention of duplicate testing, decreased likelihood of human error, and identification of abnormal results according to age, sex, and hospital standards. Some systems can send alerts for critical values directly to physicians (Marietti 2003). In addition, microbiology culture and sensitivity testing can provide treatment suggestions for the physician.

Automatic generation of specimen labels should occur when an order is placed either directly into an LIS or passed to an order entry system. Labels may include client demographic identifiers, the name of laboratory studies to be performed, and any special instruction for handling, such as "place on ice." Labels may be configured to print immediately at the client location for stat or nurse-collected specimens or in the laboratory in batch mode for laboratory-collected specimens. *Batch mode* allows the labels to be printed in groups for standard collection times, either on demand or at predefined times.

When specimens are processed by the laboratory instrumentation, the results are automatically transmitted to the LIS. The results can be viewed directly from the LIS or transmitted to another information system, such as the nursing or medical information system. Laboratory values are available immediately on completion of the testing process. If desired, printed paper copies of the results may be produced immediately at predefined locations, such as the nursing unit or physician's office, or can be printed in cumulative format for permanent chart copies. Another feature of many laboratory systems is automatic client billing for tests completed. This information may be communicated to the client billing system.

Another feature seen in many laboratory systems is the ability to integrate results collected at the bedside using portable devices. This is seen with the performance of blood glucose monitor tests in the clinical area. Results are then sent to the laboratory system immediately or sent when the blood glucose monitor is docked. This affords clinicians an integrated view of patient results and the ability to compare glucose readings taken at the bedside with glucose readings from blood specimens sent to the laboratory. While this feature is widely used and appreciated more commonly, the demand is to have LIS results available at the bedside or via mobile devices such as personal digital assistants (PDAs) where results are passed either through the laboratory or clinical information system to the PDA for review.

Another feature of some laboratory systems is the ability to use rules-based testing. A **rule** is a predefined function that generates a clinical alert or reminder. **Arden syntax** is the standard language used in the health care industry for writing rules. A rules-based LIS could automatically order a second test based on the results of an initial test. For example, if a client has an abnormal complete blood cell count value, the system will perform a differential, which is a more specific second test. Rules-based testing could also eliminate unnecessary testing after several consecutive normal results have been obtained, as when physicians order daily laboratory work. These measures save costs and the staff time of assessing the need for and performing the tests. The incorporation of rules-based technology may require the user to enter all of the information needed for specific tests. An example is weight for a creatinine clearance test to determine whether the client's renal function falls within the normal range. Another example of rules-based technology is seen when labels are printed with collection instructions such as tube color, amount needed, and directions such as "place on ice." Rules can also be used to limit tests to those covered by Medicare or other third-party payors or to determine how and where test results will be sent (Rogoski 2003).

Laboratory systems also have the potential to provide more meaningful information such as genetic predisposition toward certain diseases based on information that already exists in the hospital or laboratory database that can be useful in the diagnosis and procurement of payment from third-party payors (Rogoski 2003).

One traditionally weak area in the collection and processing of laboratory results is patient identification. Handwritten labels may be illegible for reasons of poor handwriting or spills. The use of bar coding in conjunction with an LIS to track specimens helps to eliminate this type of problem. Bar codes are either printed directly onto collection labels or affixed at the time of processing to help improve specimen tracking. This process results in improved patient safety and productivity (Marietti 2003).

Although many institutions are moving toward a paperless record, it has been common practice for staff and students to print out copies of laboratory findings for their personal reference and to communicate to other staff. The ability to send results directly to secure PDAs helps to ensure the privacy of health information because it eliminates the need for large numbers of printouts and the need to Fax sensitive information. This feature helps health care providers to comply with government requirements to safeguard client health information (Schuerenberg 2002).

Radiology Systems

A **radiology information system (RIS)** provides scheduling of diagnostic tests, communication of clinical information, generation of client instructions and preparation procedures, transcription of results and impressions, and file room management such as tracking of film location. Orders may be entered directly into the radiology system or transmitted from an order entry system. Radiology clerical staff use order information to schedule patients for testing. Once the test is complete, the radiologist interprets the findings and dictates a report. This report can be transcribed using the radiology system or a separate transcription system. The radiology system generates billing information that can be sent to the billing system. The reports are then stored within the radiology system. They may also be Faxed to the physician's office or viewed through the clinical or nursing information systems.

One example of how a radiology system might be used is seen with magnetic resonance imaging (MRI) orders. As the first step in placing an MRI order, the system generates a questionnaire that asks questions pertinent to the MRI procedure. For example, it asks whether the client is cooperative or claustrophobic, and if there are any metal foreign bodies related to previous surgeries or injuries. The nurse reviews these questions with the client, then enters the answers to each question and the order requested into the system. A radiologist reviews the order request and the questionnaire answers, and determines if the client is appropriate for testing. This procedure allows scheduling of appropriate clients only, and eliminates the time-consuming and costly scheduling and attempted testing of inappropriate clients.

More recent developments in radiology information systems include digital, filmless images as a replacement for traditional radiology films. These **picture archiving and communication systems (PACS)** allow images to be electronically transmitted and viewed using sophisticated, high-resolution monitors. The enhanced quality of these images over traditional films may result in fewer repeat procedures and improved diagnostic capability. The use of digital filmless imaging is also an integral component in the evolution of the electronic client record. Use of this technology may allow hospitals to do away with radiology images captured on film. This reduces or eliminates the large expense of radiology films, as well as handling and storage of the x-rays. In addition, PACS can provide the physician with a radiology image viewed on a computer screen within seconds after the completion of the procedure. Another benefit of a PACS is that more than one physician can view an image simultaneously in multiple locations (Gillespie 2001).

Other benefits of this technology are seen when these images are transmitted to high-acuity areas, such as emergency departments and intensive care units, where quick turnaround and immediate availability of images are critical to providing optimum client care. The use of this technology can facilitate client care in remote rural health care facilities where a radiologist may not be on-site. Images can be transmitted to a major medical center for evaluation by radiologists and other physicians. Benefits are realized in terms of cost, because it is not necessary to staff a radiologist, and improved client care when a radiologist is on staff but not available.

Implementation of a PACS system should include consideration of the following issues (Tabatabaie 2001):

- *Systems standards base.* The system should be operable without proprietary software that makes it difficult to use or upgrade.
- *Access to previous studies.* On-demand access to all prior client studies is preferable.
- *Required infrastructure.* Can the system be used with existing computers and the electronic medical record system?
- *System performance.* Are records available quickly and of sufficient quality for diagnostic purposes?

Pharmacy Systems

Pharmacy systems offer many benefits that promote cost containment and improve the quality of care. These systems can be used by a variety of health care professionals who perform activities related to the ordering, dispensing, and administration of medications. A hospital pharmacy may use an information system to access client data such as demographics, health history and diagnosis, medication history, client allergies, laboratory results, renal function, and potential drug interactions. Traditionally, pharmacists reviewed each client's medication profile, laboratory values, medical history, and progress notes manually to monitor medication disbursement and effectiveness (Amsden 2003). This is a time-intensive, laborious process. Automated systems pull in laboratory results and client information from the HISs, more quickly and accurately identifying allergy and interaction problems than a manual process. This integration of information allows pharmacists to recommend changes in parenteral nutrition formula based on laboratory abnormalities, verify that medication dosages are appropriate based on serum drug levels, avoid drugs that may impair renal function, and monitor laboratory values for possible drug toxicity. Pharmacy systems can also provide automatic alerts that can save lives. Automation of previously manual processes can result in significant cost savings.

Another benefit offered by pharmacy systems is the tracking of medication use, costs, and billing information. Automation of these functions generally improves accuracy and is more cost-effective than manual methods. In addition, this information can be manipulated and analyzed more easily for executive decision making when it is available as a computer file.

Physicians and other direct care providers may also use pharmacy systems. These systems provide on-line access to client and drug information that is critical in the drug prescription process. Pharmacy systems can provide easy access to clients' health and medication history, as well as their allergies and demographic information. Access to formulary information and on-line drug reference information helps physicians determine the most effective drug and the appropriate doses for clients. In addition, these systems can provide comparisons of costs and drug effectiveness, particularly important in the managed care arena.

Automatic Medication Dispensing in the Pharmacy Pharmacy systems can automatically dispense each client's medications in unit dose format, creating labels for each dose with the client's name and other demographic identifiers. The actual dispensing of the medications may be accomplished either with or without the intervention of the pharmacist. Some systems automatically dispense ordered medications in unit dose packages, which the pharmacy staff place in the client's medication drawer. This process can be streamlined by using robotic systems, which both collect the appropriate medications and place them in the drawers. Robotic dispensing systems are seen as a mechanism to prevent medication errors as well as reduce inventory and labor costs (Kohn, Walton-Brooks, and Henderson 2003). These systems serve to support rather than supplant the pharmacist (Barcia 1999).

Automatic Dispensing Systems on the Nursing Unit Another aspect of pharmacy systems is the use of automatic dispensing systems for use by the nurse. These systems provide a medication dispensing unit in the clinical area, generally for use by nurses who administer medications. The system is usually secured by requiring a user ID and password for access to the system and the actual medications. Features include menu-driven prompts for identifying the client, medication, dose, and number of unit doses removed. The user can also be prompted to count the current number of doses on hand when removing narcotics or other controlled substances. Automatic dispensing systems provide accurate records of medicines given in terms of what was taken from the unit and the date, time, and user who performed this activity. These records can be accessed centrally in the pharmacy to determine when supplies in the clinical area dispensing units must be replenished. In addition, this information can be used to efficiently and accurately bill clients for medications used (Barcia 1999).

Prevention of Medication Errors The National Coordinating Council for Medication Error Reporting and Prevention defines a medication error as "any preventable event that may cause or lead to inappropriate medication use or patient harm while the medication is in the control of the health care professional, patient, or consumer." The council is composed of more than

20 national organizations, including the Food and Drug Administration (FDA). The council examines and evaluates medication errors and recommends strategies for error prevention. Several other groups are also actively working on the prevention of medication errors (Meadows 2003). The Quality Interagency Coordination Task Force was formed in 2000 by the U.S. Department of Health and Human Services (DHHS) and other federal agencies, and has subsequently issued an action plan for reducing errors. In 2001 the Patient Safety Task Force was formed to improve data collection on patient safety. The lead agencies in the Patient Safety Task Force are the following:

- FDA
- Centers for Disease Control and Prevention
- Centers for Medicare and Medicaid Services
- Agency for Healthcare Research and Quality

Several agencies collect and review data collected on medication errors. The FDA reviews reports that come from drug manufacturers through the agency's safety information and adverse event reporting program, MedWatch. The Institute for Safe Medication Practices accepts reports from consumers and health professionals using collected information to publish a consumer newsletter on medication errors. Hospitals report medication errors via the MedMARX error-reporting program.

The large number of drugs on the market along with poor staffing and the high acuity levels of patients all contribute to the occurrence of medication errors (Gorman 1999). While technology can help to eliminate many errors, not all facilities will have CPOE and bar coding in place for some time yet. Medication safety is a major initiative in the present health care setting. As a consequence, the severity of medication errors in the hospital setting is the motivating force behind recent legislation and enhancements to information technology. The potential for medication errors has increased dramatically because of the large number of drug names in use. The FDA rejects all applications for similar drug names by using a computer program that searches for similar sounding names. Combining pharmacy information systems with bar code technology, as described in Box 5–4, can drastically reduce medication errors. Information systems can provide checkpoints at each phase of the medication ordering and administration process. From a pharamcy standpoint, these checkpoints may include alphabetizing drugs by chemical name; computerized dose checking; decreasing the amount of floor stock so that staff are less likely to accidentally choose the wrong drug, dose, or form for administration; improved unit dose availability from the pharmaceutical companies; final preparation of drug admixtures such as antibiotics in the pharmacy, thereby eliminating drug errors and compatibility problems with the admixture solution; availability of online drug references; delivery of only one dose at a time; and delivery of single-dose packages only (Summerfield and Lawrence, 2002).

Box 5–4   Using Information Systems to Reduce Medication Errors

Order entry and pharmacy systems, along with automated medication supply management systems, can be used to assist health care providers in reducing the occurrence of medication errors. These systems interact to provide checks and alerts throughout the medication ordering and administration process, as directed in the following examples:

1. A physician enters a medication order into the order entry system.

2. The information is automatically transmitted to the pharmacy system.

3. The pharmacy system integrates laboratory values and uses rules to ask the physician if he or she chooses to change or add medications based on laboratory values or dose for patient size or age.

4. The pharmacy system checks the patient's history and alerts the physician to any drug interactions or allergies. The physician can change the order at this time, if indicated.

5. The pharmacy system issues a warning when sound-alike medications are ordered forcing the physician and care giver to consider which drug the patient is actually to receive.

6. The order creates a requisition in the pharmacy that contains a bar code indicating the correct medication, as well as a bar code identifying the patient.

7. A robot in the pharmacy fills the medication order by matching the medication bar code on the requisition to the bar code on the medication. The medication is transported to the nursing unit.

8. The nurse scans a bar code on the patient's identification band and the bar code on the medication, administers the medication only if there is a match, and documents medications given in the bar code medication administration system. A warning will appear if insufficient time has passed since the drug was last administered.

9. The system prompts the nurse to enter pain scale, blood pressures, and pulses where appropriate.

10. The system automatically adds the nurse's electronic signature.

11. The bar code medication administration system can generate the following reports:

    • A medication due list, showing medications that need to be administered within specific time parameters, including one-time, on-call, continuous, PRN orders, and regularly scheduled medications

    • PRN effectiveness list that prompts the nurse to record the effectiveness of PRN medications

    • Medication administration history, which records nurse initials and times for medications given in a traditional medication administration record format

    • Missing dose report—prints in pharmacy to alert staff when a dose needs to be reissued; done at the time the nurse was administering meds with essentially no disruption in work flow

    • Medications not given report—lists all missed doses according to the documentation on the medication administration record.

    • Variance log—captures meds given more than 60 minutes early or late.

Box 5–5   **Other Common Clinical Systems**

- *Medical records/abstracting systems* facilitate the abstracting, or coding, of diagnoses and chart management processes. Client records may also be stored on optical disk.
- *Operating room systems* may be used to schedule procedures, manage equipment setup for individual physicians, facilitate inventory control, and provide client billing.
- *Emergency department systems* provide ready access to independent systems such as poison control. They also allow the nurse to print specific discharge and follow-up instructions based on the client's diagnosis.
- *Home care systems* allow the health care provider to access information on clients and outpatient resources, and to document care provided.

E-Prescribing *E-prescribing* is a process that allows the physician to enter a prescription into an information system. This information is electronically communicated to the client's pharmacy. This may be done using a variety of devices, including PDAs (Goedert 2002). Electronic prescriptions provide the following benefits (Cross 1996; Zurier 1995):

- Elimination of telephone authorization for refills
- Review of clients' drug histories before ordering drugs
- Reminders to order home medications for the hospitalized client
- Alerts about drug interactions
- Checking of formulary compliance and reimbursement
- Provision of a longitudinal prescription record

Electronic prescriptions require direct links between physician offices, hospitals, pharmacies, and third-party payors. Some state laws must also be changed to accommodate electronic prescription writing.

Other Clinical Systems

A number of other clinical systems address the needs of specific departments within the health care setting. Box 5–5 lists some of these systems. The rapidly changing health care environment has resulted in several requirements on the part of the clinical information system vendor. The vendor's initial support services and ability to provide ongoing support are critical success factors as the health care paradigm continues to shift (DePietro, Tocco, and Tramontozzi 1995).

Physician Practice Management Systems Physician practice management systems, which traditionally address billing and automation of administrative tasks, need to be understood and improved as part of the

---

Box 5–6   **Administrative Information Systems Used in the Healthcare Setting**

- Financial systems provide the facility with accounting functions. Accurate tracking of financial data is critical for enabling the organization to receive reimbursement for services.
- Payroll and human resource systems track employee time and attendance, credentials, performance evaluations, and payroll compensation information.
- Contract management systems manage contracts with third-party payors.
- Risk management systems track and plan prevention of unusual occurrences or incidents.
- Quality assurance systems monitor outcomes and produce reports that are used to guide quality improvement initiatives.
- Physician management systems support patient registration, scheduling, coding, and billing in the physician's office and may support results retrieval. These systems also provide better protection of patient privacy than paper records.
- Executive information systems provide administrators with easy access to summarized information related to the financial and clinical operations of the organization.
- Materials management systems facilitate inventory control and charging of supplies.

---

overall physician office computerization effort. The surge of interest in physician office access to outside data is powered by the physician's need for comprehensive clinical information (Morrissey 1997). Another advantage is that these systems help with maintaining client confidentiality and HIPAA compliance. Because health information is contained within the information system, there are fewer loose papers with client data available to be viewed by unauthorized clinical and nonclinical office staff (Rogoski 2002). Other features of these systems include the ability to track outcomes and better manage scheduling (Rivo 2000).

ADMINISTRATIVE SYSTEMS

Various administrative systems may be used in health care organizations to support the process of providing client care. Box 5–6 provides a brief review of many of these systems.

Registration Systems

The client registration system is critical to the effective operation of many other systems within the health care setting. This system is used to collect and store client identification and demographic data that are verified and updated at the time of each visit. For this reason, these may also be known as *admission/discharge/transfer (ADT) systems.* CISs use these data for the management of client care and billing purposes. The information is shared with those clinical systems that communicate directly with the registration system.

An important aspect of a registration system used in a multientity health system network is the development of a unique client identifier. This number or identification code is used to identify the client in all information systems across the organization and across all entities. This enables accurate client identification, supporting the development of a longitudinal client record that contains all clinical information available for the client.

Scheduling Systems

A scheduling system allows a health care organization to schedule clients and resources efficiently. Client demographic information must be available in the system either by direct entry or through electronic communication with a registration system. For the system to be used to schedule patient appointments, it must contain information regarding available resources. This resource information may include the following:

- Referral and authorization by patient's insurance
- Department
- Equipment
- Dates and times
- Room
- Staff
- Permits and preps
- Charging and billing information

The system uses predetermined rules for determining how resource and client information should be used to schedule a particular type of appointment. This provides the capability to schedule a patient in one location. In addition, scheduling across all facilities in an enterprise can be accomplished using one system. The benefits associated with using a scheduling system include increased staff productivity, increased client satisfaction, and cost savings to the organization (LeDonne 1997).

DECISION SUPPORT AND EXPERT SYSTEMS

Decision support and expert systems use data from both the clinical and the administrative information systems and can provide information related to clinical and administrative users. According to Turley (1993), little agreement exists on the definition of the terms *decision support systems* and *expert systems* except for the distinction of how much authority is placed in the computer system.

Decision support systems aid in and strengthen the selection of viable options using the information of an organization or a field to facilitate decision making and overall efficiency. Decision support software organizes information to fit new environments. It provides analysis and advice to support a choice. The final decision rests with the practitioner. Software can be off-the-shelf or homegrown. **Off-the-shelf software** is commercially available. The advantage to the consumer is that someone else has borne the cost for its development and testing. It is, however, geared to a general market and may not meet the needs of a particular party. **Homegrown** software has been developed by the consumer to meet specific needs usually because no suitable commercial package is available. The customer bears the cost of its development, testing, and communication with other software applications. Decision support software can provide a competitive edge and facilitate the move to managed care. Tools range from clinical practice guidelines to financial applications. An example of a decision support application is a program that assists nurses performing a skin assessment to review available alternatives, from which the best may be selected to maintain skin integrity.

    Expert systems use artificial intelligence to model a decision that experts in the field would make. Unlike decision support systems that provide several options from which the user may choose, expert systems convey the concept that the computer has made the best decision based on criteria that experts would use.

CASE STUDY EXERCISES

You are a nurse participating in the customization and implementation of a medication documentation system. Define the data that must be included in the medication order entry process and the medication administration record documentation process.

•   •   •

You are the physician liaison for the information system department. Recent federal initiatives call for the implementation of CPOE. You have the technology available, but you need to get administrative, nursing, and physician support. How would you go about this?

•   •   •

You are participating in the customization and implementation of the radiology system. Define the data that must be included in the order entry process. Define the information that the nursing staff would like to view or print from the radiology system.

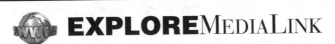

EXPLOREMEDIALINK

Multiple choice questions, case studies, and other interactive resources for this chapter can be found on the Web site at *http//www.prenhall.com/hebda*. Click on "Chapter 5" to select the activities for this chapter.

SUMMARY

- A hospital or health care information system consists of clinical and administrative systems.

- Well-designed clinical information systems can improve the quality of client care.

- Clinical information systems can extend the capabilities of health care providers.

- A nursing information system using the nursing process approach should support the use and documentation of nursing processes and provide tools for managing the delivery of nursing care.

- The use of standardized nursing languages such as NANDA, NIC and NOC, supports automation of nursing documentation and expands the utility of collected information.

- The critical pathway/protocol approach to nursing information systems provides a multidisciplinary format for planning and documenting client care.

- Other clinical systems, including order entry, radiology, laboratory, pharmacy systems, and physician management systems, give the nurse and other heath care providers the support and tools to more effectively care for clients.

- Administrative systems support the process of client care by managing nonclinical, client-related information, including demographics, codes for procedures, and insurance.

- Information systems enable decision makers to examine trends and make informed choices during these times of health care reform.

- Federal initiatives for patient safety call for the implementation of computerized physician order entry and bar code medication administration as methods to reduce error.

- Personal device assistants and wireless technology further enhance the capability of information systems to support the work of clinicians.

REFERENCES

Amsden, D. (2003). Push technology in the pharmacy. *Health Management Technology*, *24*(1), 28, 30–31.

Baldwin, F. (October 2002). It's all in the wrist. *Healthcare Informatics*, *19*(10), 57–59.

Ball, M., and Collen M. (1992). *Aspects of the computer-based patient record*. New York: Springer.

Barcia, S. M. (1999). Man vs. machine. *Health Management Technology*, *20*(9), 24.

Calabrisi, R. R., Czarnecki, T., and Blank, C. (2002). The impact of clinical reminders and alerts on health screenings. *Health Management Technology*, *23*(12), 32–34.

Clinical Information Systems. (January 28, 2002). Where are we today, where do we need to be, and how do we get there? *Modern Healthcare, 32*(4), 73.

Cross, M. (1996). Kicking the prescription pad habit. *Health Data Management, 4*(10), 82–86.

DePietro, S., Tocco, M., and Tramontozzi, A. (1995). Pharmacy systems: Keeping pace. *Healthcare Informatics, 12*(12), 29–44.

Dorenfest, S. (March 2003). Defining CPOE. *ADVANCE For Health Information Executives, 7*(3), 33–36.

Eichhorst, B. (2002). Patient-centered HIS. *Health Management Technology, 23*(4), 40.

Gillespie, G. (November 2001). Filmless radiology brightens its image. *Health Data Management, 9*(11), 55–60.

Goedert, J. (2002). Electronic prescribing: Is it just what the doctor ordered? *Health Data Management, 10*(6), 14–16.

Gorman, C. (1999). Mixed-up medusa. *Time, 154*(24), 117.

Gryskevich, R. (May 2002). Putting safety first. *Health Management Technology, 23*(5), 38.

Health informatics standards illuminated under the northern lights. (2003). *HIMSS News, 14*(7), 5.

Hendrickson, M. (1993). The nurse engineer: A way to better nursing information systems. *Computers in Nursing, 11*(2), 67–71.

Hensley, S. (1999). Leaders of the PACS in radiology. *Modern Healthcare, 29*(48), 54–58.

Hughes, S. (May 1997). Time for new thinking. *Healthcare Informatics,* 57–68.

Johnson, C. L., Carlson, R. A., Tucker, C. L., and Willette, C. (2002). Using BCMA software to improve patient safety in veterans administration medical centers. *Journal of Healthcare Information Management, 16*(1), 46–51.

Kohn, C., Walton-Brooks, D., and Henderson, C. W. (February 17, 2003). Hospitals purchase robotic drug dispensing system. *Managed Care Weekly Digest,* p. 41.

Krohn, R. (2003). Making e-prescribing work—A fresh approach. *Journal of Healthcare Information Management, 17*(2), 17–19.

Lavelle, F. W. (2002). Improved workflow through HIS. *Health Management Technology, 23*(27), 14.

LeDonne, J. (1997). Rehab facility saves $300,000 a year, reduces FTEs, with scheduling system. *Health Management Technology, 18*(7), 30.

Marshalek, G., and Cassey, S. (2003). Pain-free CPOE. *Health Management Technology, 24*(2), 24–27.

Marietti , C. (2003). Vigilance in the lab. *Healthcare Informatics 20*(5), 58.

May, S. M. (February 2003). Computerized physician order entry. *Health Care Informatics, 20*(2), 48–54.

Meadows, M. (2003). Strategies to reduce medication errors. *FDA Consumer, 37*(3), 20.

Morrissey, J. (1996). Clinical systems add market momentum. *Modern Healthcare, 26*(19), 114–132.

Morrissey, J. (1997). Retooled survey. *Modern Healthcare, 27*(1), 54.

Morrissey, J. (2001). Vendors say that they're ready to deliver. *Modern Healthcare, 31*(46), 28.

Powelson, S. A., McGahan, S. A., and Wilkinson, J. M. (July–September 2000). Where to start? Introducing Standardized Nursing Languages in educational settings. *Nursing Diagnosis, 11*(3), 135.

Prophet, C. M. (2000). The evolution of a clinical database: from local to standardized clinical languages. *Proceedings of AMIA Symposium,* 660–664.

Prophet, C., Dorr, G. G., Gibbs, T. D., and Porcella, A. A. (1997). Implementation of standardized nursing languages (NIC, NOC) in on-line care planning and documentation. *Informatics: The Impact of Nursing Knowledge on Health Care Informatics.* Amsterdam: IOS Press, pp. 395–400.

Rivo, M. L. (2000). Practicing in the new millenium: Do you have what it takes? *Family Practice Management, 7*(1), 35.

Rogoski, R. (2002). You say tomato. *Health Management Technology, 23*(10), 24–26.

Rogoski, R. (2003). LIS and the enterprise. *Health Management Technology, 24*(2), 20–23.

Saba, V., and McCormick, K. (1996). *Essentials of computers for nurses.* New York: McGraw–Hill.

Schuerenberg, B. (2002). Lab systems are joining the team. *Health Data Management, 11*(9), 61–66.

Stablein, D., and Drazen, E. (2003). Getting the most out of CPOE. *Health Care Informatics, 20*(2), 96–98.

Summerfield, M. R., and Lawrence, T. (2002). Rethinking approaches to reducing medication errors: An examination of 10 core processes. *Formulary, 37*(9), 462.

Tabatabaie, H. (November 2001). Imaging and the enterprise. *Health Management Technology, 22*(11), 14–23.

Turley, J. P. (May 1993). The use of artificial intelligence in nursing information systems. Available online at: http://www.vicnet.net.au/vicnet/hisa/ MAY93/MAY93-The.html.

Waldo, B. (1999). Closing the loop on medication errors. *Health Management Technology, 20*(11), 68.

Watson, S. (1995). Network support critical in choosing a lab system. *Health Data Management, 3*(7), 57–65.

Zurier, S. (1995). Telemedicine is bringing electronic doctors closer. *Government Computer News, 14*(21), 56.

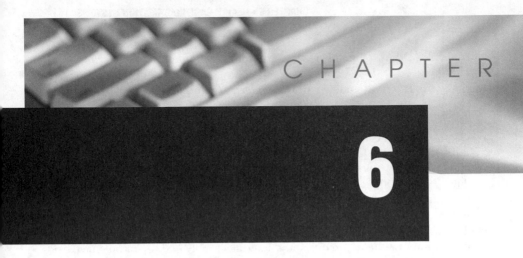

Strategic Planning

After completing this chapter, you should be able to:

- Define *strategic planning.*
- Describe how strategic planning is related to an organization's mission, goals, and objectives.
- Identify the participants in the strategic planning process.
- Understand the relationship between strategic planning for information systems and planning for the overall organization.
- Explain the importance of assessing the internal and external environments during the planning process.
- Discuss how potential solutions are derived from data analysis.

- Review the benefits of using a weighted scoring tool when selecting a course of action.
- Understand the importance of developing a timeline during the implementation phase of strategic planning.
- List tools or processes that may be used to evaluate the outcome of and provide feedback to the planning process.
- Discuss the relationship between strategic planning and information technology.

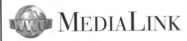

MEDIALINK

Additional resources for this content can be found on the Companion Website at *www. prenhall.com/hebda.* Click on "Chapter 6" to select the activities for this chapter.

Companion Website

- Glossary
- Multiple Choice
- Discussion Points
- Case Study: Strategic Planning Process
- Case Study: Tools for Evaluation
- Case Study: Ongoing Evaluation and Feedback
- Case Study: Scanning the Environment
- MediaLink Application: Mission and Scope
- Links to Resources
- Crossword Puzzle

Strategic planning is the development of a comprehensive long-range plan for guiding the activities and operations of an organization (Gershon 2003; Wheelen and Hunger 1995). This process includes defining the corporate mission, specifying achievable goals and objectives, developing strategies, and setting policy guidelines. This entails a determination of what products and services to offer and to what markets. This is particularly important when most organizations have more potential markets than available resources. The organizational strategic plan should guide the planning for all areas within the organization. For many businesses, including health care delivery, technology is transforming the strategic landscape and must be factored into the organization's strategic plan (Gilks 2000).

THE MISSION

The **mission** is the purpose or reason for the organization's existence and represents the fundamental and unique aspirations that differentiate the organization from others. The mission is often conveyed in the form of a mission statement that tells the organization's personnel and customers "who we are" and "what we do." The mission statement is an important tool when used to guide the planning process (Mullane 2002). An example of a mission statement is seen in Box 6–1.

The purpose of the St. Theresa Health System is clearly evident in its mission statement, which states that "the essence of our Mission and Philosophy is best depicted in our logo—St. Theresa and the words 'Healing Body, Mind and Spirit.'" This medical center's unique purpose is to provide healing for the mind and spirit, in addition to the expected purpose of physical healing. Its mission statement communicates this purpose effectively to both employees and customers.

The **scope** of an organization's mission defines the type of activities and services it will perform. The scope should be clearly identified in the mission statement so that employees and customers understand which aspects of organizational operation are most important. For example, a broad scope for a health care enterprise might be to "provide health care." The problem with such a broad scope is that the target client population is not identified, nor are the types of services that will be provided. A narrower scope provides the amount of detail necessary to appropriately guide administrators and managers in decision making. The scope of the St. Theresa Medical Center is also seen in the mission statement, which states, "the patients receive hospital or long-term care, without distinction as to their religious beliefs, race, national origin, age, sex, disability or economic status." The medical center's commitment to caring for the indigent population is clearly described in the mission statement. This scope is the basis for the development of certain goals and objectives that guide the decision makers in strategic planning.

The Mission of St. Theresa Medical Center

The Mission of St. Theresa Medical Center is the same as the Mission of St. Theresa Health System which is:

1. To establish and maintain a hospital and other health care facilities for the care of persons with illnesses or disabilities that require that the patients receive hospital or long-term care, without distinction as to their religious beliefs, race, national origin, age, sex, disability, or economic status.

2. To carry on any educational activities related to rendering care to the sick and injured or the promotion of health which, in the opinion of the Board of Directors, may be justified by the facilities, personnel, funds or other requirements that are or can be made available, including, but not being specifically limited to, the conduction of schools for the education of registered nurses and practical nurses with power to grant diplomas to graduates and residency programs for physicians in training.

3. To promote and carry on scientific research related to the care of the sick and injured insofar as, in the opinion of the Board of Directors, such research can be carried on in or in connection with the hospital.

4. To participate, as far as circumstances may warrant, in any activity designed and carried on to promote the general health of the community.

In working toward the fulfillment of these objectives, as members of the health care team, we strive to give generously of our efforts and work harmoniously together for the love of God and of our neighbor. As a result, we find that our own lives and the lives of those with whom we come in contact are being enriched and blessed.

The essence of our Mission and Philosophy is best depicted in our logo—St. Theresa and the words "Healing Body, Mind and Spirit."

GOALS AND OBJECTIVES

Identification of an organization's goals and objectives is a critical factor in fulfilling the mission. The goals and objectives explain how the mission will be realized. A **goal** is an open-ended statement that describes in general terms what is to be accomplished. Examples of goals include maintaining quality client care while promoting cost-effective operations, striving to increase market share by attracting a larger percentage of clients than their competitors, and broadening the scope of services offered. The ability to achieve defined goals is especially important in the rapidly changing health care environment as hospitals merge into large enterprises and services evolve to meet changing needs.

Objectives state how and when an organization will meet its goals. Some of the primary areas that goals and objectives may address are listed

Table 6–1
Areas of Potential Strategic Planning

Goals and Objectives	Strategy
Efficiency	Redesign work flow so that fewer people may accomplish more work.
Growth	Expand service area to include rural and outlying communities.
Utilization of resources	Train workers so that they are multiskilled.
Technological leadership	Use newer technologies to transfer information. Examples include tele-medicine, optical imaging, video conferencing, and use of the Internet.

SOURCE: Adapted from Wheelen, T. and Hunger, J. *Management and business policy,* 5th ed. (p. 21). © 1995 Addison-Wesley Publishing Company Inc. Reprinted by permission of Addison-Wesley Longman Inc.

in Table 6–1. For example, objectives that support the goal of broadening the scope of services offered may include the following:

- *Development of clinics that support and promote wellness services.* Traditionally, clinics provide treatments for various medical problems. Expansion of these services to support wellness maintenance may attract a larger market share. Some additional services that may be offered are mammography, and blood pressure and cholesterol screening.
- *Expansion of home care services.* These services might be expanded to include routine postsurgical follow-up visits as well as occupational and physical therapy.

DEVELOPING STRATEGIES

An organization's **strategy** is a comprehensive plan that states how its mission, goals, and objectives will be achieved (Gershon 2003; Michaelson 2000; Thivierge 1997; Wheelen and Hunger 1995). An examination of the mission and goals will help to define the steps that are necessary to attain them. A clear understanding of the end point is critical to the effective development of the plan. It is also important to review current strengths, weaknesses, opportunities, and threats. This includes the presence of competition. The strategic position for the organization can be determined by its reputation for quality of service and innovation, its access, the scope of services provided, and the demographics of the population served. An analysis of the current position of the organization in relation to these factors will help to determine available options. It is then possible for administration to select major initiatives to achieve their vision for the organization in light of available resources. Expediting the achievement of the mission and goals is the primary purpose of a strategic plan.

Strategic planning is led by members of the organization's upper management, including the board of directors and chief executive officer (CEO), who is ultimately responsible for the organization's strategic management. The next level of management, those who report to the CEO such as vice presidents, are also major participants in strategic planning. This should include the chief information officer (CIO). The CIO must ensure that executives understand the role that information technology plays in the organization as well as how information technology can be used to advance the goals of the organization (Clark 2002). It is the CIO's responsibility to see that upper management sees information technology as a tool to achieve organizational goals rather than just another cost center (Hoffman 2002). This involvement will help to provide direction for all information technology initiatives, establish priorities, eliminate the duplication of information systems, and ensure the wise use of information technology resources. Other lower-level managers within the organization, such as department heads, are responsible for supporting the planning process by providing information related to the current operations as well as insight into future needs of the organization. This information enables the planning team to balance the present reality against the future vision and goals. Changing economics, resources, and markets make planning more difficult, but a well-crafted strategic plan makes provisions for these changes as well as for the expenditure of time, money, and resources to carry out the plan (Thivierge 1997).

STRATEGIC PLANNING FOR INFORMATION SYSTEMS

Although the broader scope of strategic planning concerns all areas of the health care institution, one important component is the plan for information systems. Without a plan that points information systems in the right direction and helps the organization to use information systems to execute its business strategies, the organization will not be able to effectively meet its overall goals (Lederer and Sethi 1998).

The strategic planning process is often initiated by other changes that are taking place within the organization. For example, suppose a health care enterprise plans to purchase a client monitoring system to be used throughout its facilities. Other organizational changes—such as plans for construction and unit relocation, infrastructure upgrades including computer wiring and cabling, and updating the client care information systems in general—may have initiated the plans for obtaining the monitoring system. Once administrators realize the need for strategic planning for the monitoring system, they must identify the goals of the plan. These goals should be developed in accordance with the mission and goals of the organization.

Some of the goals of information systems strategic planning are discussed next. Each goal is followed by a brief explanation of how it applies to the previously described example of selecting a new client monitoring system.

- *To support business and clinical decisions.* Data management supports better decision making by providing timely and accurate information. In the example of planning for a new monitoring system, a driving force behind these plans is the need to provide physicians and nurses with accurate and complete data regarding the client's condition.

- *To make effective use of emerging technologies.* New technologies can create administrative efficiencies and attract physicians and clients. A perfect example of this can be seen with the use of PDAs and other wireless devices to collect, view, and transmit patient information from the point of care. The Internet and e-health represent other developments that change the access to and delivery of health care because patient results can be made available online from any location and patient questions addressed. These developments must be included in the strategic planning process.

- *To enhance the organization's image.* The effective use of information technologies enhances how the organization is perceived by physicians, clients, the community, and other external groups. This is especially critical in these times of competitive health care. For example, achieving state-of-the-art technology for cardiac monitoring will provide efficient and effective client care, which will enhance the organization's image.

- *To promote satisfaction of market and regulatory requirements.* Effective information systems strategic planning must include those issues related to meeting market and regulatory requirements, such as e-health, payor requirements, Joint Commission for Accreditation of Healthcare Organizations guidelines, client confidentiality, and data security. For example, when selecting a monitoring system, it is also important to determine that the system complies with safety regulations such as protection against damage from defibrillation.

- *To be cost-effective.* Cost-effectiveness is achieved when redundancies are eliminated. In the monitoring system example, this advantage is evident. If all of the critical care and monitored bed areas in the enterprise use the same monitoring system, training is cost-effective, because nurses need be trained on only one system to work in any monitored area of the hospital. Other cost benefits are seen in the need to maintain only one type of backup monitor for replacement of nonoperational equipment, as well as increased efficiency for the biomedical technicians who must maintain the monitoring equipment.

- *To provide a safer environment for patients.* There is strong initiative for patient safety at this time. A number of organizations that include government agencies, regulatory bodies, consumer groups, and professional organizations are looking into ways to improve patient safety.

STEPS OF THE STRATEGIC PLANNING PROCESS

The first step of the strategic planning process is the realization that there is a need for change. Each department in the organization should have its own long-range plan, and most departments within the organization are dependent on the management of information systems. As a result, each department comes to the information services department with its own requirements related to strategic planning. It is the responsibility of information systems to prioritize and merge these ideas together, developing a master strategic plan for the organization. This task is complicated by the rapidly changing nature of information technology and the emerging role of the Internet in health care delivery (Baldwin 1999). The fast pace of evolving technology requires periodic review and revisions of both the organization's strategic plan and the information systems department's strategic plan.

The CIO is ultimately responsible for IS strategic planning. The need to create administrative efficiencies through e-commerce, mergers and acquisitions, and requests for outcomes reporting forces CIOs to look at ways that information technology can be used to achieve strategic and operational changes (Hagland 2000). The CIO generally selects a project manager or chairperson for each major project within the overall strategic plan. The project manager may help to develop an advisory board or a strategic planning team. The strategic planning team is generally composed of top-level managers who devise the plan and present it to the CIO, who in turn presents it to the board of directors. One particularly important aspect of this process is the ability to prioritize all projects, particularly for next 2 to 5 years. This requires estimating benefits, resources, costs, and timelines for each and then reevaluating the priority of each as new developments come into play. Some recent developments that affect information technology in health care include legislation that involves patient privacy and billing as well as initiatives calling for the implementation of barcoding for medication administration, computerized physician order entry, a computerized patient record, and bioterrorism (Langer 2003; Briggs 2003; Magliore 2003). These developments will continue to have a significant affect on information technology budgets for the next few years.

Another level of strategic planning is performed by members of the project implementation team, which reports to the advisory board. This team is composed of representatives from the user departments, including managers and front-line employees who are most familiar with the activities of the department. The project implementation team should also include the analysts and programmers who will implement the system changes. The project team needs the active involvment of end users to succeed. This is particularly true because nursing staff are often opposed to change (Gillespie 2002). Frequent communication between the advisory board and the implementation team is imperative for the ongoing success of the strategic plan. This plan generally addresses a time frame covering between 3 and 5 years into the future.

Identification of Goals and Scope

Once the strategic planning teams have been identified, the actual planning process can begin. The first step is to identify the goals and scope of the project. The goals of the project must meet the needs of the users as well as support the mission and goals of the institution. The identified goals will then provide the direction for the remainder of the planning process.

In the example of selecting a cardiac monitoring system for a health care enterprise, the goals and scope of the project might be to implement a one-vendor solution. This should result in the selection of a single system that will meet the needs of all monitored areas in the organization. However, decisions should be made with input from key users. Good communication between information systems personnel and clinicians is critical to the success of any project. It is essential to elicit support from nurses and physicians in the selection of any system that they will use and to listen to their feedback (Gillespie 2002; Schuerenberg 2003). Nurses are resistant to change unless they see the potential benefits. Physicians will not use a system if it is not easy to access and use. More and more, that translates to the ability to access information from home or other locations. No system should hinder clinical staff.

Scanning the External and Internal Environments

The next step in the planning process is to **scan**, or gather information from, the external and internal environments. The **external environment** includes those interested parties and competitors who are outside of the health care institution, such as vendors, payors, competitors, clients, the community, and regulatory agencies. The **internal environment** includes employees of the institution, as well as physicians and members of the board of directors. The purpose of scanning the environment is twofold: to define the current situation and to identify areas of need.

Environment scanning is best accomplished by developing a detailed plan for collecting pertinent data. This step is often called the *needs assessment*. Information related to current trends in both health care and information technology should also be collected. Data may be collected from a variety of sources, including the following (McCormack 1996):

External Environment Scanning

- Published literature and reports
- Information from vendors
- Regulatory and accreditation requirements
- Information related to market trends

Internal Environment Scanning

- Interviews and questionnaires from managers and end users
- Observations of current technology and operations, as well as anticipated technological developments

When selecting a monitoring system, information may be obtained from vendors regarding the technologies that are currently available. All pertinent regulatory and accreditation requirements must also be investigated. A scan of the internal environment may include an inventory of equipment currently in use throughout the enterprise.

Data Analysis

After data have been collected during the internal and external environmental scans, the project implementation team must perform analysis, identifying trends in the current operations as well as future needs and expectations. Current trends in health care should be identified when considering future needs and may be related to topics such as managed care and other financial health care coverage and reimbursement considerations. Some trends to consider include the merging of hospitals into large enterprises and the growing focus on care outside of the acute hospital setting, which has resulted in an increased number of services related to wellness promotion and home care. Information technology trends such as e-health, the Internet, telemedicine, client/server technologies, and the computerized client record must also be addressed (Morrissey 1996, 2000).

In selecting a universal cardiac monitoring system, the features of each vendor's system must be evaluated, including the desirable and undesirable features of each. For example, strengths may include an easy learning curve, vendor support, integration capability, transport monitor capabilities, and screen visibility. Weaknesses may include a large number of screens for each function, busy or hard-to-read screens, slow speed of initial data entry, and unsuitable cabling requirements.

Identification of Potential Solutions

The next step in the planning process involves the identification of potential solutions, which may be in the form of system upgrades or replacements. At this point, the strategic planning team should be aware of the information system needs of the end users.

When identifying potential solutions, health care organizations must address many issues, including the following:

- *Hospitals with differing information systems may be merged together into one enterprise.* In this situation, either each organization continues to use its previous system or one system is chosen for use throughout the enterprise as a means to build a cohesive information systems strategy (Cross 1996). Several factors influence the decision to retain or adopt an information system, including costs associated with the purchase and use of software and hardware; site licenses, consulting fees, contract negotiation, maintenance and support agreements, expenses associated with training personnel to use a new system, and the availability of support staff.

* *Many hospitals use mainframe* **legacy systems,** *older vendor-based systems that have often been highly individualized to meet customer specifications.* As it is necessary to upgrade or replace these systems, CEOs and CIOs must weigh the advantages and disadvantages of alternatives that may better meet the needs of the organization. These might include retaining current systems, providing a new look and easier access to legacy software via a Web interface, new versions of vendor software, client/server or thin client technologies, outsourcing services, or using an application service provider (ASP). Box 6–2 lists several information technology considerations related to strategic planning. Box 6–3 identifies pros and cons associated with the outsourcing of services.

Selecting a Course of Action

Once all of the potential solutions have been identified, they must be analyzed and compared. One way to accomplish this task is to measure the components of the plan in terms of their ability to meet identified current and future needs. This can be accomplished by listing these needs and weighting them according to their importance. For example, essential features may be given a weighting factor of 5, and desirable but not

---

Box 6–2

Information Technology Considerations for Strategic Planning

* Does the system use open architecture?
* Is the system based on personal computer, client/server, thin client, or Internet technology?
* Does it use a graphical user interface? Is it user friendly?
* Does the software comply with HL7 standards?
* Does the system allow the user to query aggregate data and produce online reports?
* Does it support performance measurement?
* Does it support a customized view?
* Can it support expansion of features, increased numbers of users, and/or records?
* Does it allow the use of evolving technologies, such as smart cards, optical disks, interface engines, wireless technology, integrated services digital network (ISDN) communication, e-health or e-commerce, video conferencing, telemedicine, and fiberoptic networks?
* Does it support a paperless environment?
* Have criteria been developed to measure successful implementation?

SOURCE: Adapted from O'Connor, K. (1994). "Where Is your long range IS plan?," *Healthcare Informatics,* *11*(12), 64–68.

Box 6–3   **Pros and Cons Associated with the Outsourcing of Services**

Pros

- Allows the organization to focus on its core competencies
- Can shorten the timeframe to implement new applications or technology
- Better compliance with project implementation dates
- Easier to budget and manage because costs for development and implementation are shifted to the outsourcing agency
- May improve customer satisfaction because services can be delivered at the same or at a higher level as in-house services but at a lower cost
- Provides leading-edge technical skills when skilled labor resources are not available in-house
- Contract negotiations aid definition of project scope

Cons

- Limited control over data security and confidentiality
- Lack of control over application maintenance and downtime
- Insufficient advance notice of downtime
- Lack of control over when updates are implemented
- Customization may not be available
- Promises may exceed ability to deliver
- Costs can be much higher than anticipated
- Identification and resolution of system problems may be delayed
- Ability to change outsourcing services may be limited

---

essential features may be given a weighting factor of 3. Weighting of each desirable system feature should be completed before the various systems are scored.

The next step is to score the features, or requirements, of each potential system. For example, each feature may be given a score from 0 to 5, with 0 indicating that the requirement is not met, and 5 indicating that the requirement is fully met. Finally, the score is multiplied by the weighting factor for each item to determine the weighted score. The overall score is the sum of weighted scores for all items.

Figure 6–1 illustrates using a weighted score as an evaluation tool to select a hospital-wide cardiac monitoring system. This figure lists only a minimal number of the features that would actually be evaluated in this situation.

Evaluation of the various potential solutions should also include a summary of pertinent findings that have been discovered during data analysis.

Selection of a Hospital-Wide Cardiac Monitoring System

Monitoring System: _____

Evaluator: _____

Ratings (How well does the system do this?):

1 = Poor   2 = Fair   3 = Adequate   4 = Good   5 = Excellent

System Feature	Rating	×	Weighting Factor	=	Weighted Score	Comments
Operation 1. Easy to learn and operate			5			
2. Easy to set up screen			3			
Alarms 3. Easy to set alarms			3			
4. Alarm limits displayed continuously			5			
Bedside Monitors 5. Does the bedside unit work exactly the same as the central station and transport monitors?			3			
6. Can you view, control, review, and record any parameter from any bed on the network?			5			
					_____	**Overall system score** (Total of weighted scores):

FIGURE 6–1 • Example of an evaluation tool for cardiac monitoring systems

Other factors that should be considered when making a final decision include the following:

- Purchase costs versus outsourcing costs
- Ongoing maintenance and support costs
- Time required for installation
- Number of employees required to install and maintain the system
- Vendor's history and stability
- Service considerations

- Existence of national user groups
- Time and staff resources required for training

The process of strategic planning and selecting a course of action may involve time, money, and personnel resources. Nonetheless, the resources expended during this process are well worth the value of the plan that is produced, because this plan will guide the decision making of the IS department and the health care enterprise.

Implementation

The next phase in the strategic planning process is implementation of the chosen solution. The first step in the implementation process is to identify the working committee for the implementation phase. Development of a timeline is one of the initial tasks the committee will perform. Once all of the individual components of the timeline have been identified, the tasks can be assigned and initiated. Other tasks during this phase include budgeting, procedure development, and execution of the plan.

When implementing a universal cardiac monitoring system, the working committee may include representatives from the IS, purchasing, and staff development departments, as well as physicians and nurse managers. This group would first develop a timeline, prioritizing the order in which units would begin using the system. They would also be active in developing a procedure and a plan for educating staff in the use of the new equipment. Box 6–4 lists some measures to ensure a successful experience when services are outsourced.

Ongoing Evaluation and Feedback

Strategic planning is an ongoing process (DeJarnett 1999). Frequent evaluation of the current processes as well as the current and future needs must be performed. In this way, the organization is able to remain current with changing technology and health care trends. The process for identifying evaluation tools can be difficult. Measures must be adjusted to environmental changes and competitor actions as a means to help ensure success of strategic plans. One particular type of measure is benchmarking.

Benchmarking is the continual process of measuring services and practices against the toughest competitors in the health care industry. An example of benchmarking is to compare the number of IS staff required to support the clinical applications for the enterprise to that of other health care providers with similar demographic and volume statistics. When needs are no longer met, or the organization falls far below the benchmark, the process of identifying potential solutions and selecting the best option is begun again. Clinical examples of benchmarks might include the organization's cost for open heart surgery or length of stay. Benchmarking has become widespread throughout the health care industry (Hickman and Augustine 2002).

Box 6–4	Measures to Ensure a Positive Outsourcing Experience

- Define information technology functions for possible outsourcing
- Research vendor availability and capabilities
- Establish outsourcing goals and objectives
- Select the vendor that meets the requirements
- Negotiate a contract that outlines the following:
  - Term of contract and provisions for termination and renewal
  - Management of the relationship
  - Vendor and client responsibilities
  - Liabilities
  - Warranties
  - Ownership issues regarding assets/intellectual property
  - Fee structure
  - The process for staff assignment
  - Performance measures
  - Resources key to success
  - Security safeguards
  - Back-up and disaster recovery measures
  - Service level agreements inclusive of availability, response times, service quality
- Develop and use oversight procedures
- Insure against losses related to poor work

CASE STUDY EXERCISES

You are a nurse manager in a hospital that has recently merged with two other hospitals, forming a large health care enterprise. Each of the three hospitals currently uses a different clinical information system. You are a member of the strategic planning committee, which is charged with the task of selecting which of the three systems will be used throughout the enterprise. Describe the process you would use to scan the internal and external environments, as well as the types of data you would collect.

•   •   •

Develop a tool to evaluate each of the three clinical information systems for the scenario described above.

•   •   •

Your facility belongs to one of three health care delivery systems in the city. Competition is fierce. You have been asked to serve on a committee to study and recommend the retention or deletion of certain clinical services. Develop a plan for how you would do that and for how information services might facilitate that task via the use of benchmarking.

• • •

Your facility recently acquired and closed a competing hospital. All paper medical records are stored at a distant site. Records are not readily accessible. Client documentation and results were online but no longer available after the hospital closure. Some physicians never received test results for clients at the time of shut down. This had a negative impact on client care and satisfaction. How might strategic planning prevent this type of situation from occurring again?

 EXPLOREMediaLink

Multiple choice questions, case studies, and other interactive resources for this chapter can be found on the Web site at *http://www.prenhall.com/hebda*. Click on "Chapter 6" to select the activities for this chapter.

SUMMARY

- Strategic planning is the development of a comprehensive long-range plan for guiding the activities and operations of an organization.
- Strategic planning is one of the most important factors in the selection, design, and implementation of information systems, because it can save valuable resources over time and ensure that the needs of the enterprise are met.
- The strategic plan should support the mission, goals, and objectives of the organization.
- The mission is the purpose for the organization's existence and represents its unique aspects.
- Strategic planning is guided by upper-level administrators, including the CIO, but requires participation from other levels of management as well.
- Strategic planning involves the following steps: definition of goals and scope, scanning of external and internal environments, data analysis, identification of potential solutions, selection of a course of action, implementation, evaluation, and feedback.
- Strategic planning is an ongoing process.

REFERENCES

Baldwin, G. (1999). The Internet can make strategic I.T. planning precarious. *Health Data Management, 7*(12), 42, 44, 46, 48.

Briggs, B. (2003). Choose your battles wisely. *Health Data Management, 11*(4), 27–34.

Clark, F. (November 2002). The expanding role of the CIO. *ADVANCE for Health Information Executives, 6*(11), 31–32.

Cross, M. A. (1996). Building an I.S. strategy in the wake of a merger. *Health Data Management, 4*(10), 85–89.

DeJarnett, L. R. (1999). Integrated strategic measures—a new value from your IT investment. *The Executive's Journal, 16*(1), 3.

Gershon, H. J. (January/February 2003). Strategic positioning: Where does your organization stand? *Journal of Healthcare Management 48*(1), 12–14.

Gilks, J. (2000). IT strategy needs a rethink. *CMA Management, 74*(1), 52.

Gillespie, G. (2002). IT a tough sell for nursing staff. *Health Data Management, 10*(4), 56–59.

Hagland, M. (2000). The many hats of a CIO. *Healthcare Informatics, 17*(5), 69–70, 72, 74, 76.

Hickman, G., and Augustine, H. (April 2002). Optimizing your IT budget. *ADVANCE for Health Information Executives, 6*(4), 41–46.

Hoffman, T. (November 4, 2002). CIOs try new ways to demonstrate IT's value. *Computerworld, 36*(45), 6.

Langer, J. (2003). Prioritizing IT projects. *Healthcare Informatics, 20*(6), 110.

Lederer, A. L., and Sethi, V. (1998). Seven guidelines for strategic information systems planning. *The Executive's Journal, 15*(1), 23.

Magliore, M. (2003). Preparing business for biochemical attacks. *Contingency Planning and Management, 8*(4), 48–50.

McCormack, J. (1996). Strategic planning in changing times. *Health Data Management, 4*(12), 6–16.

Michaelson, G. A. (2000). Strategy to tactics. *Executive Excellence, 17*(10), 12.

Morrissey, J. (1996). A broader vision. *Modern Healthcare, 26*(10), 110–113.

Morrissey, J. (2000). Internet dominates providers' line of sight. *Modern Healthcare, 30*(15), 72, 74, 76, 78, 80–82, 84, 86, 88, 90, 92.

Mullane, J. V. (May-June 2002) The mission statement is a strategic tool: When used properly. *Management Decision, 40*, 448–455.

O'Connor, K. (1994). Where is your long range IS plan? *Healthcare Informatics, 11*(12), 64–68.

Schuerenberg, B. (2003). Docs respond to group therapy. *Health Data Management, 11*(1), 34–38.

Thivierge, B. (1997). Taking a cue from the public health professions: Applying the logical framework to strategic planning. *Technical Communication, (Special Issue: Strategic Planning), 44*(4), 390(4).

Wheelen, T. L., and Hunger, J. D. (1995). *Management and business policy,* (5th ed.). Menlo Park, CA: Addison-Wesley.

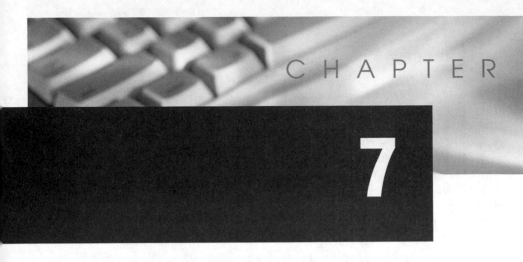

CHAPTER

7

Selecting a Health Care Information System

After completing this chapter, you should be able to:

- Define the term *life cycle* as it relates to information systems.

- List the phases of the life cycle of an information system.

- Discuss the purpose of the needs assessment.

- Identify the typical membership composition of the system selection steering committee.

- Explain the importance of using the mission statement in determining the organization's information needs.

- Identify several methods for analyzing the current system.

- Discuss the value of using a weighted scoring tool during the selection phase.

- Review the system criteria that should be addressed during the selection process.

- Describe the request for information and request for proposal documents.

- Describe the process for evaluating request for proposal (RFP) responses from vendors.

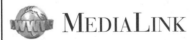 MEDIALINK

Additional resources for this content can be found on the Companion Website at *www. prenhall.com/hebda*. Click on "Chapter 7" to select the activities for this chapter.

Companion Website

- Glossary
- Multiple Choice
- Discussion Points
- Case Study: Developing a Timeline
- Case Study: "Musts" and "Wants" List
- Case Study: Request for Information
- MediaLink Application: System Selection
- Web Hunt: Vendor Selection
- Link to Resources
- Crossword Puzzle

The selection and implementation of an information system occur through a well-defined process known as the **life cycle.** This term describes the ongoing process of developing and maintaining an information system. This cycle can be divided into four main phases that cover the life span of information systems. These four phases are:

1. Needs assessment
2. System selection
3. Implementation
4. Maintenance

Figure 7–1 illustrates the relationship of these phases as circular, because needs assessment and evaluation are ongoing processes. As needs change, the organization may find it necessary to upgrade information systems periodically. The first two phases, needs assessment and system selection, are discussed in this chapter. Details regarding system implementation and maintenance are covered in Chapter 8. It is essential to develop a timeline that delineates the major events or milestones when working through the various phases of the information system's life cycle. For example, while it is desirable to complete the needs assessment and selection processes in less than 1 year, it is necessary to recognize that the process may take 1 year to complete. Therefore, it is vital to organize responsibilities around a realistic timeframe. Figure 7–2 provides a template that may be used to develop a timeline or Gantt chart for the needs assessment and system selection phases of the information system's life cycle.

NEEDS ASSESSMENT

Needs assessment is the first phase in the information life cycle (Zielstorff, McHugh, and Clinton 1988). This process is usually initiated by a person or group with a vision of the future. The needs assessment should analyze the overall needs of the organization with consideration to the strategic

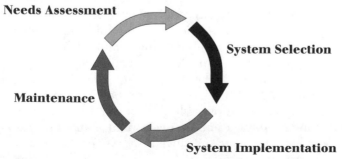

FIGURE 7–1 • The life cycle of an information system

Milestone	Person Responsible	Estimated Start Date	Completion Date
PHASE 1: NEEDS ASSESSMENT			
Develop steering committee			
Perform needs assessment:			
Identify system requirements and weighting of criteria Technical Administrative/general Registration Order entry/results reporting Medical records Accounting			
PHASE 2: SYSTEM SELECTION			
Develop the RFP Organization description System requirements Response evaluation procedures			
Evaluate RFP responses			
Conduct site visits			
Select the system for purchase			
Contract negotiations and contract signed			

FIGURE 7–2 • Sample template for developing a timeline or Gantt chart

plan. After this is done it is appropriate to look at segments within the organization (Oberst 1991). A deficit in the current method of manual or automated information handling is often recognized by people from several different groups or disciplines, such as clinical and administrative personnel who use the information, as well as programmers and other technical staff who manage the information system. Once the deficit or need is realized, a more detailed understanding of the issues must be developed.

After the selection committee discusses the current deficits and needs, they brainstorm to generate a list of possible directions for action. These actions may include minor modifications to the current manual or automated system, major enhancements to the current system, or the purchase of a new automated information system.

The analysis of identified possible actions and the decision-making process must be a collaborative effort, and is often performed by a committee that includes clinical users, information systems specialists, and administration or executive board representatives.

The Steering Committee

The steering committee is an essential component of the assessment and selection processes. Leadership of this group may affect the success or failure of the project. The committee chairperson may be a manager or director of information services or have an administrative position elsewhere in the hospital, such as chief financial officer (CFO), chief nursing officer (CNO), or medical director. The committee membership must be multidisciplinary, including representation from all departments affected by the new system and incorporating the clinical, administrative, and information system divisions. This strategy is essential for identification of all pertinent issues and reduces the possibility of overlooking potential problems (Hewlett-Packard 1990). In those health care organizations that include affiliations with other facilities, it is imperative that representation from these areas be included to address any additional needs. A general rule to follow is that any department or area that uses the information or is affected by it must have a voice in the selection process.

The structure of the steering committee must be defined early in the process. When designing the committee, it is important to consider the appropriate size of the group (Hewlett-Packard 1990). The committee should be large enough to make a good decision but small enough to be effective and efficient. At this point, it is necessary to define who has the authority to make the final decisions. For example, decision-making power may be given to a particular department, shared among a group of administrators from various departments, or shared equally among all members of the steering committee.

One strategy that is effective in larger organizations is to develop a multilevel committee. The upper level or executive board of the committee is responsible for the final decisions regarding selection. This may be a small group of high-level executives, including the chief executive officer, chief information officer, chief privacy officer, vice presidents responsible for major departments, and medical staff leadership. This subcommittee is supported by a larger group of department managers and supervisors. The committee should also include some frontline employees who will actually be using the system. These are the people who will be responsible for doing most of the groundwork and investigation during the assessment and selection processes. For this reason, it is prudent to choose committee members who are able to devote the necessary time and energy to the project. Their managers must be willing to provide them with time away from their normal responsibilities and support their involvement in the project. An effective strategy is to assign tasks to individual members or subgroups based on their expertise and knowledge. Their findings are then presented to the larger committee for discussion and approval.

Consultants

The committee should consider whether and when a consultant should be used. Consultants may be hired for assistance in any phase of the selection process, including assessing the current information system. Consultants may also be used to help with system planning, testing, security, policy and procedure development, and implementation. The effective use of consultants requires clear definition of the contractual relationship and expected outcomes as well as good communication throughout the association. The consultant should be provided with all available data regarding the current system and identified needs. The consultant's role is to analyze this information and make recommendations for action. Box 7–1 lists some of the primary qualities of an effective consultant or consulting service. On occasion, problems arise with the use of consultants that may include limited experience and knowledge of the needs and hardware and software applications under consideration as well as a lack of incentive to work toward the most useful and cost-effective solution.

Developing a Common Vision

The needs assessment committee should start the process by examining the vision and mission statements of the organization as well as the strategic plan. This will guide the committee in looking to the future and determining the organization's information needs while continuing to support the mission. From this, goals or a charge should be developed to guide the

---

Box 7–1 **Qualities of an Effective Consultant**

- Experience, including longevity and diversity
- Knowledge and understanding of the health care industry
- Good consulting skill and a proven methodology
- Good verbal and written communication skills
- Good project management skills
- Clearly defined work plan and deliverables
- Advice that will result in cost savings
- Flexibility and availability
- A fit with the corporate culture
- Leadership in a team environment
- Ability to manage expectations rather than results

Source: Adapted from Consulting Services. (July 1996). *Contingency Planning and Management*, p. 20; and Stanek, J. (May 2003). Using consultants to support your many roles. *Advance for Health Information Executives*, 48.

work of the committee. These goals must reflect the organization's purpose, scope of services, and customers. The primary goal of the committee is to identify how health care delivery can be enhanced to provide optimum client care; this can be accomplished by providing more meaningful and accurate client data. Some additional expectations of an information system might be to save time, increase productivity, contain costs, promote quality improvement, and foster staff recruitment and retention. In addition, the system must be able meet and support regulatory guidelines such as those related to Health Insurance Portability and Accountability Act (HIPAA) requirements. The committee should consider using brainstorming techniques when defining the expectations of an information system. An open-minded and creative approach will facilitate comprehensive exploration of all possibilities.

Understanding the Current System

A thorough understanding of how information is currently collected and processed is the starting point in performing a needs assessment. This is also known as assessing the internal environment. Methods for accomplishing this include questionnaires and observation of day-to-day activities (Saba and McCormick 1996). The goal is to determine what information is used, who uses it, and how it is used. Every data item used in the current paper or automated system should be analyzed. Some examples of data items include client name, sex, marital status, and diagnosis. Next, the committee must decide what information should be kept, what information is redundant, and what information is unnecessary. They should evaluate the strengths and weaknesses of the current manual or automated information system to determine the needs of the health care enterprise.

Determining System Requirements

To determine the appropriate course of action, the committee must first understand the organization's requirements for operation. One strategy for obtaining this information is to interview staff from each department or work area. The interviewer might ask what information is necessary to conduct business and what information is desired but not essential. These are often called the "musts" and the "wants." Some examples of essential information include client name, admitting physician, and insurance information. It is important to also consider those criteria that may not be necessary at the present time but might be important in the future, such as voice recognition technology. The information from numerous interviews is then compiled into a list of "musts" and "wants."

The next step is to prioritize or weight the list of "musts" and "wants" from high to low. To accomplish this task, selection committee members should develop a rating scale such as a 1-to-10 scale or rankings of low, medium, and high. Table 7–1 displays an example of some weighted "wants" and "musts" that could be identified when performing the needs

Table 7–1	Sample of Criteria Defining "Musts" and "Wants"	
Charting/Documentation Information Criteria	**"Must" or "Want"**	**Weight***
Capable of multidisciplinary charting	M	10
Able to chart medications, IVs, and treatments	M	10
Has mechanism to remind the user of undocumented activities, treatments, medications, and IVs at intervals specified by department	M	10
Automatically calculates charted IV products into intake and output	W	7
Automatically totals fluid balance by shift and 24-hour period	W	8
Able to easily switch between functions (such as charting and entering orders)	W	5

*1–10, where 10 = most important.

assessment. The criteria should also be grouped into functional categories to present a comprehensive picture of the system requirements. Some of the common categories that may be considered are listed next.

Technical Criteria. Technical criteria include those hardware and software components necessary for the desired level of system performance. Areas to consider are the following:

- *Type of architecture.* **Architecture** refers to the structure of the central processing unit and its interrelated elements. An **open system** uses protocols and technology that follow publicly accepted conventions and are used by multiple vendors, so that various system components can work together.

Examples of Criteria
  1. System maintains an open architecture environment that can continue to evolve as new technology becomes available
  2. Features ease of implementation and support of real-time integration to existing and future information systems
- *Amount of downtime.* **Downtime** refers to the period of time when an information system is not operational and available for use. Some systems have daily scheduled downtimes, during which maintenance and backup procedures are performed.

Examples of Criteria
  1. Provides 24-hour system availability with no scheduled daily downtime

2. Does not have a history of prolonged or frequent unscheduled downtimes

- *Connectivity standards.* These standards help to maximize the connectivity between application and information files, supporting system integration.

  Examples of Criteria
  1. Provides for HL7–compliant interfaces
  2. Includes the ability to interface from and to client care instruments such as monitors

- *Test environment separate from live environment.* A separate environment for the development and testing of updates and changes to the system must be available, so that the actual system (live system) can continue to operate without interference during these activities.

  Examples of Criteria
  1. Provides the ability to update the test environment without impacting the live system
  2. Provides a training environment that is separate from the live and test environments

- *Response time.* **Response time** is the amount of time between a user action and the response from the information system. For example, after the user selects a laboratory test from a menu, the system requires a certain amount of processing time before that result can be viewed.

  Examples of Criteria
  1. Ensures acceptable response time for all online transactions (1 second or less)
  2. Able to continuously track and monitor response time and provide reports containing this information

- *Support of electronic technologies.* The information system should support other technologies that will enhance client care and business operations.

  Examples of Criteria
  1. Supports various methods of data entry by the user, including touch-screen entry and voice recognition
  2. Allows the use of bar coding and scanning

Administrative/General Criteria. Administrative criteria describe how the system may be administratively controlled for appropriate and effective use of the information.

- *Security levels to comply with regulatory and legal requirements.* The Joint Commission for Accreditation of Healthcare Organizations (JCAHO), for example, regulates the confidentiality, security, and integrity of hospital systems. The HIPAA imposes requirements for the protection of patient data and penalties for noncompliance.

Examples of Criteria

1. Allows various levels of security to be defined for different user groups; each group should have access to only the information required for its client care or job duties
2. Provides an auditing utility to track and report what information has been accessed by which users

- *Online help screens.* Online help screens display instructions to assist the user with completing a specific function.

Examples of Criteria

1. Help screens must be available and easily accessed by the user
2. Help screens must be concise and easy to understand

- *Purging and restoring data.* It is important to determine how long it is necessary to maintain online access to client data before sending it to other storage devices. Sometimes it becomes essential to restore these files for the purposes of audits, and the ease of performing these procedures must be considered. Advances such as the use of imaging technology to store diagnostic images and forms must be considered when purge criteria are defined.

Examples of Criteria

1. Includes a flexible client purge process, allowing both automatic and manual purge capabilities
2. Process for restoring data that have been purged to storage to be convenient and readily accessible

- *Report capabilities.* The system should provide a report-writing software component that allows specific types of information to be extracted from the database and presented in a report.

Examples of Criteria

1. Predefined reports to be produced automatically on a set schedule
2. Users should be able to generate ad hoc reports on demand, with the capability to format them as desired
3. Reports should be available online, eliminating concerns related to printing costs, labor, distribution, storage, and disposal of confidential materials

Registration Criteria. The registration criteria are essential for ensuring that the client is properly identified for all aspects of information management.

Examples of Criteria

1. Assigns each client a unique identifier across the organization
2. Supports multiple registration sites; clients may enter the health system at a number of points of service, including the physician's office, clinics, the emergency department, or the admissions office
3. Provides the ability to change or update registration information
4. Demonstrates the ability to track a client's location within the institution, as well as to track the use of system services
5. Prevents the user from omitting required data before completing a function

Order Entry/Results Reporting Criteria. These criteria ensure that accurate entry of physician orders is accomplished in a timely and efficient manner, resulting in improved client care.

Examples of Criteria

1. Able to indicate details of orders such as frequency (for example, q6h or daily) and priority (stat, routine, and so on)
2. Notifies the user when a duplicate order is entered, and requests verification before accepting the new order. For example, the client may have a previously ordered daily chest x-ray. If a new order for a chest x-ray is now entered, the system should alert the user and request verification that this additional test is necessary.
3. Through order entry and results reporting, produces an audit trail that identifies the person who entered the order, the date/time of order entry and execution, and the status of the order (such as pending or completed)
4. Supports documentation of medications and treatments, and relates this documentation to the appropriate order
5. Automatically generates client charges for specific orders or treatments as a result of entry or completion

Medical Records Criteria. The medical records criteria should support the storage of all pertinent client data obtained from various information systems, allowing the user to access a longitudinal record of all client activities and events or visits. The system should allow inquiry about clients, using various identifiers, including social security number, name, medical record, or account number.

Examples of Criteria

1. Provides support for automatic coding, including verification of codes entered with narrative description (for example, *ICD-9-CM* and *CPT-4* codes)

2. Translates diagnosis and procedure terminology into numeric code

3. Produces deficiency lists on demand for individual records and individual physicians

Accounting Criteria. These criteria facilitate reimbursement for services rendered and help to ensure the financial stability of the enterprise.

Examples of Criteria

1. Generates summaries or detailed bills on demand

2. Allows the user to enter the client's insurance verification data, insurance plan, and charges at any time during the stay and to change the client's financial class

3. Supports physician billing and captures data for linkage to physician billing services

SYSTEM SELECTION

If the decision is made to purchase a new information system, the life cycle proceeds to Phase 2: system selection. This phase is critical to the success of the project. The extremely high purchase, installation, and maintenance costs associated with new or upgraded technology mean that the decision must be made carefully. The information gathered during the needs assessment phase is the basis for the system selection process and decision. Because it has been determined that a new system must be purchased, further information must now be gathered. Box 7–2 identifies some system selection considerations.

Additional Sources of Information

Trade shows and conferences are beneficial sources of information. Attendance at these events provides the opportunity to examine systems from various vendors in an informal atmosphere, to compare and contrast system capabilities, and to view demonstrations.

Other potentially helpful sources of information include weekly publications, trade newspapers, and monthly journals that address information and technology, and local user groups. Textbooks and reference books also provide discussions of system options. Published conference proceedings may provide insight into pertinent issues and solutions. Finally, communication via the Internet and World Wide Web can furnish additional information, including insights from other users of a given

---

Box 7–2 **System Selection Criteria**

- Overall costs
  Hardware, software, and network costs
  Implementation costs
  Support and maintenance costs
- Vendor characteristics
  Reputation
  Experienced staff and consultants
  Financial status
- Software features
  Ease of use
  Intuitive user interface, requiring minimal training
  Includes all functionality identified as "musts"
  Supports security requirements
  Supports interfaces with other applications
  Supports future growth options

---

system. This avenue may provide the most current and candid responses to questions.

Request for Information

An information systems **vendor** is a company that designs, develops, sells, and supports systems. Consideration of vendor characteristics is crucial in choosing a system that will be responsive to current needs and unanticipated changes. Characteristics to examine include service, performance, and stability (Haglind 2003). A great deal of information can be gleaned from vendors who are eager to make a sale. The **request for information (RFI)** is often the initial contact with vendors. An RFI is a letter or brief document sent to vendors that explains the institution's plans for purchasing and installing an information system. The purpose of the RFI is to obtain essential information about the vendor and its systems to eliminate those vendors that cannot meet the organization's basic requirements. One method for obtaining names of appropriate vendors is to complete reader response cards following advertisements in professional journals.

The RFI should ask the vendor to provide a description of the system and its capabilities. Often the vendor responds to the request by sending written literature. More information can be obtained by asking additional specific questions of the vendor. Some topics to consider for questioning include:

1. The history and financial situation of the company, including the extent of its investment into research and development; this provides an indication of the company's commitment to enhancing and updating the product
2. The number of installed sites, including a list of several organizations that already use the product you are considering
3. System architecture, including the required hardware configuration
4. Use of state-of-the-art technology
5. Integration with other systems. Which other systems are currently integrated with the vendor's software in other hospital sites?
6. The methods of user support provided by the vendor during and after installation
7. Future health care provider development plans
8. Procedures for the distribution of software updates

Request for Proposal

At this point, the steering committee will probably be overwhelmed with information. The next step is to evaluate this information and prepare a formal document called the **request for proposal (RFP).** An RFP is a document sent to vendors that describes the requirements of a potential information system (Cross 1996). The RFP prioritizes or ranks these requirements in order of their importance to the organization. The purpose of this document is to solicit proposals from many vendors that describe their capabilities to meet the "wants" and "needs." The vendors' responses may then be used to narrow the number of competitors under consideration.

Strategies for a Successful RFP. Because of the importance of the RFP, it must be structured to ensure successful system selection. All aspects of the document must be detailed and precise to facilitate an accurate response from the vendor. If questions are vague or poorly written, they could easily be misinterpreted by the vendor. For example, an ambiguous question might lead a vendor to indicate that the system meets a requirement when in fact it does not. It is advantageous to limit the number of requirements to those that are most important and to produce a simple and straightforward document. If an RFP is too lengthy, it will cost both the organization and the vendor a great deal of time and money to prepare and evaluate. It is difficult to evaluate a long document that is not focused on the important issues. Finally, a well-written RFP provides a framework that allows the steering committee to more accurately evaluate the vendor's proposal.

The format of RFP questions and answers may influence the authenticity of vendor responses. For example, for each question about a system feature, the RFP might offer four response choices, such as:

1. *"Yes."* If the vendor indicates that this functionality is currently available, then the vendor must also provide a written explanation of how the system performs this function.

2. *"Available with customization."* The vendor must provide an estimated cost of customization and time frame for availability.

3. *"Available in the future."* The vendor must provide an estimated time frame for availability.

4. *"No."* No further information is required.

RFP Design. Although the actual format of the RFP may vary from organization to organization, all RFPs must contain certain components that are essential for a complete and effective document. The RFP should include the following details:

- *Description of the organization.* The first objective of the RFP should be to familiarize the vendor with the organization. The RFP must describe the organization's overall environment, as well as the specific setting in which the system will function. The vendor needs to have enough information to facilitate proposal of appropriate systems and hardware configurations. The following information should be included:

  1. *Mission and goals.* The mission statement and any supporting documentation will provide the vendor with a view of the driving forces behind the selection process.

  2. *Structure of the organization.* The RFP should describe how the health care enterprise is structured, including all facilities and satellite areas that provide inpatient, outpatient, and home care services.

  3. *Type of health care facility.* The RFP should specify whether the facility is a profit or nonprofit organization and contain descriptors appropriate to the organization, such as community, university, government, or teaching facility.

  4. *Payor mix.* Additional information should quantify the proportion of clients for the various types of payors encountered. For example, the percentage of clients having private insurance, Medicare/Medicaid coverage, or health maintenance organization (HMO) membership should be indicated.

  5. *Volume statistics.* The RFP should provide volume statistics such as number of inpatient beds, average occupancy, annual

outpatient visits, emergency department visits, volume of lab tests performed, number of operations annually, and number of various categories of staff, including physicians, nurses, and technicians.

- *System requirements.* Following the description of the organization, the RFP should include a comprehensive list of the system requirements previously developed by the committee. One point to consider when defining system requirements is to avoid limiting the vendor to specific configurations, such as the type and number of devices, because the vendor may be able to suggest better solutions. The requirements should not necessitate the vendor to recreate a manual or current automated system. These limitations may prohibit the vendor from exploring improved methods of information use with the proposed technology (Metrick 2002).

- *Criteria for evaluation of responses.* Providing the vendor with an explanation of the RFP evaluation process may improve the quality of the vendor's response. If the vendors respond in the expected format, evaluating responses from multiple vendors can be more easily accomplished, and results more easily compared.

- *Deadline date.* Inform the vendor of the expected date of responses. Vendors who do not meet deadlines may be excluded.

Evaluation of RFP Responses. Once responses from various vendors have been received, the process of evaluation begins. Some initial considerations are related to how the vendor approached the RFP. For example, some questions to ask are:

- Was the response submitted by the deadline date?
- Does it represent the work of a professional team and company?
- Were the vendor representatives responsive and knowledgeable?
- Does the proposal address the requirements outlined in the RFP, or does it appear to be a standard bid?

Further evaluation is centered around the specific responses of the vendors to the requirements listed in the RFP. The prioritization and ranking of the requirements that were previously developed by the steering committee now are used to weight each item in the RFP. This produces an overall score for each vendor response. This score allows the vendors to be ranked objectively, based on their ability to meet the requirements. Vendors that are unable to meet all of the "musts" should be automatically eliminated.

The remaining vendors must now be evaluated in terms of benefits and costs. Examining the scores for the "wants" and discussing the vendor's proposed costs are components of the final decision-making process. It may be helpful to narrow the list to three finalists and then examine these more closely.

Site Visits. The use of site visits is very helpful in selecting a system. Site visits allow the system to be seen in action at a location that is comparable in size and services provided. Comparison of site visit evaluations for the top three vendors may provide additional information that will facilitate decision making.

A successful site visit often begins with the preparation of a list of questions. Asking the same questions at each site visit helps the committee draw meaningful comparisons. It is helpful to request a demonstration of the live system. This will allow observations regarding the response time. It is also beneficial to examine reports and printed documentation produced by the system, and to interview people who are actually using the system. Often, more candid information can be obtained if the vendors are not present during the interview process. Box 7–3 lists several questions that may be used during a site visit.

In addition, the vendor should provide a contact list of users from other organizations who are willing to be interviewed by phone (Cross 1996). Representatives from hospital departments may ask their counterparts in other organizations about the performance of the information system. This will provide insight into how the systems actually operate, as well as the support that the vendor provides.

Contract Negotiations. Once the decision has been made by the steering committee, the enterprise's legal and purchasing representatives carry out the contract negotiations. They may request the names of the three highest ranked vendors, as well as their RFP responses. In this way, the contract negotiations will be able to address issues not specifically included in

---

Box 7–3
Questions to Ask During a Site Visit

- How reliable is the system?
- How much downtime do you experience?
- How is the system backup accomplished, and how frequently is this done?
- Does the system use interface standards?
- How do customizations or enhancements get made to the system (in-house or by vendor)?
- How much training was required for users to learn the system?
- What do you like most about the system?
- What things would you like to change about the system?
- What features would you like to see added to the system?
- How is information access restricted, and how is security maintained?
- What have your experiences been with vendor support?

SOURCE: Adapted from *Choosing a Clinical Information System* by Hewlett-Packard Company, 1990, courtesy Hewlett-Packard Company.

the RFP responses, such as cost justification and expected implementation schedules. The end result will be the selection of one vendor and a system that will be implemented in the enterprise. After the contract is signed, the implementation phase begins.

CASE STUDY EXERCISES

You are a member of the committee that will select a clinical documentation system for nurses. Prepare a timeline for the needs assessment and system selection phases. These processes should be accomplished over a 6-month period.

• • •

Develop a list of "musts" and "wants" and assign a weight to each item. Define what your weighting scale will be.

• • •

Create a list of questions related to this system selection process that you will ask at site visits.

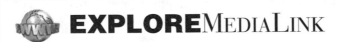

EXPLOREMEDIALINK

Multiple choice questions, case studies, and other interactive resources for this chapter can be found on the Web site at *http://www.prenhall.com/hebda*. Click on "Chapter 7" to select the activities for this chapter.

SUMMARY

- The selection and implementation of an information system occur through a well-defined process called the life cycle of an information system.

- The four phases of the life cycle of an information system are needs assessment, system selection, implementation, and maintenance.

- The needs assessment process is often initiated when a deficit in the current method of manual or automated information handling is recognized.

- The system selection steering committee is an essential component of the assessment and selection processes, and leadership as well as membership of this group may impact the success or failure of the project.

- The needs assessment process should include an examination of the vision and mission statements of the organization, because these should guide the committee in looking to the future and determining the organization's information needs.

- A thorough understanding of how information is currently collected and processed is the starting point in performing a needs assessment.

- Determination of the system requirements should address criteria related to all aspects of system performance, including technical, administrative, registration, order entry, results reporting, medical records, and accounting criteria.

- The request for information is a letter or brief document sent to vendors that explains the institution's plans for purchasing and installing an information system. The purpose of the RFI is to obtain essential information about the vendor and its system capabilities to eliminate those vendors that cannot meet the organization's basic requirements.

- The request for proposal is a document sent to vendors that describes the requirements of a potential information system. The purpose of this document is to solicit from many vendors proposals that describe the capabilities of their information systems and support services.

- A weighted scoring strategy will facilitate the evaluation of complicated request for proposal responses from vendors and will improve the ability of the steering committee to make an informed decision.

REFERENCES

Consulting services. (1996). *Contingency Planning and Management, 1*(7), 20.

Cross, M. A. (1996). RFP: Simplifying the task of selecting a system. *Health Data Management, 4*(3), 99–105.

Haglind, M. (2003). Choosing a vendor. *Healthcare Informatics, 20*(6), 87–88.

Hewlett-Packard Company. (1990). *Choosing a clinical information system.* Andover, MA: author.

Metrick, G. (2002). Selecting a product or services using the request for proposal process. *Scientific Computing and Instrumentation, 19*(12), L-8–L-12.

Oberst, B. (1991). Computerized doctor office systems: The benefit to the hospital, physician and patient. In M. J. Ball, J. V. Douglas, R. I. O'Desky, and J. W. Albright (Eds.). *Healthcare information management systems* (pp. 51–61). New York: Springer.

Saba, V. K., and McCormick, K. A. (1996). *Essentials of computers for nurses.* Philadelphia: Lippincott.

Stanek, J. (May 2003). Using consultants to support your many roles. *ADVANCE for Health Information Executives, 7*(5), 45–48.

Zielstorff, R. D., McHugh, M. L., and Clinton, J. (1988). *Computer design criteria for systems that support the nursing process.* Kansas City, MO: American Nurses Association.

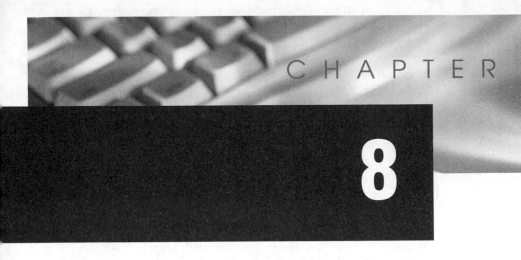

CHAPTER

8

System Implementation and Maintenance

After completing this chapter, you should be able to:

- Describe how implementation committee members are selected.

- Discuss the importance of establishing a project timeline or schedule.

- Explain the differences between the test, training, and production environments.

- List the decisions that must be addressed when performing an analysis of hardware requirements.

- Review the issues that must be addressed when developing procedures and documentation for users.

- Discuss the factors that contribute to effective training.

- Identify the components involved in "go-live" planning.

- Recognize several common implementation pitfalls.

- Name several common forms of user feedback and support.

- Explain the significance of providing ongoing system and technical maintenance.

- Recognize that the life cycle of an information system is an ongoing cyclical process.

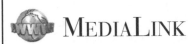
MEDIALINK

Additional resources for this content can be found on the Companion Website at *www. prenhall.com/hebda*. Click on "Chapter 8" to select the activities for this chapter.

Companion Website
- Glossary
- Multiple Choice
- Discussion Points
- Case Study: Project Timeline
- Case Study: Training and Go-Live Schedule
- Case Study: Testing
- MediaLink Application: System Implementation
- Web Hunt: Systems Life Cycle
- Links to Resources
- Crossword Puzzle

The previous chapter discussed the first two phases of the life cycle of an information system. This chapter explores system implementation and maintenance, which make up the third and fourth phases.

SYSTEM IMPLEMENTATION

Develop an Implementation Committee

The implementation phase is planned prior to the purchase of the system. Once the organization has purchased the information system, the implementation phase continues. A project leader is identified and a team of hospital staff is selected to support the project as a working committee. The steering committee chairperson or another member of the steering committee may serve as the implementation project leader. It is important, however, that the project leader be involved in the entire selection and implementation process and possess strong leadership and communication skills (Lau and Hebert 2001; Miranda, Fields and Lund 2001; Saba and McCormick 1996). This ensures that the project leader has a firm understanding of the vision, goals, and expectations for the system.

The committee membership should include technical staff from the information services department as well as clinical representatives who are knowledgeable regarding current manual or automated procedures. Each group should be represented both by managers who have the authority to make the decisions and by department staff who have knowledge and experience of day-to-day operations as well as an understanding of how those processes might be improved. Recruiting efforts should focus on people who display the characteristics that support effective group dynamics and represent all key stakeholders (Meadows 2003). In addition, the project leader should facilitate the development of effective group dynamics. Any effort that involves the implementation of a system for nurses or that will be used by nurses should include an informatics nurse. The *informatics nurse* is uniquely qualified to communicate the needs of clinical staff to information services personnel and has a working knowledge of regulatory and system requirements as well as strategic plans and budgetary constraints. The informatics nurse is also qualified to identify current problems or issues and help to choose or develop a solution. The committee members and organizational issues are every bit as important as the technology itself when implementing a new system (Lau and Hebert 2001). Box 8–1 lists some of the characteristics of a successful implementation committee.

Install the System

The initial work of the implementation committee is to develop a comprehensive project plan or timeline, scheduling all of the critical elements for

---

Box 8–1   **Characteristics of a Successful Implementation Committee**

Characteristics of Individual Members

- Communicates openly
- Uses time and talents efficiently
- Performs effectively and produces results
- Welcomes challenges
- Cooperates rather than competes

Group Characteristics

- Works toward a common goal
- Encourages members to teach and learn from one another
- Develops its members' skills
- Builds morale internally
- Resolves conflicts effectively
- Shows pride in its accomplishments
- Enhances diversity of its members

---

implementation (Fichter 2003; Hewlett-Packard 1990). This plan should address what tasks are necessary, the scope of each task, who is responsible for accomplishing each element, start and completion dates, necessary resources, and constraints (Figure 8–1). Questions asked at this stage focus on the background of the project, its goals and sponsor, key stakeholders, benefits, and budget. Clear definition of this phase of the project requires time, energy, and lots of good communication. Failure to adequately address this phase jeopardizes successful implementation. Project planning software may be helpful in developing the project timeline or schedule and a hierarchical arrangement of all specific tasks. This type of plan is referred to as a **work breakdown structure (WBS).** After the project is defined, it is imperative to work on team building, control and execution, and review and exit planning. Inadequate attention to these phases can also jeopardize implementation success.

The committee members should first become familiar with the information system they will be implementing. This can be accomplished in several ways. The vendor can provide on-site training, hospital staff can receive training at the vendor's corporate centers, or third-party consultants may be hired. Vendor training should provide the opportunity to continue to update the skills of employees and to subsequently use them as a resource throughout the implementation process (Schuerenberg 2003). Once committee members have acquired an understanding of how the system functions, they will have the knowledge needed to analyze the base

Milestone	Person Responsible	Estimated Start Date	Completion Date
PHASE 3: **SYSTEM IMPLEMENTATION**			
Develop implementation committee			
Analyze customization requirements			
Perform system modifications and customizations			
Analyze hardware requirements			
Develop procedures and user guides			
System and integrated testing			
Provide user training			
Go-live conversion preparation and backloading			
Go-live event			

FIGURE 8–1 • Sample template for a system implementation timeline

system as delivered from the vendor. Ideally the following issues are addressed during system selection but should be considered by the implementation committee before the system is installed in the event that clarification or changes are necessary (Martin 2002; Meadows 2003):

- *The technology.* It is important to consider whether the technology that is used is current and can be upgraded easily or is already obsolete. It is also necessary to have a good match between the system and the needs of the area.
- *Vendor standing.* Committee members need to consider financial solvency of the vendor for long-term service and dialog with other customers to determine their implementation issues and resolution.
- *Vendor compliance with regulatory requirements.* System customization for regulatory compliance can be expensive. It is essential to determine vendor responsibility for federal and state regulatory compliance.
- *Integration with other systems.* It is important to establish how easily the selected system exchanges information with other major systems such as medical records and financial systems.

- *Use for different types of patient accounts.* Does the system work equally well for inpatient, outpatient, and emergency care encounters?
- *Electronic medical record support.* Does the system support the electronic medical record?
- *Remote access.* Does the product permit secure access to patient data from all locations, particularly remote sites?
- *Clinician support.* Does the product support patient care?

The next step is to decide whether this system should be used as is or customized to meet the specific needs of the organization. This decision will act as the implementation strategy that will guide the committee through the implementation process.

Regardless of which implementation strategy is followed, the committee must next gather information about the data that must be collected and processed. Consideration must be given to the data that is pertinent to each function and available to the user for entry into the system. A **function** refers to a task that may be performed manually or automated; some examples include order entry, results reporting, and documentation. The output of the system should also be examined. For example, the format and content of printed requisitions, result reports, worklists, and managerial reports must be evaluated. A detailed analysis of the current work and paper flow will provide this information. Once decisions have been made regarding system design and modification, the appropriate department head should approve these specifications before the actual changes are made. Numerous changes delay implementation of the system and drive up costs.

At this point, the identified changes should be made to the system in the test environment. The **test environment** is one copy of the software where programming changes are initially made. After any changes are made, they must be tested to ensure that they display and process data accurately. Before this can be accomplished, the implementation team and all responsible managers must agree on a test plan (Gates 2002). This includes determining long-term goals and what must be tested. Testing is best accomplished by following a transaction through the system for all associated functions. In some cases vendors provide a significant cost reduction in product purchases if the buyer is willing to beta test the product. Beta testing occurs on-site under everyday working conditions. Software problems are identified, corrected, and then retested. This follows alpha testing which is an intensive examination of new software features. An example of this testing procedure might be to enter a physician's order for an x-ray into the system for a particular client. The correct printing of the requisition should be verified. Next, the results of the x-ray should be entered for this client. Both online results retrieval and printed report content should be verified. Finally, the system should be checked to make certain that the appropriate charges have been generated and passed onto the financial system. It is important to realize that the test environment is not exactly the same as the live environment, because the live environment is much larger and more complex. As a result, the findings of the system test may not always indicate how well the system will perform in the live environment. To help ensure that testing is valid, it is essential to involve more than a handful of persons from information services, the implementation committee, or a quality assurance group. Select end-users must be involved to put the test environment through the same type of stresses and rigors as occur in daily work processes.

Analyze Hardware Requirements

A separate group of tasks related to the analysis of hardware requirements must also be addressed during the implementation phase. These tasks should be initiated early in the implementation phase and continue simultaneously while system design and modifications are being completed. Some of these items include the following:

- *Network infrastructure.* The determination of network requirements, cable installation, wiring and access points, and technical standards should be initiated early in the implementation phase. The processing power, memory capacity of network components, and anticipated future needs must be addressed by the technical members of the implementation committee or other information services staff. This is particularly important because the majority of current network outages and downtime now result from cabling issues and are costly in terms of lost productivity and customer dissatisfaction (Mouton and McNees 2003). Extensive changes to network configuration are expensive and should be avoided whenever possible. Wireless technology may not be an alternative in some cases. Some functions that place a heavy demand on the network include digital imaging and archival, and telemedicine.

- *Type of workstation device.* The system may be accessed via a number of different devices. These may include a networked personal computer (PC), thin client, wireless or handheld device such as a personal digital assistant (PDA), or mobile laptop PC that uses radiofrequency technology. The committee must investigate the advantages of each option and make recommendations regarding the type of hardware for purchase and installation. Once a decision has been made regarding the type of workstation, the appropriate number of devices per area or department must be determined.

- *Workstation location strategy.* A related workstation decision is the strategy for locating and using the hardware. Several options are available. **Point-of-care** devices are located at the site of client care, which is often at the client's bedside in the emergency department, delivery room, operating room, and radiology. Another strategy involves a centralized approach, where workstations are located at the unit station. A third option is to use handheld or mobile devices that may be accessed wherever the staff finds it most convenient.

- *Hardware location requirements.* The area where the equipment is to be placed or used must be evaluated as to whether there are adequate electrical receptacles, cabling constraints, and/or reception and transmission capabilities. In addition, the work area may require modifications to accommodate the selected hardware. Another major consideration is the need to protect health information from casual view.

- *Printer decisions.* The various printer options should be examined. A choice must be made between laser printer technology, ink jet, and dot matrix, as well as specific features such as the number of paper trays and fonts. Printed output requires the same consideration for privacy of information.

Develop Procedures and Documentation

Comprehensive procedures for how the system will be used to support client care and associated administrative activities should be developed before the training process is begun. In this way, training may include procedures as well as hands-on use of the system. One approach is to examine the current nursing policy and procedure manuals and to incorporate new policies and procedures related to automation. Information regarding downtime procedures should be included, so that staff is aware of what to do in the case of planned or unexpected system downtime. It may be beneficial to develop separate documentation that includes the downtime procedures and manual requisition forms and to have this located in an easily identifiable and accessible location.

System user guides should also be developed at this point. These documents explain how to use the system and the printouts that the system produces (Saba and McCormick 1996). User guides provided by the vendor may be adequate if a limited number of modifications were made to the base system. However, if significant modifications have been made, it may be necessary to customize this documentation to reflect the system as the users will see it. In this case, user guides cannot be completed until all modifications have been completed, tested, and approved for the live system.

Another important aspect of documentation is the development of a dictionary of terms and mapping terms from one system to another. This ensures that everyone has a clear definition of terms and uses them in the same way. Data dictionaries do not contain actual data but list and define all terms used and provide bookkeeping information for managing data (Webopedia 2003). Data dictionaries help to ensure that data are of high quality.

Testing

The process of testing includes the development of a test plan, the creation of test scripts, system testing, and integrated testing. An effective test plan cannot be created until screens and pathways have been finalized and policies and procedures determined. Otherwise, the plan must be revised one or more times. The test plan prescribes what will be examined within the new system as well as all systems with which it shares data. Successful testing requires the involvement of staff who perform day-to-day work because they know the current process and expected outcomes. The test plan should include patient types and functions seen in the facility. A review is then done to identify whether functions are completed without error. Problem areas should be tested again before the person responsible for that area indicates approval and signoff. After system testing, integrated testing can start. Integrated testing looks at the exchange of data between the test system and other systems to ensure its accuracy and completeness.

Provide Training

Once all modifications have been completed in the test environment, a training environment should be established. A **training environment** is a separate copy of the software that mimics the actual system that will be used. Many organizations populate the training database with fictitious clients and make this database available for formal training classes during the implementation process and for ongoing education.

Training is most effective if the training session is a scheduled time independent from the learners' other work responsibilities and at a site separate from the work environment. This allows the learner to concentrate on comprehending the system without interruptions. Planning should address providing adequate resources to allow for the scheduling of training sessions as close as possible to the "go-live" date. In addition, learners should have a place to practice after the formal classroom instruction.

Go-Live Planning

The committee should determine the **go-live** date, which is when the system will be operational and used to collect and process actual client data. At this point, the **production environment** is in effect. The production environment is another term that refers to the time when the new system is in operation. Some of the necessary planning surrounding this event includes the following:

- *Implementation strategy.* It must be determined whether implementation will be staggered, be modular, or occur all at once. An example of a staggered implementation strategy may be to go-live in a limited number of client units but in all ancillary departments. The remaining client units would be scheduled to go-live in groups staggered over a specified time frame.

- *Conversion to the new system.* Decisions must be made regarding what information will be **backloaded,** or preloaded into the system before the go-live date. This includes identification of who will perform this task and the methodology used to accomplish it. Plans for how orders will be backloaded must be developed. For example, a "daily x 4 days" order for a complete blood cell count should be analyzed to determine how many days will be remaining on the go-live date. This number should be entered when the backload is performed. Backloading may be needed to create accurate worklists, charges, or medication administration sheets. Plans for verification of the accuracy of preloaded data should be considered.

- *Developing the support schedule.* It often is necessary to provide on-site support around the clock during the initial go-live or conversion phase. Support personnel may include vendor representatives, information system staff, and other members of the implementation committee.

- *Developing evaluation procedures.* Satisfaction questionnaires and a method for communicating and answering questions during the go-live conversion should be provided.

- *Developing a procedure to request post go-live changes.* Priority must be given to changes required to make the system work as it should. Additional changes should go before the implementation committee or hospital steering committee to determine necessity. This process helps to keep costs manageable.

Common Implementation Pitfalls

There are several common pitfalls with system implementation. Perhaps the most common is an inadequate understanding of how much work is required to implement the system, resulting in underestimation of necessary time and resources (Lau and Hebert 2001). If the initial timeline is not based on a realistic estimate of the required activities and their scope, the implementation process may fall behind schedule. Therefore, it is necessary to fully investigate the impact of the system and control the scope of the project in the early stages of planning.

Another serious problem that may occur during implementation is that of numerous revisions during design activities, creating a constantly moving target. This is sometimes known as "scope creep" or "feature creep" (Fichter 2003). **Scope creep** is the unexpected and uncontrolled growth of user expectations as the project progresses. **Feature creep** is the uncontrolled addition of features or functions without regard to timelines or budget. As needed customizations and modifications are identified, it is imperative that the appropriate user department heads approve and sign off on them before programming changes are made. Frequent changes can become very frustrating for the technical staff and result in missed deadlines. Ultimately, this can be very expensive and emotionally draining for the implementation team.

The amount and type of customization that is done to the information systems can also result in problems. To guide the implementation team, the implementation strategy must address the degree of customization that will be done. One strategy is using the system as delivered by the vendor, with minimal changes. The advantage of this strategy, which is often called the "vanilla system," is an easier and quicker implementation. In addition, future software upgrades may also be implemented with greater ease and speed. The disadvantage of using this system is that user workflow may not match the system design.

The opposite implementation strategy is to fully customize the information system so that it reflects the current workflow. Although this may seem appealing, the disadvantages include a complicated, lengthy, and expensive implementation process. A further disadvantage is seen when system software upgrades are attempted. Many of the customizations may prohibit the upgrades from being installed without extensive programming effort. As a result, the present trend in the hospital information systems industry is to recommend use of the vanilla systems as delivered by the vendors.

Other common pitfalls include failure to consider annual maintenance contracts and related costs, providing insufficient dedicated resources to the implementation committee, and a hostile culture. The vendor's purchase price for a system is only a portion of overall costs (Hudson 2002; Lasker 2003). Vendors charge additional fees for annual technical support, customization, and license fees. These charges are levied on the size of the institution or the number of users, which may or may not be concurrent. Additional costs may include hardware, operating or report software needed to support the system, site preparation, uninterrupted power systems, installation, and ongoing operating costs such as maintenance, supplies, personnel, and upgrades. Clinical representatives of the implementation committee cannot be expected to manage a full-time clinical position while contributing significant time to the implementation project. Because the end result of effective implementation is improved client care, it may be cost-effective to temporarily reassign clinical staff to the project. Project success is impeded by a hostile culture, resistance to change, and refusal to see the benefits of technology.

There may also be problems with testing. These can include poorly developed test scripts, inadequate time to retest problem areas, and the inability to get other systems to exchange data with the test system. Inadequate testing can lead to unpleasant surprises at go-live.

All too often, training suffers from inadequate allocation of time and resources. The training environment should mirror the testing environment and later the production environment. Design may not be completed when training starts. This creates a negative impression of the system among end users as well as confusion.

Finally, it is important to continually reinforce the concept that the implementation and the information system are owned by the users. If the users feel no ownership of the system, they may not accept the system or use it appropriately, nor will they provide feedback regarding potential system improvements.

MAINTENANCE

After implementation of the system, ongoing maintenance must be provided.

User Feedback and Support

One important aspect of maintenance is communication. Soon after the go-live event, feedback from the implementation evaluation should be acted on in a timely manner. This is usually the first aspect of system maintenance to be addressed. The results should be compiled, analyzed, and communicated to the users and information services staff. Any suggested changes that are appropriate may then be implemented.

Continued communication is imperative for sharing information and informing users of changes. Communication can be accomplished in a variety of ways. For example, a newsletter or printed announcement can be sent to the users, on either a regular or an as-needed basis. System messages can be displayed on the screen or printed at the user location. Focus groups or in-house user groups can be formed for discussion and problem solving.

Another form of user support is the help desk. The **help desk** provides round-the-clock support that is usually available by telephone. Most organizations designate one telephone number as the access point for all users who need help or support related to information systems. The help desk is usually staffed by personnel from the information systems area who have had special training and are familiar with all of the systems in use. Often they are able to help the user during the initial telephone call. If this is not possible, the help desk may refer more complex problems or questions to other staff who have specialized knowledge. The help desk should follow up with the user and provide information as soon as it is available. The biggest problems during go-live occur with sign-on and passwords. Users may have missed training or may not remember how to sign on to the system.

Visibility of the support staff in the user areas is another important form of support. By making regular visits to all areas, the support staff is able to gather information related to how the system is performing and impacting the work of the users. In addition, users have the opportunity to ask questions and describe problems without having to call the help desk.

System Maintenance

Ongoing system maintenance must be provided in all three environments: test, training, and production. This enables programming and development to continue in the test region without adverse effect on the training or production systems. Therefore, training can continue without interruption and the training environment can be upgraded to reflect programming changes at the appropriate time. Actual client data and workflow will not be affected in the production system until the scheduled upgrade has been thoroughly tested in the test environment.

Requests submitted by users can provide input for upgrading or making necessary changes to the system. For example, a user might request changes to standard physician orders, such as a request to delete some lab tests to contain costs, or nursing documentation related to regulatory issues or Joint Commission on Accreditation of Healthcare Organizations (JCAHO) recommendations, such as adding advanced directives documentation. Advanced directives are used to convey whether the client wishes to be intubated, ventilated, or receive CPR or other lifesaving or life-sustaining measures in the event of a medical emergency. The requesters must provide a thorough explanation of the desired changes, as well as the reason for the request. One method of facilitating this communication is to develop a request form, to be completed by the requesting users and submitted to the information services department. On receiving this form, the information services staff should determine if the change is feasible and should consider whether any alternative solutions exist. Figure 8–2 provides an example of a request for services form.

INFORMATION SERVICES REQUEST FOR SERVICES

Requested by: _____ Date: _____

Department: _____

Department Head (print) _____ Telephone #: _____

Department Head (signature) _____

Priority: ____Routine ____Urgent Date Request Needed: _____

Requirement: _____

_____

_____

_____

_____

Reason for Request: _____Cost Reduction   ____ Service Improvement

____ Client Care Improvement   ____ Organizational Requirement

____ Regulatory Requirement   ____ Other (explain)_____

Please provide other supporting details related to the reason for the request:

FIGURE 8–2 • Request for information services form

Technical Maintenance

A large portion of ongoing maintenance is related to technical and equipment issues. This maintenance is the responsibility of the information services department. Some examples of technical maintenance include:

- Performing problem solving and debugging
- Maintaining a backup supply of hardware such as monitors, printers, cables, trackballs, and mice for replacement of faulty equipment in user areas
- Performing file backup procedures
- Monitoring the system for adequate file space
- Building and maintaining interfaces with other systems
- Configuring, testing, and installing system upgrades
- Maintaining and updating the disaster recovery plan

The Information System's Life Cycle

As users and technical support staff work with the system, they may come to identify problems and deficiencies. Eventually, these faults may become significant enough that the need to upgrade or replace the system becomes evident, illustrating the cyclical nature of the information system's life cycle. Phase 1, the needs assessment phase, is initiated again, and the life cycle continues. In other words, the life cycle is an ongoing process that never ends.

CASE STUDY EXERCISES

You are the project director responsible for creating an implementation timeline that addresses the training and go-live activities for a nursing documentation system that will be implemented on 20 units and involves 350 users. Determine whether the implementation will be staggered or occur simultaneously on all units, and provide your rationale.

• • •

Create the timeline for the training and go-live schedule for this implementation.

• • •

Your present manual medication administration record is being replaced by an automated information system. Discuss the specifications you would recommend for reports that the system will generate to notify the nurse when medications are due. Determine how often the reports should print and what information they should contain.

• • •

You have been selected to develop test scripts for interface testing for a new patient care system. Develop a test script with multiple interfaces. Define the output that you should see for each system.

• • •

As the manager of the gastrointestinal laboratory in your facility, you are expanding the applications for your information system. At the present, it allows physicians to capture images and produce consults and referral letters in a timely fashion. You have been working with the vendor to expand its features to include capture of patient history. Consider the pros and cons of interchanging information collected by admitting nurses and physicians.

 EXPLOREMEDIALINK

Multiple choice questions, case studies, and other interactive resources for this chapter can be found on the Web site at *http://www.prenhall.com/hebda*. Click on "Chapter 8" to select the activities for this chapter.

SUMMARY

- One important aspect of system implementation is the development of an effective implementation committee comprising clinical and technical representatives.
- The first task for the committee is the development of a timeline for system implementation activities.
- The implementation strategy must be determined by the committee. This strategy may call for using the system as it is delivered by the vendor or significantly customizing the system to match the current work needs.
- Identified modifications are made to the software in the test environment, so that actual client data and workflow are not affected.
- The following hardware considerations must be addressed during the implementation phase: type of workstation device, hardware location, printer options, and network requirements.
- User procedures and documentation are developed during the implementation phase, and provide support to personnel during training and actual use of the system.
- Training is a key element for a successful system implementation.
- Careful consideration must be given to planning the go-live conversion activities to minimize disruptions to client care.
- The implementation committee must be aware of the common pitfalls and problems that may negatively affect the implementation process.

- Maintenance, an ongoing part of the implementation process, includes user support and system maintenance.
- The information systems life cycle is a continuous cyclical process.

REFERENCES

Fichter, D. (July/August 2003). Why Web projects fail. *Online, 27*(4), 43.

Gates, L. (2002). Extending the testing process. *Application Development Trends, 9*(10), 30–34.

Hewlett-Packard Company. (1990). *Choosing a clinical information system.* Andover, MA: Author.

Hudson, V. (2002). What's ahead for practice management vendors. *ADVANCE for Health Information Executives, 6*(8), p. 47–50.

Lasker, B. (2003). ROI × 45. *Health Management Technology, 24*(8), 42–43.

Lau, F., and Hebert, M. (2001). Experiences from health information system implementation projects reported in Canada between 1991 and 1997. *Journal of End User Computing, 13*(4), 17.

Martin, R. (2002). Choosing, implementing and evaluating a software solution. *ADVANCE for Health Information Executives, 6*(10), 51–68.

Meadows G. (2003). Implementing clinical IT in critical care: Keys to success. *Nursing Economics, 21*(2), 89–90, 93.

Miranda, D., Fields, W., and Lund, K. (2001). Lessons learned during 15 years of clinical information system experience. *Computers in Nursing, 19*(4), 147–151.

Mouton, A., and McNees, R. (July 2003). Does cabling need intelligent monitoring? *Communications News, 40*(7), 24.

Saba, V. K., and McCormick, K. A. (1996). *Essentials of computers for nurses.* New York: McGraw-Hill.

Schuerenberg, N. (2003). Going "live" in a hurry. *Health Data Management, 11*(2), 32–36.

Webopedia. (2003). Data dictionary. Available online at: http://www.webopedia.com/TERM/D/data_dictionary.html. Accessed October 11, 2003.

Information Systems Training

After completing this chapter, you should be able to:

- Outline how learning objectives are determined for each group of users.

- Identify human factors that may negatively affect training.

- Compare and contrast the merits of various teaching approaches for system training.

- Recognize factors that affect learning and retention.

- Cite advantages and disadvantages associated with hospital-based trainers, vendor-supplied trainers, and superusers.

- List content areas needed for all information system users.

- Describe methods to evaluate competence in system use.

- Review issues associated with training, including cost, staffing, computer requirements, confidentiality, realism, and teaching students.

 MEDIALINK

Additional resources for this content can be found on the Companion Website at *www. prenhall.com/hebda*. Click on "Chapter 9" to select the activities for this chapter.

Companion Website
- Glossary
- Multiple Choice
- Discussion Points
- Case Study: Ethical Computing
- Case Study: Client Confidentiality
- Case Study: Training Plan
- MediaLink Application: HIPPA eCollege
- Web Hunt: HIPAA's Impact on Health Care Systems
- Links to Resources
- Crossword Puzzle

A s information systems (IS) become more prevalent in health care settings, nurses, allied health care professionals, and support staff are forced to master computer skills as a tool for the delivery and documentation of care. Some welcome the change, whereas others fear or resent what they perceive as the forced use of computers and possible job loss following the introduction of more technology. Computer skills are acquired through study and practice. Education is key to the successful use of any information system. Effective instruction may be costly and time consuming, but the end result is greater efficiency in information handling, increased marketability of job skills, and improved quality of care. The organized approach to providing large numbers of hospital staff and health care students with the skills needed to use information systems is commonly called **training.** Some educators dislike this term because of its association with behavioral psychology, which focuses on changing the way that an animal or a person acts by rewarding desired behavior or punishing undesirable behavior. This contrasts with cognitive psychology, which concentrates on restructuring the way that a person thinks through learning to change behavior.

Instructional success may be ensured through the development and implementation of a **training plan** that addresses the following areas:

- *A training philosophy.* Training is most effective when instruction occurs at a dedicated time independent of other work responsibilities and in an environment free from interruption.

- *Identification of training needs.* Before the initiation of training, it is necessary to determine who needs to be trained, what needs to be taught, the amount of instruction needed to master the prescribed tasks, what equipment is required, and when and where training will occur.

- *Training approaches.* Instructional decisions include whether to develop or purchase class materials and how the course will be taught: for example, instructor-led discussion, self-paced modules, technology delivered training, or on-the-job training.

- *Identification of the group or persons who will coordinate or conduct training of hospital staff.* Administration may opt to use outside trainers or their own employees.

- *A timetable.* Those who draft the schedule must consider the number of users who need training before the planned date for system implementation, time required to complete training, and how soon trainees' new knowledge can be applied.

- *The budget.* Because it is time- and labor-intensive, training should be considered an investment in successful information system implementation that requires wise allocation of resources.

- *Evaluation strategies.* The ultimate success of training is measured by the ability of individuals to perform expected computer tasks. Tests and class evaluation comments may also be used. Technology delivered learning often provides a mechanism for evaluation (Newbold 1996).

A well-conceived and carefully executed training plan provides a comprehensive approach that ensures proper system use. The training plan should be in alignment with the strategic objectives of the organization (Boisvert 2000).

IDENTIFICATION OF TRAINING NEEDS

Preparation begins with identifying user needs, followed by determining training class content, class schedules, hardware and software requirements, training costs, a location for training activity, approaches used in training, and evaluation strategies.

User Needs

Needs cannot be determined until the users have been identified. This is done through administrative decisions and analysis of job responsibilities. For example, administrators decide what functions will be automated first. These may include admission/discharge/transfer activities, physician order entry, and clinical documentation. Users are the persons who perform or document automated functions or who need to access automated information. See Box 9–1 for a list of personnel who may need information system training.

Despite the fact that different types of personnel often perform some of the same functions, individual job responsibilities differ, as do laws governing professional practice. Representatives from clinical areas can help identify user classes based on job descriptions. A **user class** is a level of personnel who perform similar functions. Not all user classes perform all information system functions, nor do they need training to use all system functions. For example, licensed practical nurses (LPNs) comprise a user class. LPNs need to see and document client information, but they do not perform order entry. Registered nurses (RNs) have a larger scope of practice and a separate user class. Higher-level user classes may include functions assigned to lower classes. This allows RNs to perform functions assigned to support personnel when these personnel are unavailable.

Supplemental staff and students who rotate through institutions with information systems are also potential users. The level of automation in a given setting determines whether these groups require computer training. For example, if order entry is the only automated function, then neither students nor supplemental staff may require training. When system access is required for the retrieval of data or documentation, training is necessary

---

Box 9–1   **Who Might Need Training?**

Clinicians

- Physicians
- Dentists
- Registered nurses
- Licensed practical nurses
- Nurse practitioners
- Physician assistants
- Pharmacists
- Nutritionists
- Respiratory therapists
- Occupational therapists
- Speech therapists
- Physical therapists
- X-ray technicians
- Patient care and medical assistants

Students

- Students from all professional and technical health care programs

Support Personnel

- Admission clerks
- Dietary personnel
- Social service staff
- Home health care personnel
- Pastoral care staff
- Housekeeping personnel
- Central supply staff
- Case managers
- Infection control and quality assurance personnel
- Third-party payor certification and verification staff

---

for supplemental staff to perform their jobs and for students to acquire educational information.

Learning objectives should be based on expected user functions. An example is the trainee who must document vital signs. This trainee must learn how to access the system, record vital signs, process the vital signs, and later retrieve them for review.

Training Class Content

Once the identification of users and functions slated for automation is complete, class content and learning objectives can be determined. Training classes should address the following areas:

- *Computer-related policies.* Training is an excellent time to discuss client confidentiality, ethical computing, and sanctions for inappropriate system access. On completion of training, most institutions require employees to sign a document stating that system misuse may result in termination of employment. It is at this time that employees receive their access code. The **access code** is some form of unique identification and provides authentication of the user's identity. This can be accomplished with the user's sign-on name and a password, or with a more sophisticated form of identification such as a fingerprint on a biometric mouse. Nonemployees, such as students, may be required to sign a document stating that misused information services privileges may result in loss of clinical privileges and possible legal action. An example of misuse might include failure to properly handle and dispose of confidential computer printouts.

- *Human factors.* The implementation of an information system may present a major change in the work setting, particularly if there is minimal existing automation. Some people are uncomfortable with change and computers, and they fear job loss if they cannot adapt. These fears should be addressed at the start of training to put users at ease. A review of how automation may benefit employees provides incentive to learn.

- *Basic computer literacy.* Some people lack fundamental computer skills and knowledge. An introduction to the primary parts and function of computers lays a foundation for system training.

- *Workflow.* Automation of manual processes changes the way that work is done. Classes must outline the new process in detail to help users understand how the system works and to make the transition to information systems.

- *The steps to perform specific functions.* For example, the demonstration of order entry must show all steps required to allow trainees to enter orders.

- *Help screens and online tutorials.* Help screens and online tutorials are beneficial to users, provided that users are aware of their existence and can use them. **Help screens** list specific actions to complete a particular task. **Online tutorials** provide step-by-step instructions for how to use the software or one of its features. Online tutorials are available on the computer for referral at any time. Training classes should introduce these features and demonstrate their access and use.

- *Error messages.* **Error messages** are text communications produced by the computer to warn the user that information is missing or improperly constructed. Error messages provide an opportunity to supply missing information or to supply it in a format recognized by the information system. For example, a medication order must identify drug, dosage, route, and schedule. Failure to list any of these generates an error message. Class content should address how error messages are produced, avoided, and corrected.

- *Error correction.* Input errors result from typographical or spelling problems or incorrect choices. Errors may be corrected at the time of entry or at a later date. For example, some clinical documentation systems provide an opportunity to review and correct information before processing. Corrections are noted as made after data entry. Original entries remain as part of the record.

- *What to do when the system "freezes."* **Freezing** refers to a situation when the computer will no longer accept input or process what has been entered. Users need to know how the system should work and what to do in the event of malfunction, whether that involves referral to troubleshooting guidelines or a call to the information system help desk.

- *System idiosyncrasies.* What information systems can and cannot do is a function of programming and technical limitations. Computer programs often work differently than clinicians who perform a task manually. Major programming changes to accommodate clinicians are not always possible. For this reason, health care workers need to understand the limitations of their information system.

- *Basic equipment care and troubleshooting.* Some problems are as simple as a loose cable or cord, or an empty paper tray or toner cartridge. In other cases, lost icons, changes made to computer settings such as mouse speed or screen colors, or failure to properly log off of the system can cause difficulties. Users must learn how to deal with these problems or know who to contact for help.

- *Backup.* **Backup procedures** are alternative ways to accomplish functions normally done via the information system during downtime—times when the system is not operational or available for use. Downtime may be scheduled to perform tasks on a nightly basis or for system updates. Unscheduled downtime occurs as a result of problems. Backup procedures may not be implemented unless downtime is lengthy. Manual requisitions and paper reports of laboratory results exemplify backup procedures. Backup procedures should be introduced during training and reviewed annually or when a lengthy downtime is planned.

- *Alternative means to achieve a task.* It is often possible to accomplish a function in more than one way. Table 9–1 displays sample screen options that permit review of a client's laboratory results using any one of a variety of menu selections.

Class Schedules

Planning and scheduling class times can be challenging. Learner availability, needs, and attentiveness must be considered. Sessions of 1, 2, or 4 hours look good on paper, but it is difficult for employees to leave the clinical units and then they may feel rushed to return. It is also difficult for staff to arrive on time for sessions scheduled at the end of their shifts. Another problem occurs when workers are too tired or tense to benefit from instruction. For these reasons, dedicated training days often work best.

Class schedules must consider the available training days and the number of personnel who need instruction prior to go-live. When large numbers of people must be taught in a short period, around-the-clock training may be used. Extended class hours provide classes at times when off-shift employees are most attentive. Extra instructors may be needed to cover the additional

Table 9–1	Sample Screen Options for Reviewing Lab Results
Screen Option	**Information Retrieved**
For the most recent tests	Provides results of the most recently completed tests
For today	Lists all laboratory findings for the current date
For the previous 2 days	Shows laboratory findings from the previous 2 days
From the time of admission	Displays all laboratory findings from admission to the present time, in either chronological or reverse chronological order
From previous admissions	Lists laboratory findings by dates of previous admissions
By department, e.g., chemistry, hematology, or microbiology	Allows practitioners to quickly find a particular result, such as a wound culture

hours. Preparation time for each class must be factored into the schedule as well. Training should also occur as close to scheduled system implementation time as possible to facilitate recall and application of new knowledge. Computer instruction is most effective when provided no more than one month before the actual anticipated use in the work setting (Craig 2002).

Hardware and Software Requirements

The best way to learn how to use an information system is to train under conditions similar to working conditions. For example, learners should have the same equipment that is found in the clinical setting with a computer for their exclusive use. One workstation per individual ensures adequate practice opportunities for each person. Operation of printers and Fax machines must be included in class content when these are an integral part of unit function. No training should occur on the actual system to protect client data from inadvertent view, change, or deletion. Client data are sometimes referred to as **live data**. For this reason, many hospital information system vendors offer the capacity to support separate databases for training and for actual system use. This feature allows learners to experience how the software works with simulated client information without jeopardizing confidentiality or interfering with treatment. Different sets of simulated data may be reserved for specific user groups or functions.

Training Costs

Training is expensive primarily because of the personnel hours required to develop, present, receive, and support educational activities (Filipczak 1996). For this reason, salary costs for the following staff must be considered:

- *Trainers.* Trainers spend many hours reviewing and developing materials for the class in addition to the time spent in instruction.

- *Employees undergoing training.* Compensation for time spent in training may be at the regular hourly rate or as overtime compensation if it is scheduled in addition to 40-hour work weeks.
- *Replacement staff.* Clinical units must be staffed while regular employees undergo training.
- *Support staff.* These employees perform jobs such as typing, copying, and collating instructional materials; preparing class audiovisuals; taking reservations for classes; and documenting attendance.

Even when vendors supply training materials, time must be spent to review the suitability of these materials before use. Other expenses are the purchase of hardware and software, and the preparation of a training area. Effective training limits instruction to personnel who need system access and to the functions they need to know.

Training Center

Because client care is the top priority, no instruction should occur on the clinical units. The only permissible exceptions occur when in-services of 15 minutes or less are needed to address system updates. A dedicated training environment allows staff to focus on learning the system. A hospital site is convenient because employees are already there, travel time between clinical units and the center is nominal, and parking arrangements already exist. Unfortunately, space may not be available. Convenience of location, travel time, and parking or shuttle service are considerations with off-site facilities. Box 9–2 lists some factors to consider when selecting a training site.

No matter what site is selected, the training environment should facilitate learning through good lighting, a comfortable temperature, and good ergonomics. Chair and equipment position should minimize fatigue and repetitive stress injuries. Instructors must make an effort to create a comfortable atmosphere with frequent breaks and variations in teaching methods as a means to maintain student interest.

The training site may later serve a dual purpose because designated terminals or computers can be set up for either training or live system modes. This flexibility permits review of live data from the training area for a variety of purposes such as case management. Trainees cannot access the live system without their own unique access codes. This ability to set computers for either the training or live modes may also be used to provide additional practice opportunities for staff on the units as time permits.

Training Approaches

The overall training approach should be consistent with the institution's philosophy and reflect the fact that individuals learn at their own rate and in their own way (Abla 1995; Fender and Jennerich 1997; Glydura, Michelman, and Wilson 1995). A combination of instructional approaches improves overall retention for individuals with different learning styles. This strategy

Box 9–2   **Selecting a Training Site: Factors to Consider**

- *Space availability/cost.* Hospital space is usually limited.

- *Cabling and power supply.* Adding computer cables and power lines to an existing building is costly and may disrupt services, making an alternative site attractive.

- *Size demands.* All trainees should have their own computer or terminal to enable them to learn skills at their own pace.

- *Travel and parking.* Trainees do not want to worry about parking or travel time from the hospital to the training center.

- *Ready access versus no distractions.* On-site training eliminates travel between the hospital and an outside facility (although employees may be contacted from the unit).

- *Separation of training data and live data.* A separate training facility eliminates the chance of mixing these two types of data.

- *Setup costs.* Setup costs include cabling and wiring at any location. Off-site facilities may also require construction.

- *Maintenance costs.* Maintenance costs are determined by the decision to buy, remodel, build, or lease space.

---

recognizes individual needs and values and attempts to provide something for everybody. An example of a combination training approach may be seen with the instructor who uses a data projector to display the terminal to the class and provides written materials such as manuals, printouts of sample screens, exercises, self-tests, and a training hospital. The **training hospital** is a collection of simulated client data assembled and stored for instructional purposes in a database separate from live client data. The training hospital offers all the automated functions found in the actual system but with no access to live client information. This use of multiple media in conjunction with hands-on practice enhances learning over any single approach. See Box 9–3 for factors to consider when choosing training methods.

Many options exist for training: traditional classroom instruction, computer-based training, online multimedia, online tutorials, on-the-job training, peer training, video, job aids, and self-directed text-based courses (Filipczak 1996; Mascara, Bartos, Nelson, and Rafferty 1994). Table 9–2 outlines advantages, disadvantages, and organizational tips for each instructional approach. Although traditional classroom training is heavily used, it is resource intensive (Zielstorff 1996). For this reason the popularity of alternative approaches, such as Web-based instruction, is growing. One popular form of Web-based instruction is the **Webcast**. This format allows multiple learners to access a Web site, typically an intranet site, to attend a scheduled class. The learners are able to view a presentation online and hear the instructor speak. Webcasts generally provide some means for interaction, including questions and answers. A combination of self-paced

---

Box 9–3   **Selecting a Training Method: Factors to Consider**

- *Time.* Instructional approaches vary in the time required for development and presentation. For example, lectures can be written and revised quickly and provide content to large numbers of people at one time.

- *Cost.* Training methods vary in the number of personnel hours and money required for development and revision.

- *Learning styles.* People learn differently. For example, some people prefer to hear material, while others are visual learners. A combination of instructional methods aids overall learning.

- *Learning retention.* Repetition and the ability to apply learning via practice opportunities and application in the work setting help people to remember content.

---

and instructor-led approaches provides variety and offers the advantages associated with both methods. Case studies also help learners to work through ethical issues and apply new knowledge.

Training Materials Well-designed instructional materials are critical to successful information system training (Abla 1995; Filipczak 1996; Henry and Swartz 1995). **Learning aids** are materials intended to supplement or reinforce lecture- or computer-based training. Learning aids may include outlines, diagrams, charts, or conceptual maps. **Job aids** are written instructions designed for reference use in both the training and work settings. When vendor-supplied materials are available, they must be evaluated for quality of documentation and consistency with the current system. Vendor-prepared manuals do not usually reflect customization efforts. No training materials should be developed until system development is complete and the system works properly. User class representatives should review handouts and training materials for quality, clarity, and content before widespread training to guarantee that materials are accurate and easily understood.

Proficiency Testing

Proficiency tests are routinely included in IS training as a means to ensure that learners can perform required functions. Any instructional approach can accommodate proficiency testing (Sittig et al. 1995). Examinations may be criterion or norm referenced. Criterion-referenced measures evaluate predetermined competencies, whereas norm-referenced tools assess performance relative to other persons. Norm-referenced testing is useful in competitive hiring situations where there are more applicants than positions available. However, this type of testing is not typically used with IS training. The tasks of administering, scoring, and storage and retrieval of individual examination scores are facilitated by technology delivered learning (Vaillancourt 2000).

Table 9–2

Advantages, Disadvantages, and Tips Associated with Various Training Approaches

Training Approach	Advantages	Disadvantages	Tips for Effective Organizational Use
Instructor-led class	Flexible Easily updated Can include demonstrations Allows for individual help Can test proficiency	Often relies on lecture ↑ Class size ↓ demonstration effectiveness Consistency varies with trainer Difficult to maintain pace good for all	For each user group: • Keep a file with objectives and exercises. • Use the same presentation order. • Use generic examples unlikely to change over time. Never rely on just one trainer—leaves no paper trail for others to follow
Computer-based training (CBT)	Self-paced Interactive ↑ Retention— uses technology to teach technology 24-Hour availability Can be offered online or offline Can be done in increments Facilitates mastery learning Emulates "real" system without threat of harm	Time and labor intensive to develop and revise Requires great attention to accompanying materials Limited usefulness of vendor supplied materials without customization	Trainer serves as a facilitator Needs specific, well-prepared learning aids
Online multimedia	Interactive Stimulates multiple senses for ↑ retention Can test proficiency	Requires intense planning, resources for design, and revision Less flexible to revise	Use and revise carefully
Online tutorials	24-Hour availability Allows immediate application of learning Can test proficiency	Design and revision more involved than instructor-led training	Must have access from all locations and availability must be known
E-mail	Provides individual feedback on entry errors	All users must have e-mail Too slow for actual training	Must know how to use e-mail and have access
Video	24-Hour availability Easily revised/updated Extends resources	Not interactive Use for select content such as ethical dilemmas—not actual training	Use carefully

(continued)

Table 9–2 Advantages, Disadvantages, and Tips Associated with Various Training Approaches—*continued*

Training Approach	Advantages	Disadvantages	Tips for Effective Organizational Use
Web-based	Can be accessed from any networked PC Provides 24-hour availability Easily updated and revised	Requires knowledgeable Webmaster Requires an existing intranet that can be accessed by all employees	Include online learner assessment
On-the-job training	Individualized Permits immediate application Can test proficiency	Trainer often does not know educational principles May lose productivity of two workers Seasoned employees may pass on poor habits Difficult to achieve with many interruptions	Trainer must know basic adult education principles May work well for unit clerks, working in pairs or to learn PC applications
Peer training	Training specific to function Can test proficiency	Trainer often does not know educational principles Seasoned employees may pass on poor habits	Trainer must know basic adult education principles May work well for unit clerks, working in pairs or to learn PC applications
Superuser	Acquainted with clinical area and the information system May come from any user class Serves as communication link between user class and IS constraints	Spends time away from clinical responsibilities for additional information system training and meetings	May serve as resource persons particularly during off-shifts May assist with training other users
Job aids	↓ Need to memorize ↓ Training time ↓ Help requests	Not effective if access is limited	Requires careful planning and structure Make accessible and user friendly
Self-directed text-based courses	Self-paced Can test proficiency Lacks interaction with training hospital/system	Requires high level of motivation	Need highly structured materials

Source: Adapted with permission from Bush, A.M.P. (1993). Computer-based training: Training approach of choice. *Computers in Nursing, 11*(4), 163–164; Sittig et al. (1995). Evaluating a computer-based experiential learning simulation: A case study using criterion-referenced testing. *Computers in Nursing 13*(1), 17–24; the May 1996 issue of *Training Magazine.* Copyright © 1996. Lakewood Publications, Minneapolis, MN. All rights reserved; and Garcia (2002). Squeezing the most from your training dollars. *ADVANCE* for Health Information Executives, *6*(8), 55–56.

Box 9–4 Selecting a Trainer: Factors to Consider

- *Teaching skills and experience.* Previous experience is helpful.
- *Ability to work well with groups.* Interaction with a group differs from one-on-one communication. Most training occurs in a group setting, so this ability is an asset for system trainers.
- *Understanding user groups and their responsibilities.* Trainers may not represent every user group, but they must understand what every group does and the information they need to know to perform their jobs.
- *Training approach.* Trainers should be comfortable with the chosen approach. For example, if computer-based training is used, instructors must be acquainted with its features and help learners through it as needed.
- *Centralized versus departmental training.* Centralized hospital training presents general principles, while departmental training provides specific information related to individual responsibilities in a given area.

IS Trainers Hospital administrators decide who will conduct system training, based on cost factors and feedback from the IS department and representatives from the system selection committee. Instruction may be done by vendor-supplied personnel, consultants, or hospital employees. There are pros and cons for each approach. Vendor-supplied personnel and consultants typically know the information system well but lack knowledge of the institution's culture and procedures. Vendor-supplied trainers leave after the initial training is complete, forcing the hospital to find another means to train new employees as they are hired. Box 9–4 lists some factors to consider when selecting trainers.

Often, hospitals develop and use a core set of instructors from their own personnel ranks. These individuals receive their initial system training from the vendor and then teach staff to use the system. They often come from the following groups:

- *Hospital-wide or staff development educators.* Educators know the basic principles of adult education but may lack familiarity with specific day-to-day unit routines.
- *Clinicians.* Clinicians have expertise in their practice areas.
- *Department supervisors.* These individuals know their areas well but may not be able to leave their other responsibilities.
- *Information services personnel.* These individuals understand how the system works but lack a clinical perspective and may be unfamiliar with instructional theory.

A dedicated core of trainers helps to provide consistent instruction. Training does not end after initial system implementation; it continues as new employees are hired and additional functions are automated over the passage of time.

Superuser Another resource person is the **superuser**, a staff person who has become proficient in the use of the system and mentors others. Superusers may come from any of the user classes. Their specialized knowledge of both the system and clinical areas enables superusers to assist with training or help staff on other units. Superusers may be available on all shifts and can answer questions when IS staff are not available.

ADDITIONAL TRAINING CONSIDERATIONS

There are several issues related to training that should be addressed in every setting. These include but are not limited to the following:

- *Responsibility for training costs.* Institutions handle training costs differently. Some hospitals may charge each department a fee for training their personnel.
- *Responsibility for trainers.* Trainers frequently come from several departments. This may create confusion as to who their supervisors are or the length of their assignments. They may be temporarily assigned to the IS department.
- *Realistic training.* To be effective, training should incorporate examples seen in day-to-day practice.
- *Confidentiality.* Occasionally, simulated clients resemble actual cases or use celebrity names. This may raise concerns over confidentiality.
- *System updates.* All employees must be inserviced as additional functions are added, such as documentation of medication administration, nursing care plans, or critical pathway management. Any regulatory changes related to the use of automated patient information must also be reviewed.
- *The employee who fails to demonstrate system competence.* These situations should be handled individually. Learning time varies, and some people do not value the acquisition of computer skills. Inability to develop in this area may result in job loss.
- *Training personnel from other institutions.* As more hospitals merge, IS trainers must also teach staff from other hospitals that are at different stages of implementation.
- *Training students.* Responsibility for training and quality of clinical experiences are concerns.

Training Students

Training for students must be reevaluated periodically to keep abreast of needs and to ensure currency of information (Mascara et al. 1994). Students must be able to assess their clients and to review test results, document findings, and care on automated systems. Consideration must be given to the best ways to educate students because it is a costly undertaking in terms of time and resources. In fact, individual institutions derive few direct gains from training students unless the students seek employment within the enterprise after graduation. One IS strategy to minimize training efforts may be seen with the use of existing user classes for student use. This eliminates the need to create additional user classes and instructional materials. An example of this tactic is seen with the application of the vocational nurse user class for student professional nurses. Both of these populations demand access to client information and the ability to document assessment and care, but neither group requires order entry. Nursing assistant user functions may work well for medical assistant students.

Other options include making computer-based training available at affiliating schools or using faculty to instruct students on system use. IS training may also be incorporated into an elective course, enhancing marketability of graduates and possibly shortening their orientation period. The least satisfactory approach occurs when students receive no training or access, and faculty must enter all documentation for their students.

CASE STUDY EXERCISES

Kevin Gallagher, RN, has access to all client records on his medical-surgical unit. Consider each of the following situations:

- Kevin's mother is admitted to the unit. Is it appropriate for him to view his mother's electronic medical record? Why or why not?
- Kevin's unit clerk also has access to Mrs. Gallagher's record. Is it appropriate for her to view Mrs. Gallagher's record? Why or why not?
- Kevin's co-worker, Kaneesha, is a client on the unit assigned to another staff nurse's care. Is it appropriate for Kevin to review her chart or laboratory results? Why or why not?

• • •

Nancy Whitehorse, RN, routinely accesses client records on her medical unit. Does she violate her confidentiality statement if she performs the following actions?

1. She reviews the information and does not discuss it with anyone else.
2. She discusses information obtained from client records with other health care workers on the unit.
3. She discusses clinical cases, omitting names, in social situations.

• • •

Grace Elizaga has been given the charge of training the RNs and unit clerks from the first three client care units slated to start automated order entry at Potter's Medical Center (PMC). The target implementation date is in 2 months. A total of 93 RNs and 11 unit clerks must receive training before that time. Based on information from other agencies that have the same information system as PMC, 8 hours of training time is projected for each individual. As the nurse manager responsible for those units, you have been asked to work with Grace to develop a detailed plan to accomplish this task and submit this plan to your vice presidents of Client Care Services. Include the following in your plan and provide your rationale:

- Staffing
- Costs for your personnel
- Training start and completion dates
- Length and number of training sessions

 EXPLOREMEDIALINK

Multiple choice questions, case studies, and other interactive resources for this chapter can be found on the Web site at *http://www.prenhall.com/hebda*. Click on "Chapter 9" to select the activities for this chapter.

SUMMARY

- Education is a key factor in the proper use of an information system. Education should be guided by a teaching plan that identifies user needs and includes a teaching philosophy, desired types of educators, and a timetable for training.
- Before user needs can be identified, it is necessary to identify the users. For IS purposes, personnel levels are grouped into user classes by job description. Each class performs similar functions. For example, RNs, LPNs, physicians, and unit clerks each comprise separate user classes with different access privileges needed to do their work.
- IS training may be negatively affected by discomfort with change or computers, the training environment, the class schedule, or instructional approach.
- The need for training must be evaluated for all potential IS users, not just staff. This group may include supplemental staff and students.
- No training should occur on client units or with live client information except for short updates. This protects the integrity of live

information and provides an environment where learners can focus their attention on learning how to use the system.

- Training is a costly endeavor because it is labor and time intensive.

- IS training may be supplied by vendors or consultants or drawn from any one of the following personnel groups: hospital educators, clinicians, or IS staff.

- Superusers are personnel with additional IS training or an above-average mastery of the system or both. They serve as resource persons in their departments, answering questions and helping others to work through IS problems. Superusers may come from any user class.

- Criterion-based competence tests may be included as part of training as a means to ensure that all learners demonstrate expected computer skills.

- Some training issues include updates regarding regulatory changes, determining responsibility for costs, staffing, trainer selection and chain of command, realism in training, confidentiality, how to handle system updates, what to do with the employee who fails to develop computer skills, and how to best meet the training needs of students.

REFERENCES

Abla, S. (1995). The who, what, where, when, and how of computer education. *Computers in Nursing, 13*(3), 114–117.

Boisvert, L. (2000). Web-based learning. *Information Systems Management, 17*(1), 35–36.

Bush, A. M. P. (1993). Computer-based training: Training approach of choice. *Computers in Nursing, 11*(4), 163–164.

Craig, J. (2002). The life cycle of a health care information system. In S. Englebardt and R. Nelson (Eds.), *Health care informatics* (pp. 181–208). St. Louis, MO: Mosby.

Fender, M., and Jennerich, B. (1997). The real key to success with new technology: Understanding people. *Enterprise Systems Journal, 12*(4), 38, 40, 42, 44, 46.

Filipczak, B. (1996). Training on the cheap. *Training, 33*(5), 28–34.

Garcia, L. (2002). Squeezing the most from your training dollars. *ADVANCE for Health Information Executives 6*(8), 55–56.

Glydura, A. J., Michelman, J. E., and Wilson, C. N. (1995). Multimedia training in nursing education. *Computers in Nursing, 13*(4), 169–175.

Henry, S. A., and Swartz, R. G. (1995). Enhancing healthcare education with accelerated learning techniques. *Journal of Nursing Staff Development, 11*(1), 21–24.

Mascara, C. M., Bartos., C. E., Nelson, R., and Rafferty, D. (1994). An effective approach for providing nursing students with HIS access. In S. J. Grobe and E. S. P. Pluyter-Wenting (Eds.), *Nursing informatics: An international overview for nursing in a technological era* (pp. 563–566).

The proceedings of the Fifth IMIA International Conference on Nursing Use of Computers and Information Science. New York: Elsevier Science.

Newbold, S. K. (1996). Maximizing technology for cost-effective staff education and training. In M. C. Mills, C. A. Romano, and B. R. Heller (Eds.), *Information management in nursing and health care* (pp. 216–221). Springhouse, PA: Springhouse Corporation.

Sittig, D. F., Jiang, Z., Manfre, S., Sinkfeld, K., Ginn, R., Smith, L., Olsen, A., and Borden, R. (1995). Evaluating a computer-based experiential learning simulation: A case study using criterion-referenced testing. *Computers in Nursing, 13*(1), 17–24.

Vaillancourt, S. (May 4, 2000). *Technology delivered learning.* Presented at Tri-State Nursing Computer Network, Pittsburgh, PA.

Zielstorff, R. (1996). Training issues in system implementation. In M. C. Mills, C. A. Romano, and B. R. Heller (Eds.), *Information management in nursing and health care* (pp. 128–138). Springhouse, PA: Springhouse Corporation.

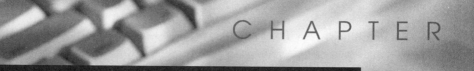

10

Information Security and Confidentiality

After completing this chapter, you should be able to:

- Differentiate between privacy, confidentiality, information privacy, and information security.
- Discuss how information systems affect privacy, confidentiality, and security.
- Relate the significance of security for information integrity.
- Review several security measures designed to protect information and discuss how they work.
- Distinguish between appropriate and inappropriate password selection and handling.

- State examples of confidential forms and communication that are commonly seen in health care settings and identify proper disposal techniques for each.
- Discuss the impact that Internet technology has on health information security.
- Discuss the implications of the HIPAA privacy and security rules for the protection of information security.

 MEDIALINK

Additional resources for this content can be found on the Companion Website at *www.prenhall.com/hebda*. Click on "Chapter 10" to select the activities for this chapter.

Companion Website

- Glossary
- Multiple Choice
- Discussion Points
- Case Study: Acceptable Computer Uses
- Case Study: Personnel Issues
- Case Study: Passwords
- Case Study: Computer Printouts
- Case Study: Handling Confidential Information
- MediaLink Application: "What is HIPAA"
- Links to Resources
- Crossword Puzzle

The recent implementation of Health Insurance Portability and Accountability Act (HIPAA) regulations heightened awareness about information security and privacy practices (Joachim 2003). Health care information systems must provide rapid access to accurate and complete client information to legitimate users, while safeguarding client privacy and confidentiality. Electronic records facilitate efficient and effective sharing of information, but the ease with which they can be accessed creates concerns over confidentiality. At the same time, health care administrators must demonstrate measures that protect information to comply with HIPAA requirements and meet accreditation criteria set forth by the Joint Commission on Accreditation of Healthcare Organizations (JCAHO). These criteria continue to evolve. The HIPAA security rule does not specify the utilization of particular technologies; instead it calls for organizations to determine threats and appropriate protective measures for information in all formats (Gillespie 2003). Protection of client privacy and confidentiality requires an understanding of the concepts of privacy, confidentiality, information privacy, and security as well as potential threats within an organization.

PRIVACY, CONFIDENTIALITY, AND SECURITY

While the terms *privacy* and *confidentiality* are often used interchangeably, they are not the same. **Privacy** is a state of mind, a specific place, freedom from intrusion, or control over the exposure of self or of personal information (Blair 2003; Kelly and McKenzie 2002; Kmentt 1987; Reagan 2003; Windslade 1982). Privacy includes the right to determine what information is collected, how it is used, and the ability to access collected information to review its security and accuracy. Anonymity may be requested by an individual because they hold public office or are a celebrity. HIPAA regulations now require that clients must be given clear written explanations of how facilities and providers may use and disclose their health information (Calloway and Venegas 2002). The movement to protect privacy is consistent with an international trend seen among industrialized nations (Australia's Privacy Legislation 2002).

Confidentiality refers to a situation in which a relationship has been established and private information is shared (Romano 1987). Confidentiality is essential for the accurate assessment, diagnosis, and treatment of health problems. Once a client discloses confidential information, control over its redisclosure lies with the persons who access it. Private information should only be shared with parties who require it for client treatment (Hill 2003). The ethical duty of confidentiality entails keeping information shared during the course of a professional relationship secure and secret from others. This involves making appropriate security arrangements for storage and transmission of private information, ensuring the equipment used for storage and transmission is secure and that measures are used to prevent the interception of e-mail, instant messages, Faxes, and other correspondence containing private information. Nurses are obligated by the American Nurses' Association Code of Ethics and state practice laws to protect patient privacy (Blair 2003). Inappropriate redisclosure can be extremely damaging. For example, insurance companies may deny coverage based on information revealed to them without the client's knowledge or consent. Inappropriate disclosure can also damage reputations and personal relationships or result in loss of employment. Most breaches of confidentiality occur as a result of carelessness and can be avoided by not discussing clients in public areas or with persons who do not have a "need-to-know," and through tight control of client records.

Information privacy is the right to choose the conditions and extent to which information and beliefs are shared (Murdock 1980). Informed consent for the release of specific information illustrates information privacy in practice. Information privacy includes the right to ensure accuracy of information collected by an organization (Murdock 1980). **Information security,** on the other hand, is the protection of information against threats to its integrity, inadvertent disclosure or availability (Griffiths 2003). Information systems can improve protection for client information in some ways and endanger it in others. Unlike the paper record that can be read by anyone, the automated record cannot easily be viewed without an access code. Poorly secured information systems threaten record confidentiality because they may be accessed from multiple sites with immediate dissemination of information. This makes clients highly vulnerable to the redisclosure of sensitive information. The HIPAA Privacy Rule focuses on the protection of the privacy of people who seek care (Blair 2003).

Consent is the process by which an individual authorizes health care personnel to process their information based on an informed understanding of how this information will be used (Kelly and McKenzie 2002). Obtaining consent should include making the individual aware of any risks that may exist to privacy as well as measures in place to protect privacy.

INFORMATION SYSTEM SECURITY

Information system security is the protection of both information housed on the system and the system itself from threats or disruption (BOMI 2001; Goedert 2002; Levy 2003; O'Daniel 2003). The primary goals of health care information system security are the protection of client confidentiality and information integrity. These goals are best met when security is planned rather than applied to an existing system after problems occur. Planning for security saves time and money and should be regarded as a form of insurance against downtime, breaches in confidentiality, losses in consumer confidence, cybercrime, liability, and lost productivity. Good security practices also help to ensure compliance with HIPAA legislation. Good security starts with a thorough assessment of assets and risks as well as necessary resources, a well-crafted security plan and policy, and a supportive organizational culture and structure. This requires administrative backing. In addition to being secure, the system must still be easily accessible for legitimate users.

Security Risks

Potential threats to information and system security come from a variety of sources (Grosh 2002; O'Daniel 2003; Reagan 2003). These can include thieves, hackers, crackers, denial of service attacks, terrorists, viruses, snatched Web sites, flooding sites with fictitious data, power fluctuations that damage systems or data, revenge attacks, fires and natural disasters, and human error. These threats may result in jammed networks, violations to confidentiality, identity theft, interruptions in information integrity, disruption in the delivery of services, monetary losses and violation of privacy regulations. Confidential client information may also be exposed through file sharing applications on employee work stations as well as unauthorized access via e-mail instant messaging, and Internet chat sites. Professionals may be hired to test the system for vulnerabilities.

System Penetration Even the best-secured systems can be penetrated (Forman 2003; Pierce 2003). The best that can be hoped for is that security strategies will minimize instances of system penetration and minimize damages. A recent survey (Tuesday 2003) found that retail, financial services, health care, and federal and local government were among the top industry sectors targeted by attackers. Significant financial losses occur annually as a result of compromised systems (Levy 2003). Barriers to effective security may include inadequate resources, money, time, and attention from management and the complexity of training as well as an increasing sophistication of users (Cyberattacks 2003).

Cybercrime is now a larger threat than physical security problems (Dearne 2002). **Cybercrime** commonly refers to the ability to steal personal information stored on computers such as Social Security numbers. Cyberattackers use widely available hacker tools to find network weaknesses and gain undetected access. Inconsistent and inadequate approaches to security risks allow entry. The main types of people who become involved in system penetration and computer crime include the following:

- *Opportunists.* Opportunists take advantage of the situation and their access to information for uses not associated with their jobs.
- *Hackers.* Hackers are individuals who have an average, or above average, knowledge of computer technology and who dislike rules and restrictions. Hackers penetrate systems as a challenge, and many do not regard their acts as criminal. Others, however, break into systems with the intent of obtaining information, creating mischief, destroying files, or making a profit. This group is sometimes referred to as *crackers* or *black hats.*

- *Computer or information specialists.* These individuals are knowledgeable about how computers work and are in the best position to commit computer crime and disable systems while avoiding detection.

Unauthorized Users Although the most common fear is that of system penetration from outsiders, the greatest threat actually comes from employees who view information inappropriately, disrupt information availability, or corrupt data integrity. Such access constitutes unauthorized use and may occur at any level within an organization. Consideration must be given to the access rights accorded to all employees, including system administrators.

Even though health care professionals have codes of ethics to maintain client confidentiality, not all professionals act ethically. This is the reason that system safeguards are needed as well. As health care alliances grow and client records become more accessible, the likelihood of unauthorized system access will increase. For the individual client, legal protection was limited in the United States until HIPAA compliance became mandatory. The Data Protection Act provides protection for confidentiality in the United Kingdom (Kelly and McKenzie 2002). Australia has taken action to protect health information as well. Consumer groups and health care professionals need to serve as advocates for health care consumers in the protection of privacy and confidentiality.

Concern for client confidentiality is not limited to the period of active treatment. Record access may occur later through loopholes that exist in automated systems (Hebda, Sakerka, and Czar 1994). These loopholes will be found by curious users and must be corrected as soon as information system (IS) personnel and administrators become aware of them. One example may be illustrated by the automated system that restricts access to client records during treatment but allows retrieval of any record or laboratory value after client discharge. Health care alliance physicians and office staff often need to see test results after the client's admission but should be able to view the results only for their clients. This type of problem represents an oversight in the design process that must be corrected. Commercial software vendors are now under greater pressure to improve the security of their products as customers use their purchasing power to exert demands (Fisher 2003). The U.S. government has started to stipulate security provisions that vendors must meet to win contracts with the government.

Sabotage The destruction of computer equipment or records or the disruption of normal system operation is known as **sabotage.** This may be a problem with IS staff, but the majority of health care users are not accorded system privileges that would permit this type of destruction. Employees who are satisfied and well informed and feel a vested interest in maintaining information and system security are less likely to wreak havoc on the system. A positive environment, a well-defined institutional ethics policy, and intact security mechanisms help to deter intentional information, or system, misuse or destruction. Consideration should be given to having background checks performed on employees who manage and maintain computer systems or are in a position to misuse information, as a means to avert this threat (Pounds 2002).

Errors and Disasters Errors may result from poor design or system changes that permit users more access than they require. This may be seen when information is restricted during the client's period of treatment but is available after discharge to any user. Errors may also arise from incorrect user entries such as inadvertent selection of the wrong client for data retrieval or documentation.

During disasters, manual backup procedures may compromise information because the primary focus is on maintaining services. One example of this is seen when paper reports of laboratory findings are not enclosed in envelopes for delivery to client care units.

Viruses, Worms, and Other Malicious Programs Viruses These are deliberately written programs that use a host computer to spread and reproduce themselves without the knowledge of the person(s) operating the computer. Viruses need normal computer operations to spread. Originally, viruses attached themselves to other computer programs. They may, or may not, damage data or disrupt system operation. Some viruses are likened to electronic graffiti in that the writer leaves his or her mark by displaying a message. Infected boot sectors of diskettes and e-mail attachments are the most common methods of infection. The boot sector of a diskette contains start-up instructions for computers. When the computer is booted, or started, from the infected diskette, the virus is spread to the computer, which then infects the hard drive and diskettes used in that machine. Another type of virus requires execution of the infected file for spread. Viruses may use a combination of these approaches and are frequently widespread at the time of detection.

Viral infection may be spread through the Internet; e-mail attachment files, shareware, and commercial software; and infected diskettes taken from one computer or network to another. The infectious period for viruses is contingent on its type. Infection may occur with each run of the infected program or during any time that the infected program is run, or the virus may remain active in the computer memory until the computer is turned off.

Viruses are not the only program types that can damage data or disrupt computing. Other malicious programs include worms, Trojan horses, logic bombs, and bacteria. See Table 10–1 for characteristics associated with each program type.

Although antivirus software can locate and eradicate viruses and other destructive programs, the best defense against malicious programs is knowledge obtained from talking with computer users and experts about problems experienced. Some people are experts in viral detection and eradication. Box 10–1 provides tips for how to avoid malicious programs.

Table 10–1

Characteristics of Malicious Programs

Program Type	Characteristics
Viruses	Require normal computer operations to spread May or may not disrupt operation or damage data
Worms	Named for pattern of damage left behind Often use local area and wide network communication practice as a means to spread and reproduce
Trojan horses	Appear to do (or actually do) one function while performing another, undesired action One common example resembles a regular system log-in but records user names and passwords to another program for illicit use Do not self-replicate Are easily confined once discovered
Logic bombs	Are triggered by a specific piece of data such as a date, user name, account name, or identification May be part of a regular program or contained in a separate program May not activate on the first program run May be included in virus-infected programs and with Trojan horses
Bacteria	Are a class of viral programs Do not affix themselves to existing programs

If a virus is contained on one machine, all diskettes used on it must be isolated. Antivirus software must be used to disinfect diskettes and computers. Suspect files should be deleted. All backup diskettes should be considered suspect. It should not be necessary to reformat the hard drive to eliminate the virus(es). Viruses, worms, and other malicious viruses are detrimental to the economy because of the loss of productivity and resources required to restore functionality (Davidson 2003; Jenkins 2003).

Additional threats to information and system security come from poor password management, sharing passwords, posting logon IDs and passwords on workstations, leaving logged-on devices unattended, and compromised handheld devices (Dearne 2003; Hatfield 2002; Jenkins 2003). Handheld devices can carry viruses and worms that may be transmitted to the hospital network from inside the firewall, threatening application, device, and network security. There also are unresolved issues with the use of wireless devices having interference as well as susceptibility to attack because passwords can be stolen by those listening in and information compromised (Arar 2003; O'Hare 2003). Improper disposal of printed reports and denial of receipt or authorship of documents also threaten information and systems as do software flaws, network misconfigurations, and targeted attacks.

Box 10–1 **How to Avoid Malicious Programs**

- Use only licensed software.
- Use the latest version of virus detection software routinely. Upload updates on a regular basis.
- Never open any file attachment from an unfamiliar source.
- Use designated machines to check all new diskettes and software for viruses before use.
- Keep copies of computer start-up instructions, including CONFIG.SYS and AUTOEXEC.BAT files.
- Maintain a list of all program files, their size, and date of creation, and review these periodically for change.
- Retain backup copies of original software, work files, and directory structure for each PC. Backup can quickly restore system setup and work. However, since most software is now available on CD-ROM and can be reinstalled quickly, backup may not be necessary.
- Have lists of vendor, purchase date, and serial number for all hardware and software items to facilitate virus tracking.
- If a virus is found, send a copy to an expert for tracking purposes.
- Watch for and download software patches that eliminate security problems.
- Ensure that system safeguards have been put into place by information technology staff. This may include programming e-mail servers to reject mail containing viruses and setting up policies related to e-mail use and educating the workforce.

SECURITY MECHANISMS

Protection of information and computer systems should receive top priority. Typically, security mechanisms use a combination of logical and physical restrictions to provide a greater level of protection than is possible with either approach alone (Pounds 2002). This includes measures such as firewalls and the installation of antivirus and spyware detection software. These measures should also be reevaluated periodically to determine which ones are still necessary (Wade 2003). An example of a logical restriction is automatic sign-off. **Automatic sign-off** is a mechanism that logs a user off the system after a specified period of inactivity on their computer. This procedure is recommended in all client care areas, as well as any other area in which sensitive data exist. The level of security provided should reflect the value of the information. Some levels of information may have no particular value and do not need protection from theft, only from unauthorized change.

Physical Security

Physical security measures include placement of computers, file servers, or computers in restricted areas. When this is not possible, equipment may be removed or locked. Physical security is a challenge for remote access. **Remote access** is the ability to use the health enterprise's information system from outside locations such as a physician's office. Secure modems and encryption are particularly useful in conjunction with remote access.

Physical security is also challenged with the growing popularity of mobile wireless devices such as notebooks, tablet PCs, and personal digital assistants (PDAs). These items may fall into unauthorized hands. Security cables, motion detectors, or alarms may be used with these devices to help ward off theft. Secure, lockable briefcases should be considered for the storage of devices not in use. In the event that mobile devices are stolen, some measure of protection can be provided by making the boot-up proccess password protected, setting passwords on individual files, storing files in zipped, password-protected folders, or encrypting the hard drive (Minagh 2002; Steers 2003). These actions are not foolproof because hard drives can be removed and copied. Daily backups and portable storage devices such as an external drive help to prevent data loss. For this reason, it is essential to conduct a risk assessment on the use of wireless devices in organizations in addition to establishing standards and policies for their use (O'Hare 2003).

Passwords and Other Means of Authentication

Access codes and passwords have long been favored as a means to authenticate access to automated records, largely because they represent a familiar, available, and inexpensive technology (Fratto 2002). A **password** is a collection of alphanumeric characters that the user types into the computer. This may be required after the entry and acceptance of an access code, sometimes referred to as the *user name*. IS administrators sometimes require this information to problem-solve or reissue passwords. The password does not appear on the screen when it is typed, nor should it be known to anyone but the user and IS administrators. Recommendations for password selection and use are given in Box 10–2. Obvious passwords such as the user's name, house number, or dictionary words are easily compromised. Strong passwords use combinations of letters, numbers, and symbols that are not easily guessed. Software is available to test and eliminate easily compromised passwords before use.

Individuals should not share passwords or leave computers logged on and unattended. System administrators must keep files that contain password lists safe from view or copying by unauthorized individuals. One compromised password can jeopardize information and the system that contains it. For this reason, users should not use the same password for access to more than one site or system. Using the same password at various sites reduces security (Spanbauer 2003). System administrators need to allow legitimate users the opportunity to access the system while refusing entry to others. One means to accomplish this is to shut down a workstation after a random number of unsuccessful access attempts and send security to check that area. Although passwords provide considerable system protection, other defenses are still necessary. These include measures to verify user identity. Figure 10–1 shows a screen shot of a logon screen.

Box 10–2 **Recommendations for Password Selection and Use**

- Choose passwords that are six to eight characters long.
- Select stronger passwords for higher levels of security.
- Avoid using the same password for more than one application.
- Do not use the browser "password save" feature.
- Use combinations of uppercase and lowercase letters, numbers, punctuation marks, and symbols.
- Do not use proper names, initials, words taken from the dictionary, or account names.
- Do not use words that are spelled backwards or with reversed syllables.
- Do not use dates or telephone, license plate, or Social Security numbers.
- Do not store or automate passwords in the computer.
- Avoid repeated numbers or letters.
- Keep passwords private.
- Change passwords frequently, with no reuse of passwords for a specified period.

Sign-on access codes and passwords are generally assigned on successful completion of system training. Passwords may be difficult for the user to recall. This leads some people to write password(s) down and post them in conspicuous places. This practice should be prohibited. Users who find it necessary to record the dozens of passwords used to access various sites and systems must store them in an area away from the computer and out of casual view. Storing passwords in a file on the computer is a problem if the device is shared by others or if the hard drive crashes or is replaced. A file-wipe utility should be used to permanently erase the drive so that password files cannot be restored. When a file is used to store passwords, it should be encrypted and password protected. Passwords must be regarded as an electronic signature.

Frequent and random password change is recommended as a routine security mechanism. This can be an arduous and unpleasant task because it is difficult for users to remember new passwords. There are, however, situations that mandate immediate change or deletion of access codes and passwords, including suspicion of unauthorized access and termination of employees. Codes and passwords should also be deleted with status changes such as resignations, leaves of absence, and the completion of rotations for students, faculty, and residents. Because IS staff can view any information in the system, all members of the department should receive new passwords when IS personnel leave. In the event that an IS employee is terminated, department door locks should be changed as well.

Disadvantages associated with the use of passwords include that they are poorly managed, frequently forgotten, and often need reset by help

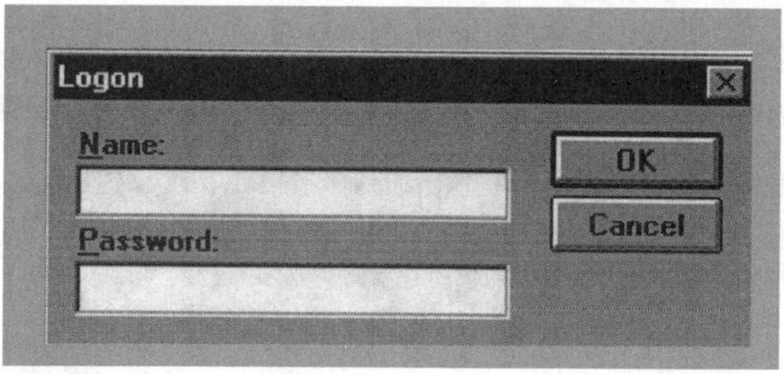

FIGURE 10–1 • Screen shot of a logon screen

desk staff; that they can be shared or stolen; the complex rules for password generation are largely unenforceable; and that the purpose of passwords is defeated when the user sets the browser to remember them (Briggs 2002a; Fratto 2002; Hatfield 2002; Paul 2002).

It is important to develop authentication policies jointly with information technology personnel, business staff, and end users. It is also critical to factor in time to install and test drivers and hardware as well as to consider the time and resources required to enroll and update users. Support costs and training times increase as the complexity of the authentication process increases (Fratto 2002). Unwieldy authentication systems can reduce staff productivity (Kohn, Walton-Brooks, Hasty, and Henderson 2003).

Firewalls

A **firewall** is a combination of hardware and software that forms a barrier between systems, or different parts of a single system, to protect those systems from unauthorized access. Firewalls screen traffic and allow only approved transactions to pass through them and restrict access to other systems or sensitive areas such as client information, payroll, or personnel data. Multiple firewalls can increase protection. Strong security policies and practices strengthen firewall protection. Once a user has passed through the firewall, controlling access to individual applications takes place elsewhere. Firewalls are not foolproof. Specialists periodically create "patches" to counter flaws in security software. It is imperative to put these into place as they become available. It is also essential to train and remind employees about their role in security (Goodwin 2003; Pounds 2002).

Application Security

Another area of concern is **application security,** which refers to protecting from harm a set of programs and the information that they store or create. Application security should be used with the client information system and other systems such as payroll records. Employees should sign off when they leave a workstation or computer, or are finished using a particular software application, because failure to do so may allow others to use their code to access information. Automatic sign-off has been designed as a security measure when employees fail to properly exit a program or step away from the computer. Improperly secured wireless networks can open large holes into previously secured wired networks and applications (Ammon 2003).

Antivirus Software

Antivirus software is a set of computer programs that can locate and eradicate viruses and other malicious programs from scanned diskettes, individual computers, and networks. The constant creation of new viruses makes it necessary to update antivirus software often. Antivirus software may come preloaded on new computers or be obtained in computer stores or over the Internet. The user must then frequently download updated virus definitions from the vendor's Web site. Some vendors automatically notify users as new virus definitions become available. Users can set up antivirus software to automatically run a virus check on the PC or server on a scheduled basis in addition to performing random checks.

Spyware Detection Software

Spyware is a data collection mechanism that installs itself without the user's permission. This often occurs when the user is browsing the Web or downloading software. Spyware can include cookies that keep track of Web use and other applications that can send valuable information such as credit card, bank, PIN, and other numbers, or personal health information stored on that computer. This is a concern for all health care providers because it threatens personal health information (PHI). No computer that is attached to the Internet is immune. Because of the security threat that this represents, spyware detection software should be utilized.

ADMINISTRATIVE AND PERSONNEL ISSUES

Ultimately, health care administrators are responsible for creating and managing the infrastructure to protect client privacy and confidentiality. This infrastructure requires a plan, policies, designated structure for implementation, and access levels (Beaver 2003). Upper management must have security awareness training and set a positive example. Next, administration must work with IS personnel to establish the following centralized security functions:

- *A comprehensive security plan.* The plan needs to be developed with input from administration, information services personnel, and clinical staff. It should delineate security responsibilities for each level of personnel as well as a timeline for the development and implementation of policy and physical infrastructure. Incorporation of computer forensics as a plan component helps to build and maintain a strong security posture (Armstrong 2002). **Computer forensics** refers to the collection of electronic evidence for purposes of formal litigation and simple internal investigations.

- *Correct, complete information security policies, procedures, and standards.* These should be published online for easy access, with e-mail notification of employees as new policies come out.

- *Information asset ownership and sensitivity classifications.* Ownership in this context refers to who is responsible for the information, including its security. Sensitivity classification is a determination of how damaging that information might be if it were disclosed inappropriately. The level of sensitivity may be used to determine what information should be encrypted.

- *Identification of security issues for managers.* Managers cannot properly safeguard information or information systems if they are unaware of actual or potential threats to either.

- *Identification of a comprehensive security program.* A well-defined security plan can avert or minimize threats. A key part of the plan is the identification of responsibility for information integrity and confidentiality. A strong plan incorporates computer forensics.

- *Information security training and user support.* Education is an important component in fostering proper system use.

- *An institution-wide information security awareness program.* Formal IS training and frequent suggestions to remind users of the need to protect information.

In reality, responsibility for system and information security is shared by health care administrators, IS and health care professionals, and all system users. Involving users in system development fosters ownership of this responsibility and facilitates the ability to trace problems, limit damage, and make corrective changes. This involvement can occur on an individual level or through an institutional security committee. Security committees should consider routine maintenance, confidentiality clauses in vendor contracts, third-party payor needs, legal issues inclusive of monitoring, ongoing security needs as the institution and system evolve, and disaster planning. The IS department should address these functions when there is no security committee. Individual users are responsible for protecting their passwords, saving and backing up work files on a regular basis, securing removable diskettes, and not leaving confidential information unattended on the computer screen or in paper form. They should also be responsible for reporting any observed unauthorized access. It may be necessary to outsource security if there are insufficient resources internally, but this decision needs to be carefully weighed (Goodwin 2003).

Levels of Access

Access should be strictly limited to a need-to-know basis. This means no personnel, including IS staff, should have routine access to confidential information unless it is required by a particular event, at which time an audit trail is established. IS personnel must be held to the same confidentiality statement that applies to other personnel.

Limits Access is determined by who needs the medical record and under what conditions and locations. Direct care providers require information on their clients. Access levels are decided by defining roles for every level of personnel. This process can be referred to as "user classes." Each user class has different privileges. Initial system access is contingent on successful completion of system training and demonstration of competence. User training should address appropriate uses of information and the consequences of information misuse. User roles and audits must be incorporated into the design of information systems to best ensure security, privacy, and confidentiality. Attempts to define user roles and implement audits into legacy systems is extremely difficult (Korpman 2002). Definition of user roles is instrumental to preventing unauthorized access to sensitive health care information. For example, nursing assistants are responsible for the documentation of hygiene, dietary intakes, vital signs, and fluid intake and output. They should not be able to access diagnostic and historical information.

User Authentication

Access by authorized individuals can be verified through user authentication. One common form of authentication is the appearance of the user's name on the screen. In the event that other staff observe a discrepancy, they have the responsibility to report it immediately. More sophisticated means of authentication include passwords used along with either a "passkey" type of device or scanned employee identification. Encrypted key-based authentication is another technology. An example is **public key infrastructure (PKI).** PKI uses an encrypted passkey that can be provided to the user in various formats, including a smartcard, token, or wireless transmitter (Lovorn 2001). The passkey provides a secret number that is verified against a registered digital certificate. The user submits the passkey information during the sign-on process, and the PKI system compares it against the registered digital certificate ID to verify a match. Digital certificates include information about the owner such as systems that they may access, level of access, and biometric measures. Digital certificates provide assurance of the identity, rights, and privileges of the user. Security tokens that resemble key chain fobs are an example of this technology. Tokens strengthen authentication because the user must use both the token and a special PIN code to gain access (Fratto 2002). PKI can provide a common infrastructure that allows access to multiple delivery systems across an organization or organizations.

Scanned employee identification may include a name badge but generally refers to biometric authentication, which is based on a unique biological trait, such as a fingerprint, voice or iris pattern, retinal scan, hand geometry, face recognition, ear pattern, smell, or gait recognition (Banham 2002, Briggs 2002b, Fratto 2002, Peck 2003). This technology is now feasible and can be very accurate. Unlike passwords or devices that can be forgotten or stolen, biometric measures are always with the individual barring major injury and cannot be lost, stolen, or used without user consent. Most experts recommend a combination approach that requires a password plus either key-based authentication or a biometric measure. Fingerprint identification is the primary measure used at the present. The quality of biometric authentication is device dependent. There is a high rate of failure of first print readings as the number of users increases. This situation may require a second or third reading. Individuals must learn the proper method of placing their fingers into scanners. Skin moisture and temperature also affect the quality of the scan. Very moist or dry skin and cold fingers negatively affect reading. Some readers can be fooled by using tape, gelatin, or other measures. Biometric authentication helps organizations to better comply with regulations and reduces the amount of time that help staff spend resetting passwords. The use of biometric measures for authentication is expected to grow as devices become easier to use, less instrusive, more reliable, and less expensive.

Other authentication devices include proximity radio systems that detect user badges within a specified distance, picture authentication packages that use pictures instead of passwords, and digital certificates. Users should have different authentication requirements depending upon the sensitivity or value of the resources that they access. Authentication can be strengthened by requiring multifactor authentication (Fratto 2002). Authentication policy outlines acceptable forms of authentication depending on multiple factors including user, resources, location, and time of day. It must also protect authentication systems from attack and sabotage. Building an authentication policy is one thing—implementing, managing, and enforcing it is another.

Personnel Issues

Personnel issues for information handling include education and policy and procedure development and implementation (Rathke 2002). Staff education is a key element for information and system security. Education for information handling and system use includes an orientation, system training, and a discussion of what is acceptable behavior. Staff should also be informed of the consequences for unauthorized access and information misuse, the use of audit trails, and ongoing measures to heighten security awareness.

Staff need to know what constitutes an incident and how it should be handled. Ongoing measures include periodic reminders that client information belongs to them and reminders about what comprises professional, legal, and ethical behavior. Yearly review of the ethical computing statement is one way to emphasize the importance of ethical behavior. Figure 10–2 displays an example of this statement. Education and monitoring activities show administrative commitment to ethical information use.

Explicit policies and procedures provide the discipline to achieve information and system security (DiFrances 2002; O'Daniel 2003). Policies and procedures should address information ethics, training, access control, system monitoring, data entry, backup procedures, responsibilities for the use of information on mobile devices and remote sites, and exchange of client information with other health care providers. Information ethics policies should do the following:

- *Plan for audit trails.* **Audit trails** are a record of IS activity. Users should know that their system access is monitored and that audit trail records will be kept for a period of years.

- *Establish acceptable computer uses.* This includes authorized access and using only legal software copies. One example of how this might be enforced is requiring licenses for all software used within the institution.

- *Collect only required data.* Limiting collection of information to what is needed, but no more, eliminates the danger of inappropriate disclosure of unneeded information and may lighten the workload.

- *Encourage client review of files for accuracy and error correction.* Client inspection of records ensures information integrity.

- *Establish controls for the use of information after hours and off-site.* As many employees and physicians work at home or complete projects on their own time, it is important to develop policies related to downloading files or carrying information off premises. Both the types of information that may be carried on mobile devices and the responsibilities of the staff member to safeguard that information must be spelled out.

Information ethics policies are most credible when practiced by top administrators and IS personnel.

System Security Management

System security involves protection against deliberate attacks, errors, omissions, and disasters. Good system management is a key component of a strong framework for security because it encompasses the following tasks:

- Monitoring
- Maintenance

ST. FRANCIS HEALTH SYSTEM
INFORMATION SYSTEM
USER SIGN-ON CODE RECEIPT

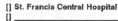

[] St. Francis Medical Center
[] St. Francis Hospital of New Castle
[] St. Francis Central Hospital
[] _____

Hospital Personnel or Hospital Based Physician Sign-On codes are confidential. Disclosure of your Sign-On code, attempts to discover another person's Sign-On code, or unauthorized use of a Sign-On code are grounds for immediate dismissal.

I, the undersigned, acknowledge receipt of my User Sign-On Code and understand that:

1. My User Sign-On Code is equivalent of my signature; (Please note that the electronic signature is recognized by the Health Care Finance Administration (HCFA) and the Commonwealth of Pennsylvania).

2. Accessing the system via my Sign-On Code, is recorded permanently;

3. If assigned a User Sign-On Code, I will not disclose this code to anyone;

4. I will not attempt to learn another user's User Sign-On Code;

5. I will not attempt to access information in the system by using a User Sign-On Code other than my own;

6. I will access only that information which is necessary to perform my authorized functions;

7. If I have reason to believe that the confidentiality of my User Sign-On Code has been broken, I will contact Information Services immediately so that the suspect code can be deleted and a new code assigned to me; and

I understand that if I violate any of the above statements, it will be referred to the appropriate authority.

I further understand that my User Sign-On Code will be deleted from the system when I no longer hold an appointment or am no longer employed at St. Francis or authorization is otherwise revoked.

I have read the above statements and understand the implications if confidentiality of Sign-On code is violated.

_____ Social Security #_____-_____-_____
Name (Please print)

Dept:_____Supervisor:_____ Position:_____

System: MIS:_____   MEDIPAC:_____   G/L:_____   A/P:_____   CYBORG:_____   OTHER:_____

Signature of Code Recipient_____ Date:___/___/____

* Trainer Signature:_____ Date:___/___/____

* Dept. Head Authorization:_____ Date:___/___/____

Issuer Signature:_____ Date:___/___/____
        Information Services

Code will not be issued without proper identification and signature in presence of issuer.
* Signature must be present prior to issuance of code.   MIS User Class:_____

FORM H-1280 Date of Origin: 2/85
        Revised: 10/95

File: Personnel Department
Physicians: Medical Staff Office

FIGURE 10–2 • Sample ethical computing statement (reprinted by permission of St. Francis Health System, Pittsburgh, PA)

- Operations
- Traffic management
- Supervision

Monitoring entails setting and enforcing standards and tracking changes (Evans 2002). It also includes observing all system activity because breeches can occur at any time without warning, and alerting managers to problems such as intruders or the introduction of a virus. Maintenance encompasses all activity needed for proper operation of hardware, including preventive measures such as testing and periodic applications of patches and replacement of select components to ensure that data are available when it is needed. Maintenance includes documentation of all configuration settings, server protocols, and network addresses and changes to any of the above, so that records are available in the event that the system must be restored. Operations management includes all activities needed to provide, sustain, modify, or cease telecommunications. Traffic management permits rerouting transmissions for better system performance. Supervision requires monitoring traffic and taking measures to prevent system overload and crashes.

Although software is available to facilitate system management tasks, the paucity of commercial packages available for management of comprehensive systems across networks forced institutions to develop in-house solutions or use outsourcing agents for customized applications. Many organizations have different staff members for network and systems management. Network staff traditionally focus on hardware and connections, whereas IS personnel track information and software use. The security officer plays a pivotal role in tracking personnel information relative to system use. It is the security officer who may assign access codes and passwords to authorized users and who deletes codes for staff no longer with the organization. Increased computing needs and limited budgets require greater staff efficiency. Wise use of system and network management tools will help to provide that efficiency, minimize the number of required support staff, reduce support costs, and improve information security.

Audit Trails

Auditing software helps to maintain security by recording unauthorized access to certain screens or records. Audits can show access of records by user or by password and all access by an individual or level of employee. Frequent review of audit trails for unusual activity quickly identifies inappropriate use. Poorly audited systems invite fraud and abuse (Kuperstein 2001). The level of control in many audit systems is not sufficient for HIPAA compliance. Optimally, audits should be able to track all access, creations, updates, and edits at the data element level for each patient record. This ability will support a consumer's right to view logs of who accessed their data, what they saw, and when it was accessed and will ensure HIPAA compliance (Korpman 2002).

Audit trail records must now be available for protracted periods. Before HIPAA, audit logs were usually kept for limited periods. Consideration must be given now to the retention period for audit logs. Department managers must be advised when audit trails indicate that their staff have accessed records without a need. Audit trails help but may still fail to demonstrate the full range of security issues (Dearne 2003).

In the event that an audit trail identifies unauthorized access, it is important to enforce written policy. At the very least, this is a verbal reprimand or possibly a notation on the employee's performance evaluation. In many institutions, however, employees are held to the statement they signed on receipt of their access code and password, acknowledging termination of employment as a possible consequence of inappropriate system use. When employees are terminated for this reason, they may be escorted off the premises by the security department. This prevents any further opportunity for unauthorized access. Audit trails may also reveal unauthorized access from outside sources, although little legal recourse has been available to punish the guilty parties until recently. There is now an increased legislative activity to prevent and punish cybercrime. The best protection is offered through improved security mechanisms.

HANDLING AND DISPOSAL OF CONFIDENTIAL INFORMATION

Although most people recognize the need to keep medical records confidential, many are less attentive to safeguarding information printed from the record or extracted from it electronically for report purposes. All client record information should be treated as confidential and not left out for view by unauthorized persons.

Computer Printouts

The primary sources of unauthorized release of information are printing and Faxing (Calloway and Venegas 2002, Preiss 2002, Ziel and Gentry 2003). All papers containing personal health information (PHI) such as prescriptions, laboratory specimen labels, identification bracelets, meal descriptions, addressograph plates or any other items that carry a patient's name or address, Social Security number, date of birth, or age must be destroyed. This may entail using shredders or locked receptacles for shredding and incineration later. Shredding onsite may offer better control as well as cost savings. Nurses may also be responsible for erasing computer files from the hard drive containing calendars, surgery schedules, or other daily records that include PHI. Disposal policies for records must be clear and enforced. For tracking purposes, each page of output should have a serial number or other means of identification so that an audit trail is maintained that identifies what each paper record is as well as the date and method for destruction and the identity of individuals witnessing the destruction. Control must be established over the materials that users print or Fax. Some institutions include a header on all printouts such as lab results that display the word "Confidential" in large letters. This reminds staff to dispose of materials appropriately.

Faxes

Sound institutional and departmental policies are needed for the use of Fax machines that consider what types of information can be sent, who should receive the transmissions, the location to which transmissions are sent, and verification of receipt (Ziel and Gentry 2003). Information should not exceed that requested or required for immediate clinical needs. Legal counsel should review policies for consistency with federal and state law. Clients should sign a release form before Faxing information. The following measures enhance Fax security:

- *Confirm that fax numbers are correct before sending information.* This helps to ensure that information is appropriately directed.
- *The use of a cover sheet.* This is a particularly important practice when the Fax machine serves a number of different users. A cover sheet eliminates the need for the recipient to read the Fax transmission to determine who gets it. The cover sheet may also contain a statement to remind recipients of the presence of confidential information. Figure 10–3 displays an example of a Fax cover sheet.
- *Authentication at both ends of the transmission before data transmission.* This action verifies that the source and destination are correct.
- *Programmed speed-dial keys.* Programmed keys eliminate the chance of dialing errors and misdirected Fax transmissions.
- *Encryption.* Encoding transmissions makes it impossible to read confidential information without the encryption key. This safeguards Fax transmissions that might be sent to a wrong number.
- *Sealed envelopes for delivery.* The enclosure of confidential information in sealed envelopes provides a barrier to discourage casual viewing.
- *Fax machine placement in secure areas.* Secure areas have limited traffic and few, if any, strangers.
- *Limited machine access by designated individuals.* Restricting access to a few people makes it easier to enforce accountability for actions and identify any transgressions.
- *Inclusion of a request to return documents by mail.* Inadvertent entry of a wrong telephone number can jeopardize sensitive information. In the event that information is Faxed to a wrong number, a request to return documents may limit further disclosure.
- *A log of all Fax transmissions.* A roster of all Faxes sent and received provides a means to keep track of what information is sent and to help ensure that only appropriate information is sent.

Electronic Files

Given that virtually all documents originate in electronic format, the destruction of paper printouts is almost incidental. For this reason, measures

ST. FRANCIS MEDICAL CENTER
FAX TRANSMITTAL FORM

ST. FRANCIS HEALTH SYSTEM

DATE: _____   NO. OF PAGES: _____
(including cover sheet)

FROM: _____

FACILITY: _____

DEPARTMENT: _____

TELEPHONE: _____   FAX: _____

TO: _____

FACILITY: _____

DEPARTMENT: _____

TELEPHONE: _____   FAX: _____

COMMENTS: _____

_____

_____

_____

_____

_____

This fax contains privileged and confidential information intended only for the use of the recipient named above. If you are not the intended recipient of this fax or the employee or agent responsible for delivering it to the intended recipient, you are hereby notified that any dissemination or copying of this fax is strictly prohibited. If you have received this fax in error, please notify sender listed above; and return the original to the above address via U.S. mail.

This information has been disclosed to you from records whose confidentiality is protected by state and federal law. Any further disclosure of this information without the prior written consent of the person to whom it pertains may be prohibited.

FIGURE 10–3 • Sample Fax cover sheet (reprinted by permission of St. Francis Health System, Pittsburgh, PA)

must be taken to ensure that confidential information contained on storage media, computers, and hard drives that is no longer needed is also disposed of properly. This method must go beyond the dumpster to include destruction of the storage media or electronically writing over files to ensure that no information can be retrieved from them. This is particularly important as equipment is often moved from one area of an organization to another and may even be donated to outside entities.

E-mail and the Internet

E-mail is discussed at length in the chapter on electronic communication and the Internet (see Chapter 4). Policy should dictate what types of information may be sent via e-mail. E-mail is a great means of disseminating information, such as announcements, to large numbers of people quickly and inexpensively. However, information that is potentially sensitive should not be sent via e-mail unless it is encrypted. Nonencrypted messages can be read and public e-mail password protection of mailboxes can be cracked. When looking at encryption, ask whether your e-mail software encrypts all messages between users, whether messages are encrypted both in transit and when stored in the mailbox, and whether messages remain encrypted when sent between different e-mail packages. Unauthorized, or dormant, mail accounts should be destroyed and firewalls used for additional protection. It is all too easy to inadvertently send out e-mail to the wrong party, attach the wrong document or include persons who do not need the information (Levy 2003; Regan 2003). Software can be used to monitor network traffic for patterns that represent client information such as lists or Social Security numbers. This same software can detect requests for files, and monitor instant messaging and Web-based mail to determine if requests come from appropriate parties or if there are problems with information going out to unauthorized recipients.

HIPAA regulations affect e-mail use and routing infrastructures. Most e-mail networks allow messages to travel through any available simple mail transfer protocol (SMTP) relay until it reaches its destination. Messages are stored at each relay and then forwarded. These relays can be hacked; encryption helps to ensure that intercepted mail cannot be read but it does not keep it secure. Security lies with access and control of decryption keys. Central administration for encryption, key management, and disclosure should be addressed via policies and training (Voelk and Geyer 2002). Another concern related to e-mail and information system security is spam. **Spam** is unsolicited e-mail that uses valuable server space and employee time and can serve as an entry for malicious programs. E-mail security software can filter out spam. The down side is that this process results in the loss of approximately 10% of legitimate mail (Briggs 2003).

Monitoring e-mail is important to avoid legal liability and maintain network security, employee productivity, and the confidentiality of information (Migliori 2003).

Web-Based Applications for Health Care

There is a high level of concern over the security of health information transmitted via the World Wide Web. The debate over whether the Web is safe enough to use for health information is likely to continue for some time. Technology and know-how can provide adequate security. Economic concerns may diminish safeguards. Internet use for health care information over the Web continues to grow. Protection of health information can be ensured by spelling out liability for its compromise and insurance.

Electronic Storage

Increased access to information through an ever-increasing number of interconnected storage devices and networks also creates additional concerns over security (Clark 2003). Security threats to stored information mirror those that may affect any network. Unauthorized access to information is a major threat that can be curtailed through careful management of the interfaces between systems. It is crucial to ensure that authorized users can access information when they need it but that sufficient security measures are in place to prevent unauthorized access. These measures include requirements for user identification and encrypted passwords to access the various components of the network such as switches.

Confidential information may also be copied from the system in the form of electronic records. Administrators may download these records for report purposes. Once the records are no longer needed, electronic copies of sensitive data should receive the same treatment as any other data that have met its purpose. In this case, file deletion or shredder software is recommended. **File deletion software** overwrites files with meaningless information so that sensitive information cannot be accessed (Davies 1998).

CASE STUDY EXERCISES

In the course of conversation, your nurse manager tells you that she loaded a copy of the spreadsheet program she uses on her home office PC onto one of the unit PCs so that she can work on projects at both locations. Your institution has a well-publicized policy against the use of unauthorized, unlicensed software copies. As a staff nurse, what should you do? Explain your response.

• • •

You notice several of the new residents playing computer games on the nursing unit. You had not been aware of these games previously. What, if any, action should you take? Explain your rationale.

• • •

To remember her computer system password, university nursing instructor Pat Pawakawicz taped her password to the back of her name pin. When Ms. Pawakawicz lost her name pin recently, it was turned into hospital security and subsequently the IS department with her password still attached. When Ms. Pawakawicz picked up her name pin, she expressed intent to use the same password. Is this an appropriate way to treat a password? Should she use the same password again? Provide your rationale. What, if any, legal ramifications might there be for Ms. Pawakawicz regarding use of her password by unauthorized users?

• • •

The administration at St. John's Hospital takes pride in their strong policies and procedures for the protection of confidential client information. In fact, St. John's serves as a model for other institutions in this area. However, printouts discarded in the restricted access IS department are not shredded. On numerous occasions, personnel working late observed the cleaning staff reading discarded printouts. What action, if any, should these personnel take relative to the actions of the cleaning staff? What action, if any, should be taken by IS administration? Provide your rationale. If current practices are maintained, are there any additional potential risks for unauthorized disclosure of client information? If you answer yes, identify what these risks might be.

• • •

The secretary on 7 Tower Oncology receives a Fax transmission about a client consult. The Fax was intended for a physician's office in the adjacent building. She places the Fax in the out bin of her desk to be delivered later by volunteers. No in-house mailer was used. Is this action appropriate? Explain why or why not.

 EXPLOREMEDIALINK

Multiple choice review questions, case studies, and other interactive resources for this chapter can be found on the Web site at *http://www.prenhall.com/hebda*. Click on "Chapter 10" to select the activities for this chapter.

SUMMARY

- The primary goals of health care information system security are the protection of client confidentiality and information integrity.
- Privacy and confidentiality are important terms in health care information management. Privacy is a choice to disclose personal information, while confidentiality assumes a relationship in which private information has been shared for the purpose of health treatment.
- Information privacy is the right to choose the conditions under which information is shared and to ensure the accuracy of collected information.
- Threats to information and system security and confidentiality come from a variety of sources, including system penetration by thieves,

hackers, unauthorized use, denial of service and terrorist attacks, cybercrime, errors and disasters, sabotage, viruses, and human error.

- Planning for security saves time and money and is a form of insurance against downtime, breaches in confidentiality, and lost productivity.

- Security mechanisms combine physical and logical restrictions. Examples include automatic sign-off, physical restriction of computer equipment, strong password protection, and firewalls.

- Ultimately, health care administrators are responsible for protecting client privacy and confidentiality through education, policy, and creating an ongoing awareness of security.

- One aspect of system security management includes monitoring the system for unusual record access patterns, as might be seen when a celebrity receives treatment.

- Health information on the Internet requires the same types of safeguards provided for information found in private offices and information systems.

- All chart printouts, forms, and computer files containing client information should be given the same consideration as the client record itself to safeguard confidentiality.

REFERENCES

Advani, D. (May 15, 2003). The new face of authentication. *Network Computing, 14*(9), 70.

Ammon, K. (October 16, 2003). Internet vulnerabilities. Statement of Mr. Kenneth Ammon, President of NetSec Corporation before the Committee on House Government Reform.

Arar, Y. (2003). Five reasons not to go wireless. *PC World, 21*(11), 140.

Armstrong, I. (August 2002). Computer forensics: Detecting the imprint. *SC Magazine.* Available online at http://www.scmagazine.com/ scmagazine/2002_08/cover/cover.html. Accessed November 24, 2003.

Australia's privacy legislation: A guide for nurses (2002). *Australian Nursing Journal, 10*(2), 24.

Banham, R. (2002). The eyes have it. *CFO–IT, 18*(11), 45–46.

Beaver, K. (2003). The 21 best ways to lose your information. *Contingency Planning & Management, 8*(1), 66.

Blair, P. D. (2003). Make room for patient privacy. *Nursing Management, 34*(6), 28.

BOMI Institute for Today's Facility Manager. (2001). Building an effective security program. *Today's Facility Manager,* pp. 89–91. Available online at http://www.facilitycity.com/tfm/tfm_01_10_news3.asp. Accessed November 24, 2003.

Briggs, B. (2002a). One finger vs. many passwords. *Health Data Management, 10*(4), 32, 34.

Briggs, B. (2002b). E-health demand may finally catch up with supply. *Health Data Management,10*(12), 30–52.

Briggs, B. (2003). New recipe for canning "Spam." *Health Data Management, 11*(9), 70, 72.

Calloway, S. D., and Venegas, L. M. (2002). The new HIPAA law on privacy and confidentiality. *Nursing Administration Quarterly, 26*(4), 40.

Capitol Hill on the case. (2003). *PC World, 21*(11), 158.

Clark, E. (2003). Storage security: Under lock and key. *Network Magazine, 18*(1), 70.

Cyberattacks become more advanced. (October 21, 2003). *USA Today.*

Davidson, M. A. (September 17, 2003). Computer virus protection. *FDCH Congressional Testimony.*

Davies, E. (February 16, 1998). Great tool for the paranoid. *Fortune, 137*(3), 129.

Dearne, K. (April 30, 2002). Business ignores hacking dangers. *The Australian.*

Dearne, K. (October 28, 2003). Hire a hacker. *The Australian.*

DiFrances, J. (2002). Protect your organization's proprietary information. *Solutions, 25*(7), 44.

Evans, A. (2002). Server and network monitoring. *ADVANCE for Health Information Executives 6*(9), 22–26.

Fisher, D. (September 29, 2003). Muscling greater security. *EWeek, 20*(39), 1.

Forman, M. A. (April 2003). Cyber security challenges. FDCH Congressional Testimony before the Committee on House Government Reform Subcommittee.

Fratto, M. (2002). Control the keys to the kingdom. *Network Computing, 13*(18), 36.

Gillespie, G. (2003). CIOs coming in for a pit stop in the HIPAA compliance race. *Health Data Management, 11*(8), 34.

Goedert, J. (2002). CIOs eye HIPAA's privacy and security rules. *Health Data Management, 10*(9), 50–52, 54, 56, 58.

Goodwin, B. (June 3, 2003). Businesses need both local and central IT security officers. *Computer Weekly,* 16.

Griffiths, D. (April 22, 2003). Treat IT security as if the law required it. *Computer Weekly,* 44.

Grosh, I. (September/October 2002). Are you a target for computer hackers? *Contigency Planning & Management, 7*(6). Available online at http://www.contingencyplanning.com/Tools/BCPHandbook/Disruption/ComputerHacking.asp. Accessed December 9, 2003.

Hatfield, S. (2002). Security remains key concern. *ADVANCE for Health Information Executives, 6*(8), 16.

Hebda, T., Sakerka, L., and Czar, P. (1994). Educating nurses to maintain patient confidentiality on automated information systems. In S. J. Grobe and E. S. P. Pluyter-Wenting (Eds.), *Nursing informatics: An international overview for nursing in a technological era, The Proceedings of the Fifth IMIA International Conference on Nursing Use of Computers and Information Science.* New York: Elsevier Science.

Hill, J. (March 29, 2003). Speak no evil. *Lancet, 361*(9363), 1140.

Jenkins, C. (October 21, 2003). Viruses eating into IT budgets. *The Australian.*

Joachim, D. (2003). Hospitals get HIPAA. *Network Computing, 14*(13), 54.

Joint Commission on Accreditation of Healthcare Organizations (1996). *Medical records process.* Chicago: Accreditation Manual for Hospitals.

Kearns, D. (2000). Biometrics not an invasion of privacy. *NetworkWorld.* Available online at http://www.nwfusion.com/columnists/2000/0522kearns.html.

Kelly, G., and McKenzie, B. (2002). Security, privacy, and confidentiality issues on the Internet. *Journal of Medical Internet Research, 4*(2), e12. Available online at http://www.jmir.org/2002/2/e12/. Accessed November 2, 2003.

Kmentt, K. A. (Winter 1987). Private medical records: Are they public property? *Medical Trial Technique Quarterly, 33,* 274–307.

Kohn, C., Walton-Brooks, D., Hasty, S., and Henderson, C. W. (June 30, 2003). US Air Force Academy hospital utilizes new authentication system. *Managed Care Weekly Digest,* 31.

Korpman, R. A. (2002). This is not your parents' security system. *Health Management Technology, 23*(11), 16.

Kuperstein, M. (2001). One and done. *Health Management Technology, 22*(12), 22–23.

Levy, C. (2003). Secure content collaboration with information rights management. *Econent, 26*(10), 36.

Lovorn, J. (2001). The power of PKI. *Health Management Technology, 22*(12), 20–21.

Meranda, D. (1995). Administrative and security challenges with electronic patient record systems. *Journal of AHIMA, 66*(3), 58–60.

Migliori, M. (2003). E-mail and Internet monitoring. *Contingency Planning & Management, 8*(1), 32–33.

Miller, D. (1993). Preserving the privacy of computerized patient records. *Healthcare Informatics, 10*(10), 72–74.

Minagh, C. (February 11, 2002). Three points on protecting your laptop. *GP: General Practitioner,* 50.

Murdock, L. E. (1980). The use and abuse of computerized information: Striking a balance between personal privacy interests and organizational information needs. *Albany Law Review, 44*(3), 589–619.

O'Daniel, M. (October 20, 2003). Keeping sensitive information safe. *New Straits Times.*

O'Hare, M. (2003). Security of wireless devices. *ADVANCE for Health Information Executives, 7*(7), 23–28.

Paul, N. (April 22, 2002). Three points on passwords. *GP: General Practitioner,* 55.

PC Week executive: Guide to data security. (1995). *PC Week, 12*(14), E7+.

Peck, B. (2003). ℞ for password headaches. *Health Management Technology, 24*(1), 50–52.

Pierce. F. (2003). Biometric identification. *Health Management Technology,* *24*(5), 38–39.

Pounds, S. (May 15, 2002). FBI expert offers tips on cyber-security at Fort Lauderdale, Fla., Conference. *Palm Beach Post, The (FL).*

Preiss, J. (September 2002). Shredding safeguards for paper records. *ADVANCE for Health Information Executives, 6*(9), 27–30.

Reagan, M. (2003). Electronic eye can protect your health information. Accessed 6/04/2003. Available online at http://www.advance forhie.com/common/Editorial/Editorial.aspx?CC-15124.

Romano, C. (1987). Confidentiality, and security of computerized systems: The nursing responsibility. *Computers in Nursing, 5*(3), 99–104.

Rothke, B. (2002). Parts of the plan. *SC Magazine. 13*(8), 26.

Safran, C., Rind, D., Citroen, M., Bakker, A. R., Slack, W. V., and Bleich, H. L. (1995). Protection of confidentiality in the computer-based patient record. *M.D. Computing, 12*(3), 187–192.

Saldanha, C., and Hayes, G. (June 16, 2003). Are patients ready to share data? *GP: General Practitioner,* 51.

Seltzer, L. (November 6, 2003). Weakness reported in wireless security protocol. *E-Week.*

Spanbauer, S. (2003). Can you pass the PC World password safety test? *PC World, 21*(10), 170.

Steers, K. (2003). Boot passwords put your PC under lock and key. *PC World, 21*(9), 168.

Tuesday, V. (April 21, 2003). Security log. *Computerworld, 37*(16), 35.

Voelk, R., and Geyer, A. (2002). Get a grip on email security. *Healthcare Informatics, 19*(4), 50.

Wade, W. (2003). Yesterday's data safeguards waste money, Ernst says. *American Banker, 168*(185), 13.

Windslade, W. J. (1982). Confidentiality of medical records: An overview of concepts and legal policies. *Journal of Legal Medicine, 3*(4), 497–533.

Ziel, S. E., and Gentry, K. L. (2003). Ready? HIPAA's here: Once the HIPAA privacy rule takes effect on April 14, you'll have to exert even more care than usual in guarding the confidentiality of patient information. *RN, 66*(2), 67.

System Integration

After completing this chapter, you should be able to:

- Discuss the importance of network integration for health care delivery.

- Explain what an *interface engine* is and how it works.

- Identify several integration issues, including factors that impede the process.

- Discuss the relevance to system integration efforts of the data dictionary, master patient index, uniform language efforts, and clinical data repository.

- Consider how standards for the exchange of clinical data affect integration efforts.

- Review the benefits of successful information system integration for health care providers and health care professionals.

- Define the role of the nurse in system integration efforts.

- Understand how Web-based tools can provide an alternative method for obtaining patient information from diverse information systems.

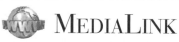 **MEDIALINK**

Additional resources for this content can be found on the Companion Website at *www.prenhall.com/hebda.* Click on "Chapter 11" to select the activities for this chapter.

Companion Website

- Glossary
- Multiple Choice
- Discussion Points
- Case Study: Integration Issues & Benefits
- Case Study: Master Patient Index (MPI)
- MediaLink Application: Improving Information Flow
- Links to Resources
- Crossword Puzzle

Most hospitals and health care providers have automated information systems in some, if not all, of their major departments. Historically, financial systems were implemented by an organization first, followed by registration, laboratory systems, order entry, pharmacy, radiology, and monitoring systems (not necessarily in that order). Some of these systems may have been implemented as stand-alone systems. Most departments select the information system that best meets their needs or that hospital administrators approve for reasons of cost, vendor promises, or the preexistence of other products by the same vendor in the institution. It is rare for all departments in a given health care institution to agree that one vendor's product meets their information system needs. As a consequence, most institutions have several different systems that do not readily communicate or share data. Each of these systems may be highly customized to meet individual department and institutional specifications. This customization, however, complicates integration. Integration needs have increased dramatically as single institutions and providers use more systems internally and as they join with other institutions to form enterprises, alliances, and networks. In addition, integration must be achieved before the electronic health record (EHR) can be realized.

Integration is the process by which different information systems are able to exchange data in a fashion that is seamless to the end user. The physical aspects of joining networks together are not nearly as complicated as getting unlike systems to exchange information in a seamless manner. Traditionally, communication between and among most disparate systems has been the result of costly, time-consuming efforts to build interfaces (Koob 2000). In other words, interface programs are the tools used to achieve integration. An **interface** is a computer program that tells two different systems how to exchange data.

Without integration, providers cannot realize the full advantages of automation, since sharing data across multiple systems is limited and redundant data entry by various personnel takes place. When this occurs, the likelihood of errors is increased. This situation is unacceptable in a time when managed care forces institutions to realize the benefits of automation to compete in today's health care delivery system. Box 11–1 lists some benefits associated with integration.

INTERFACES

Interfaces between different information systems should be invisible to the user. Many vendors claim their products are based on open systems technology which is the ability to communicate with other systems. The reality is that there is little incentive for vendors to market products that readily work with their competitors' products. Another problem is that the cus-

Box 11–1

The Benefits of Integration

- Allows instant access to applications and data
- Improves data integrity with single entry of data
- Decreases labor costs with single entry of data
- Facilitates the formulation of a more accurate, complete client record
- Facilitates information tracking for accurate cost determinations

tomization of vendor products by individual providers precludes off-the-shelf interface solutions.

This necessitates costly and time-consuming design of custom interfaces. Another problem with customized interfaces is pinpointing the responsibility for problems. Each vendor responsible for developing an interface tends to blame the other for any difficulties encountered. Without a determination of responsibility, problem resolution is delayed and no one can be held accountable for the cost of solving the problem. All too often the institution must absorb the costs for this process; yet competition in a managed care environment does not permit this luxury. In addition, the timely flow of information is critical to cost-cutting measures and institutional survival.

There are two general types of interfaces: point-to-point and those using integration engine software. A **point-to-point interface** is an interface that directly connects two information systems. Communication and transfer of data take place only between these systems. Historically these were the first types of interfaces used in health care.

More recent technology uses **interface engine** software to create and manage interfaces. This provides the ability to transfer information from the sending system to one or many receiving systems and allows users of different information systems to access and exchange information both in real-time and batch processing. **Real-time processing** occurs immediately, whereas **batch processing** typically occurs once daily. In this situation, data are often not processed until the end of the day and therefore are not available to users until that time. Although batch processing was very common in the past, the current trend is toward real-time processing.

The interface engine provides seamless integration and presentation of information results. Interface engines work in the background and are not seen by the user. This technology allows applications to interact with hardware and other applications. Interface engines allow different systems that use unlike terminology to exchange information. This is done through the use of translation tables to move data from each system to the **clinical data repository,** a database where collective data from all information systems are stored and managed. The clinical data repository provides data definition consistency through mapping. **Mapping** is the process in which terms defined in one system are

---

Box 11–2 **Interface Engine Benefits**

- Improves timeliness and availability of critical administrative and clinical data
- Decreases integration costs by providing an alternative to customized point-to-point interface application programming
- Improves data quality because of data mapping and consistent use of terms
- Allows clients to select the best system for their needs
- Preserves institutional investment in existing systems
- Simplifies the administration of health care data processing
- Simplifies systems integration efforts
- Shortens the time required for integration
- Improves management of care, the financial tracking of care rendered, and efficacy of treatment

---

associated with comparable terms in another system. The major impact of using interface engines is that mappings for multiple receiving systems can be built for each sending system. For example, a client registration system can send registration transactions to the interface engine, which then forwards them on to any number of ancillary systems such as laboratory, radiology, and pharmacy. Each of these systems is able to receive updated client health care and demographic information, eliminating the need to manually register the client in the ancillary system. Box 11–2 discusses some of the benefits associated with the use of interface engines.

Interfacing of laboratory orders and results provides another example of how the interface engine is used in a hospital setting. On admission, the client's demographic information is entered in the hospital registration system, and portions of these data are transmitted to the clinical data repository via the interface engine. When a laboratory order is entered into the order entry system, the appropriate client demographic information is retrieved from the clinical data repository and used by the order entry system. After the order is entered, the order information may be transmitted via the interface engine to the clinical data repository and the laboratory system. When testing is complete, the results are transferred via the interface engine from the laboratory system to the clinical data repository. At this point, they are available for retrieval using the order entry system or another clinical information system.

Interface engines require new skills in the information services department. Staff may now include an integration analyst who will identify initial and ongoing interface specifications, coordinate any changes that will impact interfaces, and maintain a database for translation tables. This analyst must ascertain that data integrity is intact for all data to be sent correctly through the interface engine.

INTEGRATION ISSUES

Integration is a massive project within institutions and enterprises. It generally requires more time and effort than originally projected. Several factors contribute to this situation. First, vendors frequently make promises about their products to make a sale; often these promises cannot be delivered. Second, merged institutions may prefer to keep their own systems rather than accept a uniform standard that would be easier to implement. The strategy adopted in this situation may require further negotiation and additional programming. Third, as each department and institution tries to retain its own identity and political power, it is difficult to come to an agreement on a common data dictionary, data mapping, and clinical data repository issues. Another issue is that integration brings a number of concerns for individuals, including changes in job description, learning new skills, the fear of job loss, and the general fear of change. Box 11–3 identifies several factors that may impede the integration process.

THE NEED FOR INTEGRATION STANDARDS

The need to exchange client data is rapidly increasing in response to the demands placed by managed care as well as consumer demands for improved levels of health care. To derive the utmost benefit from data, it must

---

Box 11–3 **Factors That Slow Integration**

- *Unrealistic vendor promises.* Vendors may promise that their information system easily interfaces with other systems. Many customers find they face difficult, lengthy, and costly integration efforts after they have already purchased the system.

- *Unrealistic institutional timetable.* This is often based on a lack of understanding of the complexity of the integration process.

- *Changing user specifications.* As the integration process proceeds, users frequently request additional capabilities or change their minds regarding initial specifications.

- *Lack of vendor support.* Vendors may not provide enough support and assistance to facilitate the integration efforts.

- *Insufficient documentation.* Information regarding existing systems and related programming is imperative for achieving successful integration.

- *Lack of agreement among merged institutions.* Individual facilities within a merged enterprise may wish to continue use of their existing systems. This means there are more systems to integrate.

- *All components of a vendor's products may not work together.* Although difficulties are expected in attempts to integrate competing vendor's products, there may also be problems in integrating products developed by the same vendor.

have a consistent or standard meaning across institution, enterprise, and alliance boundaries, facilitating the exchange of client data. This is the basis for developing a data dictionary within an enterprise and a uniform language for use on a national and global scale. It is becoming increasingly important for hospitals and information system vendors to adopt and use uniform standards for the electronic exchange of clinical information (Ball and Farish-Hunt 2003). Use of uniform standards will provide safer and more efficient health care delivery systems and also play a critical role in compliance with government health care regulations.

Data Dictionary

The **data dictionary** defines terminology to ensure consistent understanding and use across the enterprise. Terms defined in the data dictionary should include synonyms found in the various systems used within the enterprise. This may be achieved, in some cases, through the use of the interface engine. For example, a term or data element may be a diagnosis or a laboratory test such as potassium. Potassium may be known in the nursing order entry system as "potassium" but be called "K" in the laboratory system. The use of the data dictionary and interface engine facilitates integration and allows for the collection of aggregate data.

Master Patient Index

The integration process may require enhancements to the data dictionary, the clinical data repository, and the master patient index. The **master patient index** (MPI) is a database that lists all identifiers assigned to one client in all the information systems used within an enterprise. It assigns a global identification number for each client and allows clients to be identified by demographic information provided at the point of care. The MPI may use first and last names, birthdates, Social Security numbers, and driver's license numbers. It cannot rely on a single type of number such as the Social Security number, because of duplicates and the fact that some people, such as noncitizens, may not have one. When the MPI cannot match records based on demographic data, all possible matches are provided for the user to view and select. The MPI is a critical component in supporting successful integration. Not all health care enterprises have a data dictionary, a clinical data repository, or MPI, or these components may be in various stages of development. The move toward creating a lifetime patient record creates the need to access client encounters across time. This is particularly important in a multi-institutional enterprise. The MPI, data dictionary, and clinical data repository are tools that support this effort.

The MPI saves work because vital information can be obtained from the database rather than rekeyed with each client visit. This decreases the possibility of making a mistake and eliminates the inadvertent creation of duplicate records. As a result, the registration clerk now plays a greater role in the maintenance of data integrity.

Some of the key features of an effective MPI include the following:

- It locates records in real time for timely retrieval of information.
- It is flexible enough to allow inclusion of additional identification.
- It is easily reconfigured to accommodate network changes.
- It can grow to fit an organization of any size.

Uniform Language

One step in the integration process is the development of a uniform definition of terms, or language. This is essential for the easy location and manipulation of data. Many efforts to develop uniform languages are under way in the health care arena. For example, the National Library of Medicine has developed the Unified Medical Language System (UMLS), which includes the Uniform Nursing Language. In addition, the American Nurses Association sponsors the Congress of Nursing Practice Steering Committee on Databases (ANA revises criteria 1996). This group addresses issues including nursing classification schemes, uniform data sets, data elements, and national databases. One of its primary goals is to develop a mapping system to link various classification schemes. This would allow the development of national data sets for use by nursing.

There are several nursing classification systems currently in place, with the most prominent being the following three (Butcher 2004). North American Nursing Diagnosis Association (NANDA)—now NANDA-International is an organization that has developed a system for classifying nursing diagnoses or statements that identify client care problems that nurses are licensed to treat independently (Thede 1999). Nursing Intervention Classification (NIC) is a classification system developed at the University of Iowa to categorize interventions based on clinical judgment and knowledge that nurses perform to improve client outcome (Butcher 2004). Nursing Outcome Classification (NOC) allows nurses to measure client outcome status at any point in the continuum of care. This information can be used as input for revising the plan of care. NANDA, NIC, and NOC are designed to be used together as one large system for classifying nursing care (Thede 1999).

These allow the collection of data related to nursing care, providing many benefits such as the following:

- Collection and analysis of nursing care data for documentation in the client record
- Support of the development of an EHR by classifying and categorizing nursing data
- Facilitation of the evaluation of client care

In addition to nursing, coding systems are used in other areas of health care to communicate information about medical diagnoses and procedures performed. This information is most commonly captured using the **ICD-9/ICD-10** and **CPT-4** systems. ICD-9 (International Classification of Disease – Ninth Revision) provides a classification for surgical, diagnostic, and therapeutic procedures (Thede 1999). This information is used for hospital billing and third party payment throughout the United States. *ICD-10* is an enlarged version of *ICD-9* that is generally used in Europe at this time. The *ICD-9/ICD-10* systems are published by the National Center for Health Statistics. Another commonly used classification is *CPT-4 (Current Procedural Terminology – Fourth Revision)*, which is published annually by the American Medical Association. This system lists medical services and procedures performed by physicians and is used for physician billing and payor reimbursement.

SNOMED (Systemized Nomenclature of Human and Veterinary Medicine) is a classification system created by the College of American Pathologists (Thede 1999). This system includes signs and symptoms of disease, diagnoses, and procedures and is meant to represent the full integration of all medical information in an electronic medical record.

Data Exchange Standards

In addition to the uniform definition of terms, integration standards facilitate the exchange of client data by providing a set of rules and structure for formatting the data. A major standard for the exchange of clinical data for integration is Health Level 7 (HL7). HL7 refers to both an organization and its standards for the exchange of clinical data. The mission of the organization is to provide standards for the management and integration of health care data (Schulten 2003). In particular, these standards address definitions of data to be exchanged, the timing of the exchanges, and communication of certain errors between applications. HL7 provides a structure that defines data and elements and specifies how the data are coded. The structure of the data element must follow HL7 rules, such as those specifying the length of the fields and the code nomenclature. Use of HL7 standards in individual applications will improve the integration of these applications with other applications or systems. Benefits include easier and less costly integration within an organization and more accurate and useful data integration nationally and globally. Integration efforts and the development and use of integration standards, including HL7, are taking place at many levels. For example, integration is seen beyond the hospital setting in the form of integrated delivery systems (IDS). Although efforts are under way to develop both national and international health data networks, competition does not now encourage this type of information sharing. Standards may be in place but not necessarily be used. Another factor is that HL7 standards may be somewhat modified by information system vendors to support various applications. These variations must be addressed during the integration process.

HL7 standards are not the only standards that have been evolving to fit the changing health care model. Other organizations have also been instrumental in supporting the development of standards and in helping to define data exchange. These organizations include the Institute of Medicine and the National Committee on Vital and Health Statistics (NCVHS) (Gillespie 2003a). This advisory committee to the U.S. Department of Health and Human Services promotes standardization of code sets, nomenclatures, and terminology for inclusion in a standard clinical vocabulary. The major goal of this group is to enable health care organizations and their information systems to speak the same language. They are reviewing many existing codes sets such as *CPT* and ICD-9 (International Statistics Classification of Diseases and related health problems), NANDA (nursing diagnosis definitions and classifications), NIC, NOC, and SNOMED (Systematized Nomenclature of Medicine), with the goal of creating one standard clinical vocabulary.

BENEFITS OF INTEGRATION

One major benefit of integration and the ability to exchange client data is the development of the electronic health record. In this case, integration allows data from many disparate information systems to be accessed from one point by the user, providing a complete record for each client. The clinical data repository is a key element of the EHR. It provides a storage facility for clinical data over time. The data in the clinical data repository may be generated from various systems and locations. For example, laboratory data may be generated by a laboratory system and may be collected in an acute, ambulatory, or long-term care setting. Other data may be included from clinical systems such as radiology, pharmacy, and order entry. Decision support applications that use clinical repository data can be used at other facilities if data from all facilities can be mapped to the data dictionary. One of the stumbling blocks to the creation and maintenance of the clinical data repository may be poor documentation regarding term definitions in the individual systems collecting the data. Figure 11–1 depicts an example of mapping with laboratory test terms.

Hospitals and health care enterprises also benefit from integration. Using integration strategies will permit data exchange within each hospital and across health care networks or enterprises, allowing them to find trends in financial and clinical data. Integration can open up a realm of possibilities for new ways to chart data trends, such as by provider, by diagnosis, or by cost. In this way, health care providers can obtain improved information, making them better able to react to market changes and maintain a competitive edge.

Integration of related systems such as Radiology Information System (RIS), Picture Archiving Communication System (PACS), and the EHR provides clinicians with a greatly enhanced view of diagnostic radiology information that can be accessed from many points within the hospital or remotely. This integration provides the abilty to view an electronic text report

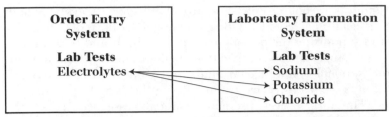

The order entry system lists a test called Electrolytes. The laboratory information system does not list a test called Electrolytes but lists its individual component tests. Before the interface engine can allow exchange of data, the relationships between the tests listed in both systems must be established by mapping.

FIGURE 11–1 • Mapping of laboratory test terms

related to a radiology examination from the EHR and then seamlessly view the associated electronic images from the PACS sytems. A standard client identifier used by all the organizations' information systems is key to creating this type of integration (Gillespie 2003b).

The lack of data integration is a barrier to effective data reporting and analysis (Merlo and Freundl 1999). For example, executive information needs may require data regarding all aspects of an obstetric client's care, including prenatal care, risk factors, complications before admission, length of hospital stay, and cost of the entire episode of care. Some of this information may be stored in an independent information system in the physician's office. Other data may be found in the hospital clinical information system and in the financial system. Without effective integration of clinical, financial, and administrative data, it is difficult to provide a complete system information base for management and decision support.

Another benefit of integration is that it facilitates data collection for accreditation processes. For example, Joint Commission on Accreditation of Healthcare Organizations (JCAHO) requirements call for the ability to provide aggregate data. These requirements include the following:

- Uniform definition of data
- Uniform methods for data capture
- Ability to provide client-specific as well as aggregate data

These information standards allow JCAHO to compare data within and among health care enterprises.

INTEGRATION IMPLICATIONS FOR NURSING

There are also particular concerns for nursing in relation to system integration. A primary consideration is that nursing involvement is essential in the interface design phase. Nurses must be involved in identifying and defining data elements that an interface may be able to supply. One way to ensure this is to recruit staff nurses to provide input during the interface design.

Another concern is ensuring that data will be collected in only one system and shared via the interface engine and clinical data repository with all other systems requiring it (Merlo and Freundl 1999). This eliminates redundant effort while ensuring data integrity. For example, a client's allergies should be identified and documented by a nurse and entered into a clinical information system. This data are then transmitted to the clinical data repository via the interface engine, where it is available for retrieval by other systems that may require it, such as a pharmacy system.

Nursing can also benefit from integration and data exchange. For example, trends in client care data and cost analysis can be used to justify nursing staffing levels in the hospital setting. In addition, integration provides a tool to build nursing knowledge.

EMERGING INTEGRATION SOLUTIONS

The traditional integration process is an enormous project that is costly and may require many years to complete. An emerging solution for providing interim access to data from disparate systems involves the use of Web-based tools and a hospital's intranet or the Internet (Turisco 1999). These tools often require a Web browser, security clearance, and an intranet or Internet connection. Most of these tools allow view-only access to various diverse applications used within the enterprise. Some may provide a minimal level of update capability. Access to client data from many systems is managed by the use of a common patient identifier, or MPI, which will allow the user to identify the client only once and then view that client's information from a number of separate information systems. Although this Web-based approach provides immediate data access, it is not a replacement for integration between information systems. Its value is that it requires minimal maintenance effort, while remaining a low-cost interim solution.

CASE STUDY EXERCISES

You have been selected as a member of the Integration Project Team, which is charged with identifying ways that system integration could improve information flow. You work on an inpatient unit that uses a stand-alone nursing documentation system that is not interfaced or integrated with any other hospital information system. Identify the implications of this situation, and suggest integration options that could improve information flow.

• • •

You are working to identify elements in your health care enterprise that could be used for a master patient index (MPI). List five basic elements and describe how each could be used for an MPI.

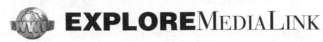

EXPLOREMEDIALINK

Multiple choice review questions, case studies, and other interactive resources for this chapter can be found on the Web site at *http://www.prenhall.com/hebda*. Click on "Chapter 11" to select the activities for this chapter.

SUMMARY

- An interface is a computer program that tells two different systems how to exchange data.

- Most health care providers have a variety of automated information systems that do not readily share data unless major efforts are made to build interfaces.

- Integration is the process by which different information systems are able to exchange data without any special effort on the part of the end user.

- The creation of networks to exchange data between systems and the process of integration are essential in today's health care information world, where an institution or enterprise may have multiple disparate clinical information systems.

- The interface engine is a software application designed to allow users of different information systems to exchange information without the need to build direct customized interfaces between systems.

- Other processes that facilitate the move toward integration and the exchange of client information include the clinical data repository, mapping, the data dictionary, the master patient index, uniform language efforts, and data exchange standards.

- The clinical data repository is a database that collects and stores data from all information systems.

- Mapping of terms establishes the relationship between terms defined in one system and those used in another.

- The data dictionary defines terms used within an enterprise to ensure consistent use.

- The master patient index lists all identifiers assigned to one client in all information systems and assigns a global identification code as a means to locate all records for a given client.

- Standardization of clinical terms through a uniform language is one means to facilitate the exchange of information across health care enterprises. The Congress of Nursing Practice Steering Committee on Databases and the National Library of Medicine (through its Unified Medical Language System) are working on uniform language issues.

- Some commonly used nursing classifcation systems are NANDA, NIC, and NOC.

- Health Level 7 is a standard for the exchange of clinical data that provides rules and structure for how data are formatted.

- Integration improves data integrity and access for caregivers, eliminates redundant data collection, and improves data collection for staffing, for finding financial trends and client outcome trends, and for meeting requirements of regulatory and accrediting organizations.

- Integration is a necessary component for the development of the electronic health record and for integrated delivery systems.

- An interim solution to the costly and time-consuming process of integration is the use of Web-based tools to access client data from various systems using the hospital's intranet or the Internet.

REFERENCES

ANA revises criteria for evaluating nursing vocabularies, classification systems. (November/December 1996). *The American Nurse*, 9.

Ball, M., and Farish-Hunt, H. (2003). Standards at center stage. *Healthcare Informatics*, *20*(11), 52–54.

Bazzoli, F. (1996). Providers point to index software as key element of integration plans. *Health Data Management*, *4*(9), 61–65.

Butcher, H. (2004). Nursing's distinctive knowledge. In L. Haynes, T. Boese, and H. Butcher (Eds.), *Nursing in contemporary society: Issues, trends and transition to practice* (pp. 71–103). Upper Saddle River, NJ: Pearson Prentice Hall.

Hebda, T., Czar, P., and Mascara C. (2004). Information technology. In L. Haynes, T. Boese, and H. Butcher (Eds.), *Nursing in contemporary society: Issues, trends and transition to practice* (pp. 163–183). Upper Saddle River, NJ: Pearson Prentice Hall.

Gillespie, G. (2003a). NCVHS to extol a standard vocab. *Health Data Management*, *11*(5), 50–58.

Gillespie, G. (2003b). Trying to form a more perfect union. *Health Data Management*, *11*(11), 26–34.

Hammond, W. E. (June 1996). Politics and standards. *HL7 News*, 13.

Koob, L. (2000). Integrating data is key to enhancing information systems. *Ophthalmology Times*, *25*(1), 13–14.

Merlo, J., and Freundl, M. (1999). Overcoming the barriers to cross-continuum information integration. *Healthcare Financial Management*, *53*(6), 35–38.

Schulten, C. (2003). The mission of Health Level 7. *Healthcare Informatics*, *20*(9), 68.

Thede, L. Q. (1999). *Computers in nursing: Bridges to the future.* Philadelphia: Lippincott.

Turisco, F. (1999). Using internet technology to extend access to legacy systems. *Healthcare Financial Management, 53*(5), 86.

The Electronic Health Record

After completing this chapter, you should be able to:

- Define the term *electronic health record (EHR)*.

- Define the term *computer-based patient record (CPR)*.

- Discuss the similarities and differences between the EHR and the CPR.

- Understand the 12 characteristics of the CPR, as defined by the Institute of Medicine.

- Discuss the benefits associated with the EHR.

- Review the current status of the EHR, including impediments.

- List several concerns that must be resolved before implementation of the EHR.

- Define *community health information network (CHIN)*.

- Describe the current status of CHINs in the United States.

 MEDIALINK

Additional resources for this content can be found on the Companion Website at *www. prenhall.com/hebda*. Click on "Chapter 12" to select the activities for this chapter.

Companion Website

- Glossary
- Multiple Choice
- Discussion Points
- Case Study: Designing the EHR
- Case Study: External Sources
- Case Study: Implications of Electronic Client Information
- MediaLink Application: An Electronic Medical Record Program
- Links to Resources
- Crossword Puzzle

R equirements for the management of health care information are evolving—transforming the ways that health care providers store, access, and use information. The traditional paper medical record that reports client status and test results no longer meets the needs of today's health care industry. Paper records are episode-oriented with a separate record for each client visit. Key information, such as allergies, may be lost from one episode to the next jeopardizing patient safety. Another drawback to paper records is that only one person can access the record at any given time. As a consequence of this fact, health care providers waste time looking for paper records and treatment may be delayed. Paper records cannot incorporate diagnostic studies that may include images and sound, nor do they make use of decision support systems. The electronic health record (EHR) has the potential to integrate all pertinent patient information into one record as well as improve the quality of health information, patient safety, contain costs, support research, and contribute to the body of health care knowledge (Aspden, Corrigan, Wolcott, and Erickson 2004; IOM 2003; Dochterman and Jones 2003).

DEFINITIONS

Numerous terms have been used over the years to describe the concept of an electronic health record. This situation has created confusion about the terminology and definitions related to the EHR. Some of the other terms frequently used include electronic medical record (EMR), computer-based patient record (CPR), and CPR system, as described later.

The **electronic health record (EHR)** is a "secure, real-time, point-of-care, patient-centric information resource for clinicians" (Healthcare Information and Management Systems Society [HIMSS] 2003, p. 2). It provides access to the client health record information at the time and place that clinicians need it. In addition, it provides evidence-based decision support, it automates and streamlines the clinician's workflow, and it supports the collection of data for uses other than direct client care. This includes billing, quality management, outcomes reporting, resource planning, and public health disease surveillance and reporting. HIMSS is in the process of developing a document, *HIMSS Electronic Health Record Definitional Model*, which outlines the definitions, attributes, and requirements for assessing the extent to which an organization is using an EHR. The attributes of the EHR, as identified in this document, include the following:

1. Provides secure, reliable real-time access to client health record information where and when it is needed to support care
2. Captures and manages episodic and longitudinal EHR information
3. Functions as clinicians' primary information resources during the provision of client care

4. Assists with the work of planning and delivery of evidence-based care to individual and groups of clients

5. Captures data used for continuous quality improvement, utilization review, risk management, resource planning, and performance management

6. Captures the patient health-related information needed for medical record and reimbursement

7. Provides longitudinal, appropriately masked information to support clinical research, public health reporting, and population health initiatives

8. Supports clinical trials and evidence-based research

In July 2003, the Department of Health and Human Services announced the formation of the EHR Collaborative (*www.ehrcollaborative.org*). This group of founding stakeholder organizations is charged with the task of facilitating rapid input from the health care community to support the adoption of standards for the EHR. Member orgranizations include the following:

• American Health Information Management Association (AHIMA)
• American Medical Association (AMA)
• American Medical Informatics Association (AMIA)
• American Nurses Association (ANA)
• College of Healthcare Information Management Executives (CHIME)
• eHealth Initiative (eHI)
• Healthcare Information and Management Systems Society HIMSS
• National Alliance for Health Information Technology (NAHIT)

The EHR Collaborative sponsored a series of open forum meetings in August 2003 and synthesized the input received into the "Final Report: Public Response to HL7 EHR Ballot 1." This report is available online at *www.ehrcollaborative.org*. The health care industry is developing a functional model and industry agreed-on standards. Once completed, the nationally agreed-on standards for the EHR will affect the entire health care community. For example, the following areas will be affected:

• Hospitals
• Physicians
• Payers
• Researchers
• Pharmacies
• Public health agencies
• Patients

Older terminology related to the EHR include the EMR and the CPR. Waegemann (2003) explains the relationship of these terms, many of which are still used today. The EHR is the generic term for all electronic health care systems. It has since become the favored term for the lifetime computerized record. The CPR is a lifetime client record that includes all information from all specialties, while the EMR is the electronic medical record for one episode. The PCR (patient-carried record) is the client's health record on a portable card that is carried by the patient. The EPR is the electronic client record but does not necessarily contain the lifetime record, focusing on relevant information for this episode of care.

The EMR is an electronic version of the client data found in the traditional paper medical record. The six basic components of the EMR include the following:

- Clinical messaging and e-mail
- Results reporting
- Data repository
- Decision support
- Clinical documentation
- Order entry

EMR result reporting and data repository components include unstructured data, which are data that do not follow any particular format and often are provided as a text report. Examples are reports produced by transcription services including history and physical assessments, consultation findings, operative reports, and discharge summaries. The EMR also includes structured data, which are data that follow a predefined format and are often presented as discrete data elements. Structured data are often obtained from automated ancillary reporting systems; a primary example is laboratory results from an automated laboratory information system. Another type of data that may be included in the EMR is electronic imaging produced by diagnostic studies, including tomography, ultrasonography, and magnetic resonance imaging. Although the EMR is often confused with the CPR, the EMR is generally defined as one component of the EHR. The CPR is a comprehensive lifetime record, while the EMR is the record for a single treatment episode. The classic definition and attributes of the CPR, as identified by the Institute of Medicine (IOM), provide the basis for today's understanding of the EHR.

HISTORICAL DEVELOPMENTS

The IOM identified the following 12 major components of the CPR, which they consider the "gold standard" attributes (Andrew and Bruegel 2003):

1. Provides a problem list that indicates the client's current clinical problems for each encounter. A problem list should also denote

the number of occurrences associated with all past and current problems, as well as the current status of the problem.

2. Evaluates and records health status and functional levels using accepted measures. In the current competitive health care market, increased attention to measuring outcomes and quality of care are imperative, and must begin to be addressed by information system departments and vendors.

3. Documents the clinical reasoning/rationale for diagnoses and conclusions. Allows sharing of clinical reasoning with other caregivers and automates and tracks decision making.

4. Provides a longitudinal or lifetime client record by linking all of the client's data from previous encounters.

5. Supports confidentiality, privacy, and audit trails. System developers must supply multiple levels of security to ensure appropriate access to confidential client information.

6. Provides continuous access to authorized users. Users must be able to access the client record at any time.

7. Allows simultaneous and customized views of the client data for individuals, departments, or enterprises. This ability improves efficiency for the specific users by allowing the data to be presented in a format that is most useful to them. The flexibility to support multiple different and simultaneous views of client data is a feature that many vendors find difficult to achieve.

8. Supports links to local or remote information resources, such as various databases using the Internet or organization-based intranet resource. Access to pertinent information from various external sources will provide the caregiver with needed information in a timely and effective format that can be used to support client care. Examples include access to literature searches and drug information databases.

9. Facilitates clinical problem solving by providing decision analysis tools. Examples include simple support, such as timely reminders regarding health maintenance activities, and rules-based alerts that supply decision-making support for the physician.

10. Supports direct entry of client data by physicians. The question of how to provide a simple and acceptable mechanism for direct entry of data by physicians without relying on dictation continues to be a problem for vendors.

11. Includes mechanisms for measuring the cost and quality of care. This area is vitally important in providing a significant competitive edge in today's health care market.

12. Supports existing and evolving clinical needs by being flexible and expandable. Many information systems address specific areas of specialty such as emergency or ambulatory care. These systems may be difficult to customize and expand to meet the specific needs of the health care enterprise.

Most of the data included in the CPR are automated structured data. Other data formats may also be linked to the CPR, including dictation and transcription, images, video, and text. These data, and collective data from all systems, are stored and managed in the clinical data repository. This database allows retrieval of multiple elements of client data regardless of their system of origin. For example, the user may retrieve a lab result from the clinical data repository that was originally produced by the laboratory information system (LIS), along with a radiology report that was generated in the radiology information system (RIS) from a transcribed dictation. Collectively, these various systems and the clinical data repository make up the CPR.

The development of data exchange standards is instrumental for the implementation of the CPR. These standards will allow the uniform capture of data that is required to build a longitudinal record comprising integrated information systems from multiple vendors. Figure 12–1 shows some sample components of the CPR.

BENEFITS OF THE EHR

The driving forces for the development of the EHR are client safety and managed care. A well-developed EHR facilitates the provision of quality

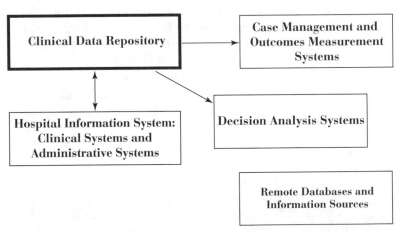

The CPR comprises the systems shown above. Client data flows between the systems as indicated by the arrows. External databases and information sources may also be accessed by the CPR, even though no client data flow to them.

FIGURE 12–1 • A Sample of EHR components

care and management of costs. The powerful framework of the CPR optimizes the collection, presentation, and communication of client data. This results in time and money savings for anyone who participates in the health care delivery process, including clients, physicians, and health care providers and payers.

The benefits of the EHR can be best understood when considering the needs of various groups of users. Some of the benefits are general, but others relate to nurses, physicians, and other care providers, as well as the health care enterprise.

General Benefits

- *Improved data integrity.* Information is more readable, better organized, and more accurate and complete.
- *Increased productivity.* Caregivers are able to access client information whenever it is needed and at multiple convenient locations. This can result in improved client care due to the ability to make timely decisions based on appropriate data.
- *Improved quality of care.* The EHR supports clinical decision-making processes for physicians and nurses.
- *Increased satisfaction for caregivers.* Caregivers are able to take advantage of easy access to client data as well as other services, including drug information sources, rules-based decision support, and literature searches.

Nursing Benefits

- Current data and data from previous events are easily compared.
- The nurse can maintain an ongoing record of the client's education and learning response across various encounters or visits.
- Baseline demographic and assessment data do not have to be repeated for each encounter.
- Data that have been entered is universally available to all who have access to the EHR.
- Data for research are more readily available and of better quality.
- Prompts are provided to ensure administration and documentation of medications and treatments.
- Automation of critical and clinical pathways is facilitated.
- When used with a common unified structure for nursing language, the electronic health record supports the development of a database that facilitates research, provides information useful to administrators and clinicians, and allows recognition of nursing work in measurable units (Dochterman and Jones 2003).

Physician Benefits

- Multiple users can access the client record simultaneously.
- Physician can easily access previous encounters.
- Chart access is faster. There is no need to wait for old records to be delivered from the medical records department.
- Better reporting tools. Trends and clinical graphics are available on demand.
- Physicians can save time and reduce liability through better documentation (Barrett 2000).
- System generated prompts can improve compliance with preventive care protocols.

Health Care Enterprise Benefits

- Client record security is improved.
- Less space is needed for record storage.
- The medical record department saves costs because of decreased need for pulling, filing, and copying of charts.
- Client eligibility for coverage in managed care settings is easily verified.
- Cost evaluation is improved based on clinical outcomes and resource utilization data (Barrett 2000).
- Facilitates compliance with regulatory requirements.

CURRENT STATUS OF THE EHR

Box 12–1 lists six qualities of a successful EHR. While many organizations struggle with the slow piecemeal conversion to electronic medical records, unintended negative outcomes may be seen. These include increased workloads and delayed information retrieval as clinicians search multiple data sources for client information (Barrett 2000).

Considerations when Implementing the EHR

Information system vendors as well as health care providers are, for the most part, aware of the pressing need to develop the EHR and are continuously working toward its evolvement. Development of an electronic infrastructure and cost are the two major impediments to the creation of a fully functioning EHR. The principal requirement is that the major participants in the health care arena, including health care facilities, payers, and physicians, must be linked electronically. This is a very costly undertaking in many cases. Other impediments include the lack of a common vocabulary, security and confidentiality issues, and resistance among caregivers.

Box 12–1
Qualities of a Successful EHR

1. Fast	The user is able to quickly enter and retrieve data.
2. Familiar	The EHR follows familiar graphical user Interface (GUI) conventions.
3. Flexible	The EHR allows personalization of documentation style, enabling it to meet the information needs of many types and categories of users.
4. Enhances Workflow	The EHR improves work efficiency and effectiveness.
5. Improves Documentation	The user sees the EHR improving the process of documentation.
6. Meets Regulatory Requirements	The EHR supports the regulatory requirements related to data content and security measures.

Electronic Infrastructure The health care facilities, payers, and physicians must all have the ability to access and update the client's longitudinal record. In other words, the various information systems that support these stakeholders must be linked electronically by the network infrastructure. Agreement must first be reached regarding the nature and format of client data to be stored, as well as the mechanisms for data exchange, storage, and retrieval. This means that all participants must use common data communication standards. First and most important is the decision regarding the recognition of a universal client identifier, such as a Social Security Number or MPI (master patient index) number, so that all client data can be associated with the correct client. Improvements in connectivity alone are not enough to support the EHR. It is also important to include components such as interoperability, comparability, decision support, and point-of-care data capture to achieve a longitudinal electronic record. (Amatayakul 2000).

Cost Another impediment to the EHR is cost (Gaillour 1999). The development of the electronic links forming the infrastructure is costly, and the allocation of fiscal responsibilities is difficult. Currently each health care enterprise or system is paying for its own EHR development. Links to other facilities and agencies are rare and for the most part limited to provider–payer arrangements. Further progress is likely to be minimal until decisions regarding cost allocation are reached.

Vocabulary Standardization There is little standardization in health care settings regarding the medical vocabulary or language used in client records. This lack of standards prevents the integrating of discrete and disparate data from multiple sources into one complete record (Waegemann,

2003). Additional progress in the development of a universal medical and nursing language will support the development of the EHR. This effort is already under way with the development of the Nursing Minimum Data Set.

A conference brought together the leaders of the NANDA and the center for nursing classification and clinical effectiveness to create a common unifying structure across the three languages NANDA, NIC, and NOC. The goal of this alliance is to advance the development, testing, and refinement of nursing language. NANDA has been integrated into SNOMED. Additional work will still need to be done but this is a significant development in the vocabulary standardization.

Security and Confidentiality Security and confidentiality concerns are critical considerations in EHR development (Mendoza 2003). The EHR system must be configured to allow access only to those who have been identified as authorized users. The system must authenticate the user's identiy with user IDs and passwords and possibly biometrics. HIPAA considerations include the need to be able to provide the client, upon request, with a log of caregivers who have accessed their chart. In addition, client information should not be available to anyone without the client's approval. Data that is communicated via the Internet must be encrytped. Firewalls must be in place when data are sent and received via the Internet to safeguard its integrity.

Caregiver Resistance Resistance on the part of caregivers such as physicians and nurses also acts as an impediment to the development and use of the EHR. The fully developed EHR necessitates mandatory use of computers by caregivers as part of their daily routine. Some individuals are unable or unwilling to use computers; this may be related to various factors such as the complexity of software, the availability of workstations, and resistance to change in the work patterns. Some physicians believe that data entry is demeaning and a waste of time and interferes with their ability to provide client care on a timely basis. In addition, they may resist perceived changes to the way they practice medicine that will be required by the EHR system (Rogoski 2003). Actual practice reveals that nearly all physicians will do some data entry, but only a few will do a lot (Gaillour 1999).

Data Integrity

Data integrity can be compromised in three ways: incorrect entry, data tampering, and system failure. In general, data integrity can be improved by implementing security measures, including the use of audit trails, as well as the development of detailed procedures and policies.

Incorrect Data Entry The client data found in the EHR are only as accurate as the person who enters them and the systems that transfer them.

Therefore, critical information, such as allergies and code status, should be verified for accuracy at each encounter. This will allow the correction of data entry errors and screen for changes that have occurred in client status. This is especially crucial because data may be entered or modified from many different encounters in the health care arena, such as hospitals, clinics, and home care visits. Data integrity is also compromised if an interface is not receiving or sending data correctly (Walizer 2003). When corrections to the data in the electronic record must be made, it is imperative to correct the data in multiple areas. The data in the source system must be corrected, as well as any receiving systems. This may involve correction using interface transactions or manual intervention.

Data Correction In addition to accidental data entry errors, it is possible for an individual to make malicious data modifications. An effective audit trail procedure permits the tracking of who entered or modified each data element, allowing appropriate follow-up measures.

Master File Maintenance The development and maintenance of various master files and data dictionaries is critical to maintining data integrity. Careful attention to initial development of the files, including documentation, will ensure that data are accurate and communicates valid information. Periodic review and validation of master files, at least annually, is necessary to maintain current and accurate data (Walizer 2003).

System Failure Hardware and software malfunctions, such as a system crash, may result in incomplete or lost data. Once the problem has been resolved, it may be necessary to verify the client data that could have been affected.

Ownership of the Patient Record

Currently, paper medical records are the property of the institution at which they are created. This institution is responsible for ensuring the accuracy and completeness of the record. With the development of the EHR, however, ownership issues become more complex. Because many providers use the same data, it is unclear who actually owns them and is responsible for maintaining their accuracy. Because the data are shared and updated from many sites, decisions must be made regarding who can access the data and how it will be used. In addition, it must be determined where the data will actually be stored.

Privacy and Confidentiality

Preservation of the client's privacy is one of the most basic and important duties of the health care provider. Because one of the key attributes of the EHR is the ease of data sharing, the client's privacy rights may not be guarded by all who have access to the record. Legislation such as HIPAA has been initiated that addresses electronic access to client records. In addition, health care providers must address client privacy rights when developing the electronic record.

Electronic Signature

The health care provider has always been required to authenticate entries into the paper medical record with a handwritten signature. This cannot be done with the EHR because all entries are electronic. An electronic signature must be used to authenticate electronic data entries (Cohen and Amatayakul 2003). A user's computer access code and/or password recognizes that individual by name and credentials and allows access to the system. The user should be required to sign a confidentiality statement before obtaining an access code, stating that no other person will be permitted to use the code. Other newer technologies, such as private encryption keys and biometric authentication, should be considered when developing an electronic signature mechanism (Tabar 2000).

Systems typically affix a date and time log to each entry, as well as the identity of the user in the form of an audit trail. The electronic signature is automatically and permanently attached to the document when it is created. This electronic signature cannot be forged or transferred to any other transaction and provides authentication of the health care provider.

SMART CARDS

One of the evolving technologies associated with the EHR is the smart card. The smart card is used to store client information such as demographics, allergies, blood type, current medications, current health problems, including recent findings, and payer or insurance provider. Some cards may also include the client's photograph. The smart card is similar in appearance to a plastic credit card. The smart cards that contain a microprocessing chip are able to store thousands more bits than a magnetic strip card (Tabar 2000). Smart cards allow client information and medical history to be accessed quickly, which may be important during an emergency. In nonemergency situations, the smart card allows the client to provide his or her history easily and accurately.

At the present time, smart cards are just beginning to be introduced in the United States; however, use is more widespread in Europe. A person carrying a smart card presents it to the health care provider at the time of treatment, and it is processed through an electronic card reader. The card provides detailed client information that is not part of an electronic network, thus ensuring accuracy and making information readily available. One of the major barriers to widespread use of the smart card is the cost (Reynolds 2003). In addition to the cost of the actual smart card, there is a cost associated with card readers. Each facility must have one or more card readers to access the information on the card. The operating system and software used by one facility's card and card reader may not be compatible with those used by other facilities, so the cards may not be able to be used by more than one organization.

CHINs

Another concept for information sharing among health networks is the CHIN, or Community Health Information Network. A CHIN can be defined as an organization that offers electronic connections that enable all providers, payors, and purchasers of care to exchange financial, clinical, and administrative information in a defined geographic location, eliminating redundant data collection and reducing paperwork (Tabar 2000). Regulatory agencies may receive information directly from CHINs. The CHIN concept emerged in the early 1990s, however, only a few communities created viable CHINs that continue to operate today. Most of these are in large metropolitan areas, such as Boston, Cincinnati, and Milwaukee. However, many other CHINs were not successful and no longer exist. The concept of community development has been a major challenge to the development of successful CHINs. Although CHINs have become somewhat out of fashion, the more recent emergence of Internet technology has led some to reconsider their viability. Figure 12–2 shows the relationship between the various CHIN participants within the community.

Information sharing within a CHIN should be accomplished in a manner that conveys data in a seamless, standardized electronic format. A

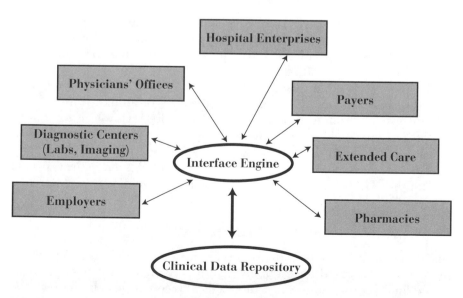

FIGURE 12–2 • Relationship between CHIN participants (Gordon 1996; copyright © *Healthcare Technology Management magazine*, HealthTech Publishing Company, East Providence, RI)

CHIN can be thought of as a network of networks, connecting the various networks of participating organizations into one large network. This allows for the retrieval of information without the user needing to know where the information actually resides. According to Bir and Zerrenner (1995), the four primary features of a CHIN are as follows:

1. *Open communications.* Open communications, facilitated by an interface engine, are necessary for providing access to the data throughout the CHIN. This provides connectivity between the computer-based patient record, various data repositories, and payer information, so that all data are available to the various participants in the CHIN.

2. *The EHR.* Access should be provided to the EHRs from all participating CHIN members.

3. *Clinical data repository.* The CHIN clinical data repository is a combination of all clinical data available from the various individual data repositories of each participating organization.

4. *Mechanisms for cost, outcome, and utilization analysis.* This type of analysis is based on information provided by the payers, as well as the outcomes recorded by the health care providers. The data can be manipulated and analyzed by decision support software, including rules-based analysis. For example, a clinical information system can suggest a treatment plan based on an analysis of the collective data from many clients available within the CHIN data repository.

In addition to providing access to client data, CHINs may also provide members with other types of services that facilitate and improve the management of client care. A list of the major services that may be available in a CHIN is given in Box 12–2.

The key factors that doomed CHINs in the 1990s were a lack of clear agreed-on objectives at the beginning and the focus on administrative transactions instead of safety and quality (Marietti 2004). However, the future of CHINs is uncertain. Some believe that this concept will be viable once industry-wide standards for the electronic health record are developed.

The CHIN concept has made an important contribution to the expectation for the EHR in terms of the ability to share information across systems.

CONSIDERATIONS FOR THE FUTURE

One of the stumbling blocks in the development of the EHR is the quest for the perfect system. Although many health care organizations have automated large portions of the patient's medical record, others hesitate to implement an EHR because they have not yet found a system that meets all of their expectations. It is suggested that these organizations implement something that can be useful today, even though it may not be perfect

Box 12–2

Information Available in a CHIN Data Repository

- Laboratory results
- Pathology results
- Radiology results
- Physician's dictation, including history and physical, progress notes, and discharge summaries
- Inpatient medication treatments
- Nursing care documentation
- Client demographic information
- Client health care insurance information
- Names of primary and consulting physicians

(Gaillour 1999). This will provide the capability to automate workflow with the goal to reduce steps and improve accuracy. Connectivity will allow the sharing of core client information across the organization. Finally, data will be available for reporting and analysis, providing the ability to benchmark client types, and individual client progress and outcomes (Barrett 2000).

A new concept with electronic records is the continuity of care record (CCR). This record is intended to improve continuity of care when clients move between various points of care. The CCR will include contributions from many types of caregivers, including physicians, nurses, physical therapists, and social workers. The record supports the patient's safety and has a positive impact on the quality and continuity of care (Tessier and Waegemann 2003).

CASE STUDY EXERCISES

You are a member of the committee charged with designing the EHR at your facility. Identify which components of nursing documentation should be retained in the clinical data repository. For example, would you want to include all client vital signs from the current hospital admission? Explain why you would include or exclude the various components.

• • •

Identify several external sources of information that would be useful as part of the EHR for access by a home health nurse.

• • •

Discuss the implications of providing nurses in a hospital setting with access to all electronic client information. Identify which types of information are appropriate for access by nurses.

EXPLOREMEDIALINK

Multiple choice review questions, case studies, and other interactive resources for this chapter can be found on the Web site at *http://www.prenhall.com/hebda*. Click on "Chapter 12" to select the activities for this chapter.

SUMMARY

- The electronic health record (EHR) is an electronic client record that includes client data, medical knowledge, and other essential health care information.
- The Institute of Medicine has identified 12 major components or characteristics of the CPR, which are designated as the "gold standard" attributes.
- The EHR offers benefits to nurses, physicians, and other health care providers, as well as to the health care enterprise.
- As of mid 2004, the EHR is still being defined and developed.
- Infrastructure, cost, vocabulary standardization, and caregiver resistance are the major impediments to the development of an EHR.
- Issues that must be considered when developing the EHR include data integrity, ownership of the patient record, privacy, and electronic signature.
- An emerging technology related to EHR development is the use of smart cards to store client information.
- Community health information networks (CHINs) are networks that allow the exchange of data among health care providers, payers, and purchasers of care within a defined geographic community.
- The four primary components of a CHIN are open communications, the computer-based patient record, a clinical data repository, and mechanisms for cost, outcomes, and utilization analysis.

REFERENCES

Amatayakul, M. (2000). Critical success factors: Steps to achieve a truly integrated information system. *Health Management Technology*, *21*(5), 14–18.

Andrew, W., & Bruegel, R. (2003). 2003 CPR systems. *ADVANCE for Health Information Executives*, *7*(9), 59–64.

Aspden, P., Corrigan, J. M., Wolcott, J., and Erickson, S. M. (Eds.). (2004). *Patient Safety: Achieving a New Standard for Care.* A report from the Institute of Medicine Committee on Data Standards for Patient Safety and Board on Health Care Services. Washington, DC: The National Academies Press. Available online at http://www.nap.edu/books/0309090776/html/. Accessed March 24, 2004.

Barrett, M. J. (2000). The evolving computerized medical record. *Healthcare Informatics, 17*(5), 85–93.

Bir, N., and Zerrenner, W. (1995). Network design and implementation of a CHIN from a hospital's perspective. Toward an electronic patient record '95. *Proceedings, 2,* 50–58.

Cohen, M., & Amatayakul, M. (2003). Electronic signatures. *ADVANCE for Health Information Executives, 7*(8), 16.

Dochterman, J. M., and Jones, D. A. (Eds.). (2003). *Unifying nursing languages: The harmonization of NANDA, NIC, and NOC.* Washington, DC: American Nurses Association.

Electronic medical records: Why their time has come. (2003). *Healthcare Informatics, 20*(9), Special advertising section, 1–8.

Gaillour, F. R. (1999). Rethinking the CPR: Is perfect the enemy of good? *Health Management Technology, 20*(4), 22–25.

Gordon, M. S. (1996). Get ready to take it on the CHIN. *Health Care Technology Management, 7*(5), 36–39.

HIMSS. (2003). *Electronic Health Record Definitional Model,* Version 1.1. Available online at http://www.himss.org/content/files/ehrattributes070703.pdf. Accessed March 24, 2004.

Institute of Medicine. (IOM) (2003). *Key capabilities of an electronic health record system.* A letter report Committee on Data Standards for Patient Safety and Board on Health Care Services. Washington, DC: The National Academies Press. Available online at http://books.nap.edu/catalog/10781.html. Accessed March 24, 2004.

Marietti, C. (2004). Health care transformation via infrastructure. *Healthcare Informatics, 21*(2). 44–50.

McFall, E. (1993). An electronic medical record—Delivering benefits today. *Healthcare Informatics, 10*(10), 76, 78.

Mendoza, E. (2003). Security considerations when choosing an EMR system. *Health Management Technology, 24*(10), 48.

Reynolds, P. (2003). Smarter than y1ou think. *Health Management Technology, 24*(12), 10–14.

Rogoski, R. (2003). Having it your way. *Health Management Technology, 24*(5), 12–16.

Tabar, P. (2000). The latest work: A glossary of healthcare information technology terms. *Healthcare Informatics, 17*(3), 75–133.

Tessier, C., & Waegemann, C. (2003). Continuity of care record. *Healthcare Informatics, 20*(10), 54–56.

The EHR collaborative report. Field response to the HL7 EHR Ballot 1. Available at www.chrcollabortive.org. Accessed August 29, 2003.

Waegemann. C. (2003) The EHR vs. CPR vs. EMR. *Healthcare Informatics, 20*(5). 40–44.

Walizer, D. (2003). Data integrity in master files. *ADVANCE for Health Information Executives, 7*(3), 18.

Regulatory and Accreditation Issues

After completing this chapter, you should be able to:

- Review important legislation for the protection of health care records, including HIPAA.

- Discuss issues related to the implementation of HIPAA administrative simplification requirements.

- Analyze the impact of HIPAA security requirements on the health care delivery system.

- Discuss the influence of major accrediting agencies and reimbursement issues on the design and use of information systems.

- Review design and implementation considerations for automated documentation systems in specialized facilities in light of legal and regulatory requirements.

 MEDIALINK

Additional resources for this content can be found on the Companion Website at *www.prenhall.com/hebda*. Click on "Chapter 13" to select the activities for this chapter.

Companion Website

- Glossary
- Multiple Choice
- Discussion Points
- Case Study: Protection of Client Record Information
- Case Study: Adherence to JCAHO Information Standards
- Case Study: CARF Standards
- Case Study: Patient Data
- MediaLink Application: JCAHO Virtual Tour
- Web Hunt: JCAHO Web Site
- Links to Resources
- Crossword Puzzle

Health care institutions deal with an increasing number of legislative and regulatory issues daily. There are local, state, and federal laws as well as watchdog agencies that safeguard private health information and monitor the quality of care delivered. Some of the organizations that perform accreditation and establish standards for health care delivery in the United States include (Saufl and Fieldus 2003):

- Joint Commission on Accreditation of Healthcare Organizations (JCAHO)
- Commission for Accreditation of Rehabilitation Facilities (CARF)
- National Committee for Quality Assurance (NCQA)
- American Medical Accreditation Program (AMAP)
- American Accreditation Healthcare Commission/Utilization Review Accreditation Commission (AAHC/URAC)
- Accreditation Association for Ambulatory Healthcare (AAAHC)
- American Association for the Accreditation of Ambulatory Surgical Facilities (AAAASF)

In addition, the Foundation for Accountability (FACCT) and the Agency for Healthcare Research and Quality (AHRQ) play important roles in ensuring the quality of health care. Accreditation entails an extensive review process that monitors performance against predetermined standards. The accreditation process certifies to the public that the facilities involved meet nationally accepted standards through a recognized program. The amount of documentation required for compliance with these various laws, regulations, and performance standards is voluminous. There is a growing recognition that information systems can and must be used to improve client safety and quality of care as well as enhance regulatory compliance through improved data capture and system prompts, thereby relieving demands on an already overburdened health care providers. This capture should occur as a byproduct of daily documentation activities (Ball, Garets, and Handler 2003; Meadows 2003).

PRIVACY AND CONFIDENTIALITY LEGISLATION

Recent polls indicate a growing public concern related to third-party access to medical records without consent (Follansbee 2002). Several large-scale breaches of client privacy have occurred when personal health information (PHI) has been accidentally posted to the Web. This necessitates measures to safeguard client privacy (Buppert 2002). Until the 1996 passage of the Health Insurance Portability and Accountability Act (HIPAA), legal protection for PHI had been poor. HIPAA, also known as the Kennedy-Kassebaum Bill, represented the first federal legislation to protect automated client records and to provide uniform protection nationwide.

This legislation called for the establishment of an electronic patient records system and privacy rules (Frank-Stromborg and Ganschow 2002; Information Policy Committee 1997). PHI refers to individually identifiable health information such as demographic data; facts that relate to an individual's past, present, or future physical or mental health condition; provision of care; and payment for the provision of care that identifies the individual. Examples include name, address, birth date, and Social Security number.

Previous attempts to legislate medical records privacy included the Individual Privacy Act, the Fair Health Information Practices Act of 1995, and the Medical Records Confidentiality Act of 1995 (Thomas 2003). However, none of these bills were passed. Table 13–1 provides a synopsis of each of these proposed bills.

The Medical Records Confidentiality Act, otherwise known as the Bennett Bill, was notable because it contained the following points (Braithwaite 1996):

- A definition of *health information trustee* as a person or entity that creates, receives, obtains, maintains, or transmits protected health information and any employee, agent, or contractor of same
- Conditions for the inspection and copying of protected information
- Provisions for the correction or amendment of protected health information
- Time limits and additional constraints over disclosure of information
- Authorization and accountability for disclosure of information, including electronic disclosure
- Stiff sanctions for inappropriate access or use of health-related information

Although the Bennett Bill did propose safeguards for health care information, the American Civil Liberties Union (ACLU) and several consumer rights groups opposed the bill because they thought it did not adequately address client control over the use and dissemination of health information. Other critics thought that its wording would prevent legitimate exchange of client information between institutions (Barrows and Clayton 1996; Braithwaite 1996). Box 13–1 lists some principles identified by the ACLU for the formulation of a health information privacy policy.

The Privacy Act of 1974 protected federally managed records, such as those of Medicare and Medicaid, and mandated that federal agencies develop, implement, and disclose their plans for maintaining the security of stored data (Frawley 1995; Hebda, Sakerka, and Czar 1994; Robinson 1994; Rothfeder 1995). Veteran Affairs and Administration hospitals published their plans. There was no similar federal mandate for private institutions and providers at this time. As a result, European agencies refused to transmit medical information to the United States.

Table 13–1	Previous Attempts at Legislation to Protect the Privacy of Medical Records
Title	**Synopsis**
Individual Privacy Protection Act of 1991	Designed to amend the Privacy Act of 1974, increasing the minimum amount of civil damages when records are not properly maintained Provided penalties for violations of privacy rights Established an individual privacy protection board
The Fair Health Information Practices Act of 1995	Required health care providers, information service organizations, benefit plan sponsors, and health researchers to allow individuals to examine their own records Set forth provisions concerning the use and disclosure of protected information Established penalties for violations of the act
Medical Records Confidentiality Act of 1995	Designed to ensure medical record privacy Defined *health information trustee* Established circumstances for disclosure Required trustees to establish safeguards and to maintain records of disclosures not related to treatment Established penalties for failure to comply with the act
Medical Privacy in the Age of New Technologies Act of 1997	Established safeguards for health information Restricted the use and disclosure of information Proposed civil and criminal sanctions for failure to comply with the act
Fair Health Information Practices Act of 1997	Required health care providers to allow individuals to examine their records Restricted the use of protected information to the purpose for which it was collected or for which disclosure authorization has been obtained Mandated the establishment of standards for electronic document transmission, receipt, and maintenance Established civil and criminal penalties for violations of the act Authorized research on protecting health information

SOURCE: Adapted from "Legislative information on the Internet," Thomas, 1997. On the Internet at: *http://thomas.loc.gov/home/thomas.html.*

It is important to note that the Privacy Act of 1974 was enacted before widespread computer use. As a result, protection of medical records varies, from state to state, necessitating that practitioners be familiar with the regulations of the states in which they practice. Some states had regulations, statutes, and case laws that recognized the confidentiality of medical records and limited access. Breach of confidence might lead to disciplinary action for health care professionals by their state boards for licensure. Other states had criminal sanctions against violations of client confidentiality, but enforcement and quantification of damage were difficult.

Several groups besides the ACLU have a strong interest in privacy issues for medical records; these include the Center for Democracy and

Box 13–1	American Civil Liberties Union (ACLU) Principles for Formulating a Health Information Privacy Policy

- Strict limits on access and disclosure of all personally identifiable health data
- Individual control of all personally identifiable health records, with no disclosure without informed consent
- Security measures that protect against unauthorized access or misuse by authorized persons
- No access to personally identifiable health information for employers or potential employers
- Individuals have the right to access, copy, and/or correct any information contained in their own medical records
- Full notification of clients of all uses of their health information
- Establishment of a private right of action and government enforcement to prevent or correct wrongful disclosures or information misuse
- Establishment of a federal system to ensure compliance with privacy laws and regulations

SOURCE: Adapted from "Privacy, confidentiality, and electronic medical records" by R. C. Barrows and P. D. Clayton, 1996, *Journal of the American Medical Informatics Association, 3*(2), 139–148; and *Toward a new health care system: The civil liberties issues,* an ACLU Public Policy Report, 1994.

Technology, the Electronic Privacy Information Center (EPIC), and the Center for Patient Advocacy, among other professional organizations and regulatory bodies. Each group maintains its own Web site.

The Health Insurance Portability and Accountability Act

HIPAA (Public Law 104-191) was passed into law by Congress in 1996. This act had the following objectives (Haramboure 1999; Hellerstein 2000):

- To ensure the portability of health insurance
- To prevent health care fraud and abuse
- To ensure the security and privacy of health information
- To enforce health information standards that will improve the efficiency of health care delivery, simplify the exchange of data between health care entities, and reduce cost
- To reduce the paperwork associated with processing health care transactions

HIPAA Standards HIPAA affects all aspects of health information management, including privacy and security of patient records, coding, and reimbursement (Frank-Stromborg and Ganschow 2002). The broad scope and complex nature of HIPAA resulted in an extensive definition of its rules. This was accomplished in steps since its enactment in 1996. All of the final rules are now out (Gillespie 2003). The Clinton Health Security

Act provided the framework for the national standards created by HIPAA (Annas 2003). The Department of Health and Human Services (DHHS) developed the privacy rule after Congress failed to do so within the time-frame prescribed by HIPAA. It was released for public comment in 1999 and published in 2000 and then modified and published in final form in 2002. The deadline for compliance was April 14, 2003, for most providers. Some small health plans were given until April 14, 2004, to achieve compliance (Final Privacy Rule 2002). The DHHS Office of Civil Rights is responsible for implementing and enforcing the privacy rule with respect to voluntary compliance and civil monetary penalties. The privacy rule attempts to ensure that PHI is properly protected while allowing the flow of data needed to promote high-quality care and protect the public's health and well-being. HIPAA sets a minimum level of protection (Annas 2003). It does not override state laws that are more stringent in their provisions.

The HIPAA privacy rule affects all organizations and individuals involved in the delivery of health care. Organizations, including hospitals, physician offices, home health agencies, and nursing homes and all individual clinicians, instructors, students, and volunteers, now have additional responsibilities and must examine current policies and practices to comply with the provisions of this legislation. Also affected are payers, employers, data services, clearinghouses, regulatory agencies, and information system vendors, Medicare, and Medicaid. HIPAA affects individual care providers, including physicians, nurses, and other clinicians. Others who have direct or indirect access to client information are also be affected. Examples include utilization review staff as well as housekeeping and maintenance personnel.

HIPAA Privacy Rule Compliance HIPAA mandates call for both administrative and technical procedures to protect privacy (Lawson, Orr, and Klar 2003). Administrative procedures include information access controls, contingency plans, formal mechanisms for processing records, security configuration and management, security incident procedures, security management processes, security training, certification of compliance, chain-of-trust partner agreements, and termination procedures. Certification of compliance is implicit with the act of filing a claim as this indicates that the organization has met Medicare and Medicaid statutes and regulations (Nowicki and Summers 2001). The certification process confirms the ability of software products and users to submit readable transactions but does not guarantee payment of claims. Chain-of-trust partner agreements are required when a provider exchanges individually identifiable client information. These agreements must include language that certifies HIPAA compliance (Maddox 2003). Certification may be met when an organization certifies itself and audits every business partner in its chain of trust. Business partners in this chain can include all payers, providers, employers, and clinical service vendors such as independent laboratories and radiology or therapy departments. Certification may also be obtained through third-party reviewers.

Technical security mechanisms include audit controls, authorization controls, data authentication, communication and network controls, encryption, and various types of authentication for event reporting, integrity controls, message authentication, message integrity, and user authentication. Compliance requires a supportive infrastructure. This requires consideration of the project scope, incorporation of HIPAA into the strategic plan for the entire system, review and revision of policies and procedures, designation of a privacy officer, and implementation of a security plan and system safeguards (Buppert 2002; Welker and Podleski 2003, Wilson 2003). The chief nurse executive, informatics nurse, and representative clinicians all share a responsibility for health information privacy and confidentiality and should be actively involved in the development of strategies to achieve compliance (Follansbee 2002). As an advanced practice clinician, the informatics nurse understands clinical processes, information systems, and the significance of relevant legislation. This makes the informatics nurse ideally suited to serve as a member of the HIPAA team. There must also be representatives from medical records, information systems, accounting, client intake and registration, risk management, public relations, ancillary services, human resources, and the compliance office. Designation of a chief privacy officer assigns accountability for HIPAA compliance. The privacy officer is responsible for the following areas:

- Periodic risk analysis to review current systems and procedures and overall compliance
- Identification of changes that must be made, including system changes, to improve compliance
- Formulation of a plan to carry out needed revisions
- HIPAA training
- Communication and education of all staff regarding system revisions and updates to policies and procedures
- Implentation of a mechanism to track requests to view PHI and maintain that documentation
- Means to archive privacy policies and procedures, privacy notices, disposition of complaints, and other documentation required by the privacy rule for 6 years after their creation or last effective date

Gard (2002) notes that with proper security systems in place that include encryption, passwords, and unique client identifiers, electronic records may be more secure than paper records. Box 13–2 lists examples of current security measures that should be evaluated for HIPAA compliance.

One very visible requirement of the privacy rule is the requirement that all health care consumers must receive a privacy notice. The content of this notice must address the following:

Box 13–2	Evaluation of Current Security Measures for HIPAA Compliance

Examples of Security Measures That Should Be Evaluated

- *Determine what types of data are stored on PCs and storage media such as diskettes.* Do they hold patient data?

- *Secure workstations.* Do workstations require a unique sign-on for each user? Are workstations and point-of-care devices protected from theft?

- *System security.* Is there an auto–log-off procedure in place?

- *Evaluate network security.* Is your network protected from unauthorized access?

- *Update your hardware and software inventories.*

- *Examine physical features in accordance with security requirements.* Identify location of backup media and workstations in relation to public access.

- *Printout security.* How are paper reports containing patient information disposed of?

- Ways in which PHI may be used or disclosed
- Responsibility of providers to protect privacy, provide a notice of privacy practices, and abide by the terms of the notice
- Description of individual's rights, including the right to complain to HHS and the provider in the event that the individual believes that his or her rights have been violated
- Point of contact for further information and complaints

HIPAA also includes requirements for electronic signature standards if an organization chooses to use them. The electronic signature standard is applicable only with respect to use with the specifics defined in the Health Insurance Portability and Accountability Act of 1996.

Electronic or digital signatures include an encrypted digital tag added to an electronic document (Tabar 2000). This technology has the following features:

- User authentication that guarantees the user's identity
- Provides evidence that supports the validity of the signature
- Ensures the integrity of the message

HIPAA Security Rule Compliance The final security rule was published February 2003. The date for compliance has been identified as April 2005. This rule mandates safeguards for the physical storage, maintenance, transmission, and access to PHI to ensure its confidentiality, data integrity, and availability when required for treatment (Amatayakul 2002a). Like the privacy rule, it specifies administrative, technical, and physical procedures to keep protected health information secure. It applies only to PHI, not to all individually identifiable information. The security rule requires covered entities to appoint a security officer, just as the privacy rule requires the appointment of a privacy officer (Lawson, Orr, and Klar 2003). Security readiness involves people and processes, as well as information technology. Covered entities must conduct a risk analysis and then determine the security measures that best meet their needs (Amatayakul 2002b). These may vary by the size of the office and the transactions that take place there. Physician offices may elect different disaster recovery measures than large health care systems. Critical gaps should be addressed first. These may include simple solutions such as locking storage areas or emptying confidential trash more frequently. Compliance with HIPAA security and privacy rules is closely linked. Changes in the final security rule include a requirement to encrypt PHI transmitted via open networks (Goedert 2003a). Organizations and providers should not wait until compliance with the final security rule is required to address security issues.

The HIPAA legislation includes descriptions of the various penalties for noncompliance, which can be severe. For example, the penalty for violating transaction standards is up to $100 per person per violation and up to $25,000 per person per violation of a single standard per calendar year. Penalties for wrongful disclosure of client information include large fines as well as possible imprisonment.

HIPAA Issues One of the greatest issues related to HIPAA is the removal from the final privacy rule of the requirement for written client consent before the circulation of PHI by hospitals or other providers involved in routine uses of information for treatment, payment, or other health care (Tieman 2002). This generated concern over possible abuse of information. There are also concerns related to how HIPAA affects daily clinical practice. Clients must now receive a privacy notice that includes a clear written explanation of the allowable uses and disclosures of their PHI and they must be notified of their rights to see and amend health data and learn who has seen their health care records. Providers, in turn, must make a good faith effort to obtain written acknowledgement that each client has received a copy of the provider's privacy notice and maintain an audit log of all parties who have requested access to a client record or PHI. Authorization, rather than consent, is requested for the disclosure of information for nonclinical and reimbursement issues. Authorization differs from consent because it is specific to the release of PHI for a specific purpose and expires on a particular date. Individual clinicians must take reasonable efforts to avoid disclosure during care and to protect written, spoken and recorded information (Amatayakul 2002b; Lepar 2003; Rovner 2002). One example to protect PHI is the use of a password selected by the client in order for information to be given out for inquiries. Clients can then disclose the password to individuals who may secure information concerning their condition.

Other protective measures include the elimination or modification of sign-in sheets, locking up medical records when cleaning crews and other workers come in, exercising care when sending Faxes, reconfiguring offices and nurses stations to remove charts and x-rays from casual view, not posting client names outside rooms or on assignment boards that can be viewed by the public, turning monitor screens so they cannot be viewed by outsiders, and respecting the rights of individuals who opt out of the hospital directory.

HIPAA allows the use or disclosure of PHI without authorization or permission when required by law and for public health activities such as controlling disease, abuse, violence, Food and Drug Administration tracking, and for work-related illnesses. PHI may also be shared in the following instances:

- Audits or investigations by health oversight agencies
- Judicial and administrative proceedings
- Law enforcement
- As needed by funeral directors and coroners
- To facilitate donation/transplantation of tissues
- Research
- Essential government functions such as combat
- Worker's Compensation

The removal of PHI from information removes it from HIPAA's privacy requirements (Frank-Stromborg and Ganschow 2002; DHHS 2003).

Other Privacy Legislation

Several pieces of legislation have been introduced since the enactment of HIPAA that address privacy and confidentiality. The Medical Records Privacy Act of 1997 proposed medical record privacy and the right for a client to access private automated information with the capability to allow or deny the release of information and limit the extent of disclosure (Curtin and Simpson 1999). The Health Care Personal Information Nondisclosure Act of 1998 denied client access to his or her own medical record if it could cause mental harm (Curtin and Simpson 1999). Several bills have been introduced in recent years that address the privacy of health information. Much of this legislation sought to do one of the following: 1) provide additional protection for the privacy of private health information, 2) provide additional control over the disclosure of health care information, or 3) delay the dates for compliance with HIPAA regulations. On a related, but somewhat different vein, the Identity Theft Prevention Act sought to halt the practice of using Social Security numbers as identifiers by requiring the Social Security Administration to issue all Americans new Social Security numbers within 5 years after the enactment of the bill (Thomas 2003).

ACCREDITATION AND REIMBURSEMENT ISSUES

Several agencies have a major affect on health care providers. Accreditation or approval determines whether providers receive funding, enhances the provider's image, instills confidence in the quality of services rendered, and attracts qualified professionals. This process has direct implications for how documentation and information systems are structured. These agencies may be subdivided into accrediting bodies and agencies that dictate reimbursement criteria. Several accrediting bodies exist. JCAHO and CARF fall into the first group, with Medicare and Medicaid and other third-party payors in the second group, as well as ambulatory payment classifications (APCs). Each is discussed next.

Joint Commission for Accreditation of Healthcare Organizations

The mission of JCAHO is to "improve the safety and quality of care delivered to the public through the provision of health care accreditation and related services that support performance improvement in health care organizations" (JCAHO 2003). JCAHO recently strengthened its focus on client safety and the safe administration of medications (Cudney 2002; Grissing and Rich 2002). Once limited to acute care facilities, JCAHO standards now exist for ambulatory, long-term, home health, mental health, and hospice care, as well as managed care. JCAHO accreditation benefits providers by helping them to meet all, or portions of, state and/or federal licensure and certification requirements. JCAHO accreditation also expedites third-party payment and provides guidelines for the improvement of care, services, and programs. Other benefits include community confidence in the organization and improved staff recruitment and retention.

JCAHO standards shape organization practice and documentation, thereby affecting information system documentation design (JCAHO 1996). When accreditation standards change, documentation must reflect additional requirements. Furthermore, JCAHO introduced information management standards for health care organizations in 1994. A brief description of JCAHO information standards follows:

1. Measures that protect information confidentiality, security, and integrity, inclusive of:
   - Determining user need for information access and level of security
   - Easy, timely retrieval of information without compromising security or confidentiality
   - Written and enforced policies restricting removal of client records for legal reasons
   - Guarding records and information against loss, destruction, tampering, and/or unauthorized use

2. Uniform definitions and methods for data capture as a means to facilitate data comparison within and among health care institutions.

3. Education on the principles of information management and training for system use. This may include education about the transformation of data into information for subsequent use in decision support and statistical analysis.

4. Accurate, timely transmission of information as evidenced by the following characteristics:
   - Twenty-hour availability in a form that meets user needs
   - Minimal delay of order implementation
   - Quick turnaround of test results
   - Pharmacy system designed to minimize errors
   - Efficient communication system

5. Integration of clinical systems (i.e., pharmacy, nursing, laboratory, and radiology systems) and nonclinical systems for ready availability of information.

6. *Client-specific data/information.* The system collects, analyzes, transmits, and reports individual client-specific data and information related to client outcomes that can be used to facilitate care, provide a financial and legal record, aid research, and support decision making.

7. *Aggregate data/information.* The system generates reports that support operations and research and improve performance and care. For example, information may be provided by practitioner, client outcomes, diagnosis, or drug effectiveness.

8. *Knowledge-based information.* Literature is available in print or electronic form.

9. *Comparative data.* The system can extract information useful to compare the institution against other agencies. Deviations from expected patterns, trends, length of stay, or numbers of procedures performed may be noted.

Information standards may be demonstrated through the presence of the following: planning documents, institutional and departmental policy and procedures, data element definitions and abbreviations, observations, continuing education outlines and records, interviews with administrators and staff, and meeting minutes. A scoring system notes the degree to which each standard is met. Scoring criteria can be found in the JCAHO's accreditation manual.

Commission on Accreditation of Rehabilitation Facilities

CARF is another health care accrediting body (CARF 2003). In addition to its focus on the improvement of rehabilitative services to people with disabilities, CARF provides accreditation in the following service areas: adult day services, assisted living, behavioral health, services for the visually handicapped, employment and community services, and opioid treatment. CARF provides a template for operations as well as a tool for evaluation. CARF is a private, nonprofit organization that uses input from consumers, rehabilitation professionals, state and national organizations, and third-party payors to develop standards for accreditation. Although similar in purpose and structure to JCAHO, CARF places a greater emphasis on the following factors:

- Accessible services
- Comprehensiveness and continuity in individual treatment plan
- Input from consumers about CARF and its decision making
- Safety of persons with disabilities and their evacuation in the event of an emergency
- Postdischarge outcomes

Like JCAHO standards, CARF standards shape institutional practices and documentation requirements. This may necessitate changes in automated documentation systems to comply with CARF standards.

Reimbursement Issues

Medicare, Medicaid, and other third-party payors dictate reimbursement criteria to health care organizations. Health maintenance organizations (HMOs) also have numerous criteria that must be met for the reimbursement of services. Failure to demonstrate client need for a service may result in denial of that service or reimbursement for that service. For example, Medicare will pay for a client's care in a transitional or subacute care unit only if the client has a preceding hospital stay. It also requires a demonstrated daily need for skilled services. Documentation plays an essential role in this process. At the present, 3% to 5% of net revenues are lost as a result of payment denials from insurance companies (Goedert 2003b; Straight Talk: New Approaches 2002). Automated documentation systems should support entry of information about client need through initial screen design and the use of prompts to elicit needed information. Automated systems can also remind providers of remaining days of coverage for each client, as well as services not covered by Medicare, Medicaid, or their third-party payors. And last, information systems can be used to help track claims and report denials.

APC describes reimbursement criteria for ambulatory procedures for Medicare patients that became effective in August 2000 (CMS 2002; Fee 2002; Micheletti 2000; Straight Talk: Be Aware 2003). Similar to diagnosis-related groups (DRGs) on the inpatient side, APCs were designed to promote efficiency in the delivery of services and to save money. There are specific coding guidelines for ambulatory reimbursement and guidelines for managing APC compliance. APC compliance requires verification of the integrity of the charge description master (CDM) to address issues of overlapping charges and duplication of charges for services and to develop appropriate management reports to facilitate reimbursement. The CDM is a master list of charges for all procedures, tests, and visits to the provider. Failure to code and bill properly risks lost revenue and non-compliance. Revenue may be lost with double coding, missed coding, charge-capture problems, missing modifiers, and denials. This is particularly problematic because APC coding is primarily done by clinicians rather than by coders who have had extensive training in the process. The information services staff must work closely with the clinicians and coders to maintain an updated CDM in the information system.

HIPAA Electronic Data Interchange (EDI) and Transactions Rule

The CMS published regulations in August 2000 mandating all providers, insurers, and middlemen involved in health care claims submission, referrals, eligibility verification, and the transmission of other client-related information to use a common format to send and receive electronic information by October 2002. An act of Congress extended that deadline to October 2003 (Goedert November 2003c; Feds clarify 2003; Maddox 2003; Morrissey September 29, 2003). CMS extended that deadline again when it announced that it would continue to process nonstandard claims for an unspecified period of time as many providers petitioned for an extension. Paper claims are exempt from this requirement. While many providers have submitted claims electronically for several years, others have delayed making changes in their computer systems. It make take several more years before this standard is fully met. Providers also have the option to buy and maintain a HIPAA-compliant practice management system (PMS) or use a claims clearinghouse to meet this standard. Either of these options may prove to be cost effective.

QUALITY INITIATIVES

At the present, there are no U.S. government mandates for specific uses of information technology in health care, but several agencies are looking for ways to provide incentives for providers to invest in systems that can improve client safety (Clancy 2003; Clancy and Simpson 2002; Providers 2003; Putting 2003). The U.S. Agency for Healthcare Research and Quality (AHRQ) exemplifies one such organization. AHRQ funds studies that identify preventable injuries and complications, and demonstrate how technologies like decision-support systems, electronic medical records and data warehouses, and computer models can improve care. Electronic data warehouses can be used to track quality indicators for best practices of care based on client outcomes. AHRQ maintains the National Quality Measures Clearinghouse (NQMC). NQMC is a Web-based resource that allows users to search for measures that target a particular disease/condition, treatment/intervention, age range, gender, vulnerable population, setting of care, or contributing organization and to compare quality measures to determine which best suit their needs. The intent is to provide information on the most up-to-date, clinically proven measures (AHRQ 2003; Morantz and Torrey 2003).

The National Committee for Quality Assurance (NCQA) is a private, nonprofit organization dedicated to improving health care quality. NCQA accredits and certifies health care organizations and manages the evolution of Health Plan Employer Data and Information Set (HEDIS), a set of standardized performance measures that health plans use to measure and report on their performance (NCQA Shifts 2003). NCQA introduced a Web-based Interactive Survey System (ISS) that is expected to change the way in which health care organizations are reviewed, making the process faster and more efficient while providing organizations with more immediate feedback.

The Leapfrog Group is another organization with a focus on client safety and quality of care. This consortium of Fortune 500 companies and other large private and public health care purchasers first focused on three client safety practices to reduce preventable medical errors—computer physician order entry (CPOE), evidence-based hospital referral, and intensive care unit (ICU) physician staffing. Leapfrog uses its purchasing leverage to reward entities that meet or demonstrate progress toward meeting its standards. Clinicians need to play an active role in the success of CPOE through active involvement in the selection of a system and vendor that actually meet the criteria defined by the Leapfrog Group (Meadows and Chaiken 2002).

The Institute of Medicine (IOM) is an advisory body to the national academies. The IOM launched a concerted, ongoing effort focused on assessing and improving the nation's quality of care in 1996. This effort is now in its third phase, which focuses on operationalizing the vision for health care described in its landmark *Quality Chasm* report. A recent IOM report entitled *Patient Safety: Achieving a New Standard for Care* (Aspden, Corrigan, Wolcott, and Erickson 2003) reiterates the need to develop a health care information technology infrastructure because information is key to providing safe care. Unfortunately, the IOM is an advisory body and has no power to implement the changes needed to create this infrastructure.

SPECIAL FACILITY ISSUES

Specialized facilities have unique needs with implications for automated documentation systems. Not all of these needs are covered by JCAHO accreditation. State regulations, including mental health legislation, play an important role in dictating standards for information systems. No attempt is made here to address each type of facility, but pertinent considerations are noted.

Geriatric and Long-Term Facilities

Because of long stays and high client ratios for each nurse, documentation in nursing homes and long-term facilities must be concise, while addressing specific problems for this client population. Many institutions have developed their own forms to expedite this process and address required areas in accord with the mandated frequency of charting for reimbursement. For example, monthly comprehensive summaries on each resident are required. Box 13–3 identifies areas that a monthly summary might include. Figure 13–1 displays a sample documentation screen from an automated summary. When long-term or skilled beds (beds occupied by clients who require specialized nursing care) are located within an institution with automated documentation, additional screens are needed to meet the special needs of this population. Automation can speed updates, provide prompts to ensure appropriate response, decrease entry errors on *ICD–9* reimbursement codes, and generate automated plans of care. Screen design of documentation requires an increased emphasis on psychosocial functioning and several other areas. JCAHO, Medicare, and Medicaid requirements are driving forces in documentation design.

Box 13–3   Minimum Data Set for Nursing Home Resident Assessment and Care

- Identification and background information
- Cognitive patterns
- Communication/hearing
- Vision patterns
- Physical functioning and structural problems
- Continence in last 14 days
- Psychosocial well-being
- Mood and behavior patterns
- Activity pursuit patterns
- Disease diagnoses
- Health conditions
- Oral/nutritional status
- Oral/dental status
- Skin condition
- Medication use
- Special treatment and procedures
- Identification information
- Resident information
- Discharge information

Section B. Cognitive Patterns

1 Comatose
- ❑ Yes (skip to Section E)
- ❑ No

2 Memory
Short-term—recall after 5 minutes
- ❑ OK
- ❑ Problem

Long-term
- ❑ OK
- ❑ Problem

3 Memory/recall ability
- ❑ Current season
- ❑ Location of own room
- ❑ Staff names/faces
- ❑ That he/she is in a nursing home
- ❑ None of the above

4 Cognitive skills
for daily decision
making
- ❑ Independent
- ❑ Modified independence—some difficulty with new situations
- ❑ Moderately impaired—poor decisions, requires supervision
- ❑ Severely impaired—never makes decisions

5 Indicators of delirium/
disordered thinking
- ❑ Less alert, easily distracted
- ❑ Changing awareness of environment
- ❑ Episodes of incoherent speech
- ❑ Periods of motor restlessness or lethargy
- ❑ Cognitive ability varies over course of day
- ❑ None of the above

6 Change in cognitive status
- ❑ None
- ❑ Improved
- ❑ Deteriorated

FIGURE 13–1 • Sample screen shot from an automated summary for a nursing home resident

Psychiatric Facilities

Each state has its own public health and mental health legislation and regulations that affect information system design. For example, regulations relative to the use of restraints vary from state to state. Documentation must comply with state law as well as JCAHO requirements. Important points for charting on the application of restraints, for example, include date and time applied, reason for use, type of restraint applied, length of time the client remains in restraints, neurovascular status distal to the restraint, and frequency of assessments done on the client in restraints. Policy must be established that includes these areas and identifies a maximum length of time that a client may remain in restraints without a renewal order from a physician. This policy should be reflected in time limits on doc-

Documentation of Restraint Application/Assessment

Time applied: __:__ (Maximum time policy identifies for removal automatically shown)
Time scheduled for release: __:__
Reasons for use: (indicate all that apply)
❑ Behavior harmful to self/to others
❑ Necessary to prevent injury
❑ Assaultive behavior
❑ Increased agitation
❑ Impulsive behavior
❑ Other (Specify): _____

Type of restraint applied:
❑ Soft wrist
❑ Waist
❑ Jacket posey
❑ Geriatric chair
❑ Locked leather wrist
✓ One
✓ Two
❑ Locked leather ankle
✓ One
✓ Two
Time restraints removed: __:__
Neurovascular status distal to restraints:
-Pulses: may select from predetermined responses or indicate "other" and describe
-Color: may select from predetermined responses or indicate "other" and describe
-Sensation: may select from predetermined responses or indicate "other" and describe
Frequency of nursing assessments: __:__

FIGURE 13–2 • Suggested screen design for restraint use in an automated documentation system

umentation screens. Seclusion policies should be basically the same. Figure 13–2 shows a suggested documentation screen for restraint use and seclusion.

There also is a greater tendency for interdisciplinary documentation in psychiatric care, due to the need to provide adequate system and record access to many different personnel. Nursing staff, psychiatrists, psychologists, social workers, and recreational therapists require access to psychiatric client records regardless of the unit to which the client is admitted.

CASE STUDY EXERCISES

You are teaching an undergraduate course titled Nursing Informatics. One class session is scheduled for a discussion on the protection of client record information. How would you summarize the current status of legislative safeguards in the United States? What, if anything, would you suggest that students might personally consider to improve this situation?

• • •

You have been appointed to the Clinical Information Systems Committee, which is charged with looking at ways that automation can facilitate data collection for the next JCAHO accreditation visit. List examples of how your community hospital demonstrates adherence to JCAHO information standards, and state your rationale for why you feel these examples display compliance.

• • •

You are the general nursing information systems liaison person at Wilson Rehabilitation Institute. CARF accreditation is coming up. What would you do to ensure that your automated documentation is in compliance with CARF standards? Explain your rationale.

• • •

You are instructing new health care employees during orientation regarding HIPAA. A question is asked regarding how family members receive information on a delusional client. Discuss how you would deal with the issue and how you would provide additional safeguards over the disclosure of health care information.

• • •

You are part of a research team studying CVA treatments. Discuss how you use patient data and how data is de-identified.

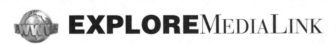

EXPLOREMEDIALINK

Multiple choice review questions, case studies, and other interactive resources for this chapter can be found on the Web site at *http://www.prenhall.com/hebda*. Click on "Chapter 13" to select the activities for this chapter.

SUMMARY

- Legislative, regulatory, and accreditation issues and quality initiatives place excessive demands on health care providers to safeguard, track, provide, and manage information. Information systems can and must facilitate this process.
- Several pieces of legislation address health record privacy and confidentiality, most notably, HIPAA legislation.

- HIPAA affects all aspects of information management, including reimbursement, coding, security, and client records.

- HIPAA compliance requires a broad approach that incorporates administrative and technical procedures. Education, the development and enforcement of policies, and process changes are key factors.

- Accrediting agencies such as JCAHO and CARF, Medicare and Medicaid regulations, third-party payor demands, state and federal laws, and ambulatory payment classifications dictate documentation requirements.

- Electronic claims submission now must meet standards set forth by HIPAA. These standards were established to streamline the claims submission process.

- Information systems and the design of automated documentation must incorporate safeguards for information privacy as well as standards for quality of care imposed by accrediting agencies.

- Automated documentation can facilitate the collection of data for accrediting bodies, third-party payors, and state and federal requirements.

- Special care facilities have documentation requirements that require additional automated screen design.

- There are several bodies that focus on quality and safety in the delivery of health care. These include, but are not limited to, AHRQ, NCQA, the Leapfrog Group, and the IOM. All recognize the potential of information technology to help ensure client safety.

REFERENCES

AHRQ. (2003). AHRQ launches new Web-based quality measures resource. Available online at http://www.ahcpr.gov/news/press/pr2003/nqmcwebpr.htm. Accessed January 2, 2004.

Amatayakul, M. (2002a). Security project plan. *Journal of Healthcare Information Management, 16*(1), 12–13.

Amatayakul, M. (2002b). Risk assessment and serendipitous effects of HIPAA. *Journal of Healthcare Information Management, 16*(4), 7–11.

American Civil Liberties Union. (1994). *Toward a new health care system: The civil liberties issues.* An ACLU Public Policy Report. New York: American Civil Liberties Union.

Annas, G. (April 10, 2003). HIPAA regulations—A new era of medical-record privacy. *The New England Journal of Medicine, 348*(15), 1486–1490.

Aspden, P., Corrigan, J. M., Wolcott, J., and Erickson, S. M. (Eds.). (2003). *Patient safety: Achieving a new standard for care.* Washington, DC: Institute of Medicine of the National Academies.

Ball, M. J., Garets, D. E., and Handler, T. J. (February, 2003). Leveraging IT to improve patient safety. Available online at http://www.himss.org/content/files/whitepapers/PatientSafetyWhitePaper122602.pdf. Accessed November 29, 2003.

Barrows, R. C., and Clayton, P. D. (1996). Privacy, confidentiality, and electronic medical records. *Journal of the American Medical Informatics Association*, *3*(2), 139–148.

Blair, P. D. (2003). Make room for patient privacy. *Nursing Management*, *34*(6), 28–29, 60.

Braithwaite, W. R. (1996). National health information privacy bill generates heat at SCAMC. *Journal of the American Medical Informatics Association*, *3*(1), 95–96.

Buppert, C. (2002). Safeguarding patient privacy. *Nursing Management*, *33*(12), 31–36.

CARF. (2003). What is CARF? Available online at http://www.carf.org/consumer.aspx?content=content/About/FAQ.htm#CARF. Accessed December 7, 2003.

Centers for Medicare and Medicaid Services. HIPAA Administrative simplification—security. Available online at http://www.cms.hhs.gov/hipaa/hipaa2/regulations/security/default.asp.

Clancy, C. (2003). AHRQ: A tradition of evidence. *Healthcare Management Technology*, *24*(8), 26–28.

Clancy, C., and Simpson, L. (2002). Looking forward to impact: moving beyond serendipity. *Health Services Research*, *37*(4), xiv–xxiii.

CMS. (2002). Advisory panel on ambulatory payment classification groups established health care financing administration solicits nominations. Available online at http://cms.hhs.gov/media/press/release.asp?Counter=389. Last modified on October 30, 2002. Accessed December 17, 2003.

Cudney, A. E. (2002). JCAHO: Responding to quality and safety imperatives. *Journal of Healthcare Management*, *47*(4), 16(p).

Curtin, L., and Simpson, R. (1999). Privacy in the information age. *Health Management Technology*, *20*(8), 32–33.

Department of Health and Human Services. (2003). *OCR privacy brief: Summary of the HIPAA privacy rule.* Available online at http://www.hhs.gov/ocr/privacysummary.pdf. Last revised May 2003. Accessed December 7, 2003.

Feds clarify HIPAA compliance plans. (2003). *Health Data Management*, *11*(10), 26.

Fee, D. N. (September 2002). Success with APCs: Despite their complexity, APCs offer providers opportunities to increase payment for outpatient services. *Healthcare Financial Management*, *56*(9), 68.

Final privacy is good, but need security rules too. (2002). *Health Management Technology*, *23*(10), 10.

Follansbee, N. M. (2002). Implication of the Health Insurance Portability and Accountability Act. *Journal of Nursing Administration 32*(1), 42–47.

Frank-Stromborg, M., and Ganschow, J. R. (2002). How HIPAA will change your practice. *Nursing*, *32*(9), 54–57.

Frawley, K. (1995). Achieving the CPR while keeping an ancient oath. *Healthcare Informatics*, *12*(4), 28–30.

Gard, C. (2002). How private are your medical records? *Current Health 2*, *29*(3), 30(2p).

Gillespie, G. (2003). CIOs coming in for a pit stop in the HIPAA compliance race. *Health Data Management, 11*(8), 34.

Goedert, J. (2003a). It's time to "address" the final security rule. *Health Data Management, 11*(4), 16.

Goedert, J. (2003b). Getting claims paid in a HIPAA world. *Health Data Management, 11*(10), 68.

Goedert, J. (2003c). Electronic transactions: Standards aren't common. *Health Data Management, 11*(11), 36–42.

Grissing, M., and Rich, D. (2002). JCAHO: Meeting the standards for patient safety. *The Journal of the American Pharmaceutical Association, 42*(5 Suppl 1), S54–S55.

Haramboure, D. (1999). An industry unready for HIPAA's proposed privacy legislation. *Health Management Technology, 20*(8), 16–17.

Hebda, T., Sakerka, L., and Czar, P. (1994). Educating nurses to maintain patient confidentiality on automated information systems. In S. J. Grobe and E. S. P. Pluyter-Wenting (Eds.). *Nursing informatics: An international overview for nursing in a technological era.* The Proceedings of the Fifth IMIA International Conference on Nursing Use of Computers and Information Science. New York: Elsevier Science.

Hellerstein, D. (2000). HIPAA and health information privacy rules: Almost there. *Health Management Technology, 21*(4), 26–31.

Information Policy Committee National Information Infrastructure Task Force (April 1997). Options for promoting privacy on the National Information Infrastructure. Available online at http:/www.iitf.nist.gov/ipc/privacy.htm.

Joint Commission on Accreditation of Healthcare Organizations (1996). *Medical records process.* Chicago: Accreditation Manual for Hospitals.

Joint Commission on Accreditation of Healthcare Organizations. (2003). About us. Available online at http://www.jcaho.org/about+us/index.htm. Accessed December 17, 2003.

LaRochelle, B. (1999). Fundamental and trade-offs of IT security. *Health Management Technology, 20*(8), 18–21.

Lawson, N. A., Orr, J. M., and Klar, D. S. (2003). The HIPAA privacy rule: An overview of compliance initiatives and requirements: The privacy rule contains a maze of mandates and exceptions requiring that entities covered by HIPAA need the best of health care counsel. *Defense Counsel Journal, 70*(1), 127.

Lepar, K. (July 2003). Nursing and HIPAA. *ADVANCE for Health Information Executives, 7*(7), 16–17.

Maddox, P. J. (2003). HIPAA: Update on rule revisions and compliance requirements. *MedSurg Nursing, 12*(1), 59.

McCourt, A. E. (1993). *The specialty practice of rehabilitation nursing: A core curriculum* (3rd ed.). Skokie, IL: The Rehabilitation Nursing Foundation of the Association of Rehabilitation Nurses.

Meadows, G. (2003). Streamlining regulatory compliance through clinical systems. *Nursing Economics, 21*(4), 196.

Meadows G., and Chaiken, B. P. (2002). Computerized physician order entry: A prescription for patient safety. *Nursing Economics, 20*(2), 76–77, 87.

Micheletti, J. A. (2000). APC environment poses new compliance risk. *Health Management Technology, 21*(6), 54–56.

Morantz, C., and Torrey, B. (2003). AHRQ launches Web-based quality measures resource. *American Family Physician, 67*(7), 1626.

Morrissey, J. (October 13, 2003). HIPAA unplugged: Troublesome burden of claim transactions sidetracks progress in adopting other cost-cutting standards. *Modern Healthcare, 33*(41), 8.

Morrissey, J. (September 29, 2003). Stopping the clock. *Modern Healthcare, 33*(39), 14.

NCQA shifts to Web-based survey. (July 31, 2003). *US Newswire,* p1008212n4868.

Nowicki, M., and Summers, J. (2001). Managing impossible missions: Ethical quandaries and ethical solutions. *Healthcare Financial Management, 55*(6), 62.

Proposed standards for privacy of individually identifiable health information. (2000). U.S. Department of Health and Human Services. Available online at http://aspe.os.dhhs.gov/admnsimp/pvcsumm.htm.

Providers turn to it to reduce health-care errors. (October 8, 2003). *InformationWeek,* pNA.

Putting a clamp on medical mishaps: Data warehouses and picture-archiving systems can reduce patient risks. (October 13, 2003). *InformationWeek,* pNA.

Robinson, E. N. (1994). The computerized patient record: Privacy and security. *M.D. Computing, 11*(2), 69–73.

Rothfeder, J. (1995). Invasion of privacy. *PC World, 13*(11), 52+.

Rovner, J. (May 6, 2002). Some advice on consent: Legislators and providers need to look closer at the reality of medical privacy. *Modern Healthcare, 32,* 21.

Saufl, N. M., and Fieldus, M. H. (2003). Accreditation: A voluntary regulatory requirement. *Journal of Perianesthesia Nursing. 18*(3), 52–59.

Straight talk: Be aware: Medicare's ambulatory payment classification poses significant risks in both lost revenue and noncompliance. (April 28, 2003). *Modern Healthcare, 33*(17), 41.

Straight talk: New approaches in healthcare. Are you in denial over your denials? Enhance your revenues with denial management. (November 25, 2002). *Modern Healthcare, 32*(47), 31.

Tabar, P. (2000). The latest work: A glossary of healthcare information technology terms. *Healthcare Informatics, 17*(3), 75–133.

Thomas, Legislative information on the Internet. (2003). Available online at http://thomas.loc.gov/home/thomas.html.

Viswanathan, H. N., and Salmon, J. W. (2000). Accrediting organizations and quality improvement. *The American Journal of Managed Care, 6*(10), 1117–1130.

Welker, J., and Podleski, J. M. (2003). Preparing the front office staff to carry out HIPAA privacy procedures. *The Journal of Medical Practice Management, 19*(2), 67–70.

Williams, A. W. (September 9, 2003). Compliance with EDI rule. *A S H A Leader, 8*(16), 13.

Wilson, M. (2003). Mobilizing the right resources to achieve HIPAA compliance. *Journal of Healthcare Information Management, 16*(2), 5–7.

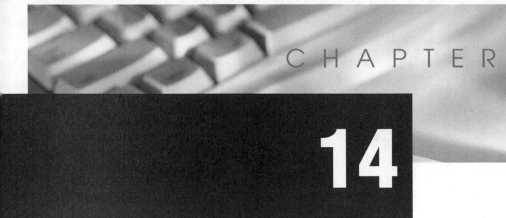

CHAPTER

14

Contingency Planning and Disaster Recovery

After completing this chapter, you should be able to:

- Discuss the relationship between contingency planning and disaster recovery.

- Outline the steps of the contingency planning process.

- Review the advantages associated with contingency planning.

- Identify events that can threaten business operation and information systems (IS).

- Discuss how information obtained from a mock or an actual disaster can be used to improve response and revise contingency plans.

- Discuss legal and accreditation requirements for contingency plans.

 MEDIALINK

Additional resources for this content can be found on the Companion Website at *www.prenhall.com/hebda*. Click on "Chapter 14" to select the activities for this chapter.

Companion Website

- Glossary
- Multiple Choice
- Discussion Points
- Case Study: Physical Vital Record Inventory
- Case Study: Internal Disaster
- Case Study: Environmental Disaster
- Case Study: Vendor-Supported Applications
- Case Study: Using Post-Disaster Feedback to Improve Planning
- MediaLink Application: Contingency Plan
- Web Hunt: Use of Computer Systems in Planning for Disasters
- Links to Resources
- Crossword Puzzle

Until recently, disaster planning focused primarily on the recovery and restoration of data. However, as reliance on timely access to data grows, so does the recognition of the importance of contingency planning for all organizations dependent on timely access to and processing of information for continued operation. This is no less true for health care agency information systems, networks, and freestanding personal computers (PCs). Lost or damaged data have a negative impact on business processes, impedes the delivery of safe care, reduces productivity, and undermines public confidence (Iverson 2003; Price 2003; Sussman 2002). Lost data are costly to recreate and threaten the survival of a business or health care delivery system in a highly competitive environment. While it is obvious that the primary focus of health care delivery must be the well-being of the clients, it is also essential to protect the technology and data that support their care (Spath 2002). Health care providers must determine how a disaster may affect the delivery of services, and identify strategies to ensure availability of information and continuity of care on a 24-hours-a-day, 7-days-a-week basis.

WHAT IS CONTINGENCY PLANNING?

Contingency planning is the process of ensuring the continuation of critical business services regardless of any event that may occur. This includes the continuity of all of its business-critical applications, its data, and its Web, database, and file servers. A contingency plan is a critical aspect of an organization's risk management strategy and is instrumental to its survival should a disaster occur (Midgley 2002). Contingency planning began as disaster recovery, but increased dependence on automation for daily operations created a shift toward more detailed planning to maintain daily functions (Kirchner and Ziegenfuss 2003; Smalley and Glenn 2003; Zein, Cohn, and Broadway 2002). Contingency planning is sometimes referred to as **business continuity planning (BCP).** It combines information technology disaster recovery planning with business function recovery planning. The development of the plan is the most difficult aspect of business continuity (McCormick 2003). Disaster planning was largely the providence of IS personnel. The broader scope of contingency planning now requires the expertise of operations staff and IS experts (Wold and Vick 2003).

A disaster is an occurrence that disrupts or disables necessary business functions, necessitating immediate action (Rike 2003). Disasters strike without warning. For this reason, every institution needs to develop a plan that anticipates potential system problems, implements measures to avoid problems whenever possible, and institutes measures to maintain the security of client information under adverse or unexpected conditions. Disaster plans also provide an alternative means to support the retrieval and processing of information in the event that the information system fails. Disaster recovery plans enable the retrieval of critical business records from storage, restore lost data, and allow organizations to resume system operations, but this process may take 48 hours or longer to accomplish (Regard 2003). There also is another difference between restoration and business continuity (McCormick 2003; Price 2003); restored data do not typically show the relationship between how information is created and used.

Plans should ensure uninterrupted operation or expedite resumption of operation after a disaster while maintaining data integrity and security. Plans need to encompass the multiple vendor platforms found in most organizations and address the implications for other agencies of an inoperable system. For example, if a health care information system is down for a lengthy period of time, information will not be available to third-party payors and suppliers. A comprehensive plan actually consists of separate plans for each of the following areas:

- *The emergency plan.* Provides direction during and immediately after the incident.
- *The backup plan.* Maps out steps to ensure the availability of key employees, vital records, and alternative backup facilities for ongoing business and data processing operations.
- *The recovery plan.* Restores full operational capabilities.
- *The test plan.* Uncovers and corrects defects in the plan before a real disaster occurs.
- *The maintenance plan.* Provides guidelines ensuring that the entire plan is kept up to date.

Consideration of each of these areas as separate plans may provide for better division of responsibility and increased awareness of significance.

The security officer should have a key role in disaster planning. This starts with a basic understanding of the plan development process to help direct the effort. Part of the security role is the protection of information. This is particularly important with federal mandates and accreditation requirements.

STEPS OF THE CONTINGENCY PLANNING PROCESS

The **first step** in contingency planning is a **business impact assessment or analysis (BIA).** This is the process of determining the critical functions of the organization and the information vital to maintain these operations as well as the applications and databases, hardware, and communication facilities that use, house, or support this information (Disaster Resource Guide 2003; Rike 2003). Interviews with employees in each area establish the following:

- Description, purpose, and origin of the information
- Information flows
- Recipients, or users, of the information

- Requirements for timeliness
- Implications of information unavailability

The importance of information dictates the priority given to maintaining its continuity. The BIA identifies threats and risks and includes a workflow analysis to determine interdependencies. General policy and procedures, hardware and software, troubleshooting, backup, training, testing, and overall costs must be weighed. Interviews with department heads help to identify the most appropriate strategies to be used to maintain or recover business functionality and sequencing for restoration (Jackson and Dec 2003; Wold and Vick 2003). Data flowcharts help to ensure that all critical processes are documented. Each company must select its criteria for business recovery timeframes based on its own perspective (Zein, Cohn, and Broadway 2002).

Even after information critical to system users has been identified, it is important to realize that critical information is more than the information required for direct client care. Individual areas within the institution have vendor contracts, personnel files, financial or claim documentation, important e-mail, permits, building blueprints, regulatory compliance documentation, equipment manuals, and reporting data in a variety of formats and places. Approximately 60% of an organization's valuable information assets are not protected because it resides on PCs, laptop computers, and personal digital assistants (PDAs) that are not backed up regularly or solely in paper format (Hickman 2003; Olson 2002). Much of this information would be difficult or time consuming to replace. For this reason, each area should develop a disaster plan and complete a physical vital records inventory such as the one depicted in Figure 14–1. This inventory should specify:

- Volume and description of information
- Format; for example, whether it is maintained on paper, disk, or tapes
- When the information was created, its use, and how it relates to other records
- When the information is transferred to storage or destroyed
- Equipment used to store critical information
- Consequences for the loss of this information

The **second step** is the planning process. This is broken down into several phases:

1. *Secure top management support and commitment resources.* This is critical because administrative support is essential to the development of a viable plan, which in turn can make the difference between an organization's demise or survival.

2. *Select the planning committee.* Agency staff may develop a contingency plan, but consultant expertise on the team can develop a plan more quickly, objectively, and knowledgeably because no one individual can know everything needed to

Make one copy of this page for each record listed. When parentheses appear, select one response from within them.

Record name:
Scheduled and Unscheduled Meds Due lists/Parenteral Therapy lists

Purpose of record:
Used to administer medications to patients

Who is responsible for this record:
HIS*-generated document based on MD orders

Media (paper, fiche, mainframe, etc.):
HIS paper document

Where is the record stored:
HIS system, on nursing units for 24 hours

Volume/frequency of change:
Many times/day

Retention requirement:
24 Hours

Originating office:
Nursing units

Location of any copies:
Nursing units/outdated copies

The record is: (irreplaceable, unique/difficult to replace/not hard to replace)

The record is: (essential for business/not essential but important/not important)

How would you obtain this record if your copy were destroyed?
If HIS system available, reprint; if not, go through each patient's chart

How would you re-create the information on this record?
Through patient's chart and current hard copy of Patient Care Plans

How long after a disaster could you work without this record?
Few hours—would use documents available

How is this record protected from destruction? (not protected, sprinklered office area, fireproof cabinet, duplicates kept in other locations, sprinklered warehouse, mainframe computer files, easily re-created, etc.)
HIS backups—paper documents not protected

Duplication and off-site storage is: (already being done/should be done/is not necessary)
Already being done—HIS

Are you prepared to supply input data, or work in progress, to allow the rerun of your critical applications from the last off-site backup?

Who is in charge of removing/restoring this record if it is damaged? What provisions have been made to restore/remove damaged records? What is the relocation destination? Who will transport damaged records and what is this person's 24-hour telephone number and security clearance?

* HIS, hospital or health care information service.

FIGURE 14–1 • Example of a physical vital records inventory sheet

implement an effective plan for a large, complex system. For this reason, each section of the plan should be authored by the parties with the greatest expertise in the area (Bell 2003; Miano 2003; Wilson, Corcoran, and Eckles 2003; Zein, Cohn, and Broadway 2002). The chief information officer should play a major role on the committee and in the development of the plan (Spath 2002).

3. *Risk Assessment.* During this phase, the planning committee identifies the following information:

   a. Types and probabilities of various types of disasters; risks range from low to high (Herbig 2003)

   b. Potential impact of a particular disaster scenario

   c. Estimated costs of lost/damaged information/records and lost time and customer goodwill

   d. Costs to replace and restore records, equipment, and facilities, as well as to hire or replace staff, versus the costs to develop and maintain the disaster plan

   e. Risk of the worst-case scenario striking the organization

4. *Set processing and operating priorities.* During this phase, the committee determines the equipment and telecommunication links and vital records needed to perform daily business functions and viable alternatives in the event that these are not available.

5. *Data Collection.* This phase entails a determination of available resources. This includes external resources such as backup and duplication systems, recovery services, and internal resources. Internal assets include staff information; inventories of vital records, equipment, supplies, or forms; policies and procedures; contact lists for staff, vendors, and other service providers; a review of security systems; and an evaluation of facilities for potential problems.

6. *Writing the plan.* A common mistake is to assign the responsibility for writing the plan to an individual who already has a full workload or who lacks authority to confront managers about the criticality of information in their areas. If the task is tackled internally, it needs to be divided among persons with expertise in specific areas. A successful plan must be well organized, up to date, concise, and simple to follow. Software tools are available to aid the process; these include personal software or office productivity tools, enterprise software, and Web-based tools. Office productivity tools are readily available, but plans tend to get locked away on desktops with issues of version control and contact lists, and pager and telephone numbers that are not kept up to date. Enterprise software offers a proven track record but may be expensive, difficult to install and learn, and antiquated in design. Web-based software is easy to use and provides version control and free access to extensive

information and instant, interactive communication. It offers wide dissemination, the ability to incorporate questionnaires and surveys, automated contact management, and security. The plan must catalog all strategies needed to sustain delivery of services and to test the plan.

Well-documented systems and procedures are essential for the continuity of operations and disaster recovery. Although each institution and system is different, the plan should identify the following (Spath 2002):

- Planning process description
- Purpose of the plan
- General system policies and procedures, including who can declare a disaster, the mechanism for calling a disaster, and the distribution and maintenance of the plan
- Emergency telephone tree/call schedule (inclusive of telephone, cellphone, and pager numbers) and the length of time required for each identified person to arrive, whether the person is an employee, or any other individual key to the recovery process
- Alternative communication methods, such as cellphones and pagers
- Responsibilities for each administrator
- Floor plans for water, gas, and oxygen lines and exits
- Cable, electrical, and telecommunication diagrams
- System configurations inclusive of server configurations and port connections
- Schematics for backup systems and schedules
- Outline of what users should do in the event of a disaster, including their responsibilities with manual systems and restoration efforts
- Projected timeline for system restoration
- Troubleshooting and problem resolution
- Data backup, security, and restoration procedures
- Insurance documents
- Repair procedures
- List of basic resources required to perform services, including equipment and software vendors, and restoration and storage services
- Vital record inventory that includes, but is not limited to, vendor/service provider and warranty information
- Provisions for nonclinical vital record access, backup, and, if needed, appropriate restoration techniques for each type of storage medium used
- Vendor service agreements along with identification numbers

- Mechanism to store and retrieve passwords and software from a protected site
- Locations of all operations
- Auditing procedures

Documentation must be explicit because staff come and go. For example, instructions should provide details on responsibilities and where staff will report in an emergency. Key information, such as persons responsible for implementing the plan and their roles, must be kept up to date. Documentation should include goals for the implementation of suggested and/or required changes.

The **third step** of contingency planning is the implementation of the strategies identified to maintain business continuity, delivery of client services, and restoration of lost or damaged data. This includes the implementation of policies and procedures as well as contracts with vendors and various service providers necessary to ensure business continuity in the presence of a threat or disaster.

The **fourth step** in contingency planning is evaluation. Once developed, the plan should be carefully reviewed for weak spots. This includes consideration of the reliability, adequacy, compatibility, and appropriateness of backup systems, facilities, and procedures. The plan should be evaluated annually and when major changes occur in system processes. Training for team members should occur at this time. An actual test of the plan should be done in sections after peak business hours and evaluated for effectiveness. Strategies and methods must then be determined to test and evaluate the plan annually, if not more often, to determine if it is workable, documentation is appropriate, and staff are trained. Actual disaster or outage situations provide an excellent test opportunity (Kirchner and Ziegenfuss 2003).

ADVANTAGES OF CONTINGENCY PLANNING

It is not always possible to avoid a disaster or to provide 100% protection against every threat, but a good plan can anticipate problems and minimize losses incurred by damage (Pelant 2003). A good plan is clear and concise and does the following (Miano 2003; Midgley 2002):

- Identifies vulnerabilities within the organization and strategies for correction
- Provides a reasonable amount of protection against interruption in services, downtime, and data loss
- Ensures continuity of the client record and delivery of care
- Expedites reporting of diagnostic tests
- Captures charges and supports billing and processing of reimbursement claims in a timely fashion

- Ensures open communication with employees and ensures customers of availability of services or interim arrangements
- Provides a mechanism to capture information needed for regulatory and accrediting bodies
- Helps to ensure compliance with HIPAA legislation and Joint Commission for Accreditation of Healthcare Organizations (JCAHO) requirements
- Establishes backup and restoration procedures for systems, databases, and important files
- Allows time for restoration of equipment, the facility, and services

In short, an effective disaster plan saves money up front and over time through limiting loss of data, equipment, and services. Any agency that requires information integrity and availability cannot afford to be without a disaster plan. A good plan can make the difference between institutional survival or demise when the likelihood of bankruptcy increases with each moment those data are unavailable.

DISASTERS VERSUS SYSTEM FAILURE

Hazards come from a variety of sources, including environmental disasters, human error, sabotage and acts of terrorism and bioterrorism, high-tech crime, operating system or application software bugs, viruses, overtaxed infrastructure, power fluctuations and outages, and equipment failure (Midgley 2002; Wiles 2004). Table 14–1 lists some IS threats. A thorough appraisal by IS personnel can minimize the risk of damage from various situations.

Environmental Disasters

Environmental disasters may be natural or man-made. Plans must anticipate the predictable and the unpredictable, inclusive of climate, location, building features, internal hazards such as fire or smoke damage, and utility service. Many hospitals and providers lack the infrastructure to accommodate and support information systems. Often the system and data are housed in areas threatened by potential plumbing leaks or exposure to dangerous materials, such as oxygen, anesthetic agents, or other hazardous chemicals. Both the security of the IS power supply and availability of backup power to sustain uninterrupted computer operation must be considered. The hospital utility lines may be at risk because of their location, particularly if construction is under way and power or telephone lines have not been marked and protected from inadvertent damage.

Human Error

Human error is one of the largest contributing factors to data loss along with mechanical failure. Both account for 75% of all data loss (Margeson

Table 14–1	Threats to Normal System Operation

Threat	Examples
Accidents	Brown outs and power outages/grid failures File corruption Transportation accidents Chemical contamination Toxic fumes
Natural disasters	Avalanche Floods Earthquakes Hurricanes Tornadoes Blizzards Epidemics
Internal disasters	Hardware or software errors Water line breaks Construction accidents Fire Sabotage Theft Ex-employee violence
Malicious or violent acts	Hackers Bombs Terrorism and bioterrorism Civil unrest Armed conflict

2003; Sussman 2002). Examples of human error include accidental file deletion, failure to follow proper backup procedures, file overwrite, the introduction of viruses or vandalism, theft, and loading incomplete programs. An example of the latter might include a vendor software update that was inadequately tested before distribution.

Sabotage, Cybercrime, Terrorism, and Bioterrorism

Both current and former employees pose the greatest risk to IS in terms of their capabilities to change data and damage systems because of their special knowledge and access. For this reason, random unannounced background investigations of employees with access to sensitive and critical IS organizational information should be considered as a means to avert sabotage, inadvertent disclosure of PHI, and wrongful system use, such as, identity theft and credit card fraud (Marcella 2004).

On a national and international level, it is essential to consider the impacts of terrorism and bioterrorism on the delivery of care and the potential effects on Information Services. Can the IS handle mass casualities without significant degradation or loss of service or even aid in the detection of suspicious patterns? Threats that once seemed remote are now considered high risk. These include explosions, radiation, and biological warfare (Chandler and Wallace 2002).

System or Equipment Failure

System or equipment failure may occur in the absence of any of the preceding environmental disasters. System failure may result from the failure of a component part or parts. Central processing unit (CPU) crashes, cabling and software problems, and even loose plugs may cause difficulties. When feasible, spare parts such as hubs, patch cables, extra printers, PCs, and servers as well as trained support staff should be available to troubleshoot system problems, avert downtime, and initiate recovery. Redundancy in system design raises the initial system cost but increases IS reliability. A well-executed physical system prevents many problems or makes them easier to discover. A review of the facility, system, policies and procedures, and disaster plan conducted quarterly can identify vulnerable areas. A review should also be done whenever major changes are introduced. Box 14–1 lists areas for consideration.

CONTINUITY AND RECOVERY OPTIONS

The 24-hour-a-day operations of health care providers make continuity of services essential. This focus should guide the selection of computer services, hardware and software for day-to-day operations, backup, and recovery, yet most current strategies are not well suited to meet the stringent requirements of 24-hours-a-day, 7-days-a-week availability (Puttagunta 2002). Hardware redundancy is the first line of defense in providing continuous systems; hardware redundancy allows operations to continue even when individual components fail. This redundancy may be accomplished via redundant processors and disk arrays in one location or at two separate locations of the same agency or another facility. An increasing number of organizations now split their information technology between two locations for added protection (Cope 2002; Winkler 2002). A second data processing site requires sufficient space for equipment and staff, especially if it may double as a backup data center (Davies 2003). Functional requirements include mainframe and or server capacity, printers, storage devices, sufficient cabling, power, UPSs, air conditioning and space for a help desk, and operations center and test room. Online replication of data is an integral part of business continuity providing data availability, averting disaster, and reducing costs and recovery time (Desmond 2002; Zalewski 2003). Connecting storage devices to a redundant network provides multiple data paths, which helps to protect data damage.

Box 14–1 Suggested Areas for Review to Avert System Disasters

- Documentation
- Network access controls
- Physical security
- Archived data
- Vital records
- Backup procedures
- Recovery procedures
- Backup equipment
- Backup facility
- Organizational contingency plan
- Network diversity
- Communications links
- Spare parts inventory
- Backup services
- LAN configurations
- Personnel availability
- Off-site storage
- Operations personnel
- Technical personnel
- Vendor service and maintenance agreements
- Vendor contingency plans
- Antivirus updates

Backup and Storage

Data availability, recovery time, disaster avoidance, retention requirements, and costs determine the best backup and storage options for a given organization (Stephens 2003; Zalewski 2003). Continuous delivery of services is the goal, but solutions to achieve zero downtime are expensive. For this reason, organizations must determine data storage requirements and acceptable recovery time on a system-by-system basis. These decisions help to determine media choices. The most common antidisaster protection methods include automated backups, off-site media storage, data mirroring, remote data replication, and snapshots of data at prescribed intervals (Iverson 2003). Data mirroring is the creation of a duplicate online copy. This technique eliminates wait time but may also replicate corrupt data. Best practices for long-data retention include the selection of standardized file formats, good management of metadata, the selection of media intended for long-term storage and proper housing, and regular inspection and maintenance of stored media. **Metadata** is a set of data that provide information about how, when, and by whom data are collected, formatted, and stored (Morgenthal and Walmsley 2000). It is essential to the creation and use of data repositories. Backup allows restoration of data if, or when, they are lost. Losses may occur with disk or CPU crashes, file deletion, file corruption secondary to power or application problems, or overwritten files.

Fast data recovery minimizes the worst consequences of downtime, including a tarnished image and financial losses. Networked storage area networks (SANs) and electronic vaulting provide the type of protection needed to ensure business continuity. Electronic vaulting sends backups over telecommunication links to secure storage facilities. This approach eliminates labor costs and the need to physically transport tapes. It also improves data integrity and shortens recovery efforts (Regard 2003). Electronic vaulting may be provided by commercial enterprises that provide backup services for customers. Customers receive backup software at their site and at a central, remote file server. The customer dials to the remote server to back up data. Each customer has a separate account, and file access is limited to authorized persons. Remote backup service (RBS) staff protect both data and data integrity. Data retrieval, when needed, is limited only by the speed of the communication link. RBSs also provide reports to show which files have been backed up. Tape and other older media do not support fast data recovery efforts. There are also issues surrounding failed backup.

Backup may fail because of faulty software, bad network connections, worn tapes, or poor storage conditions. For this reason, backup should be verified and periodically tested. Advancements in technology and changes in the costs of backup options and storage media provide more options to maintain business continuity and backup and storage. Newer tape drives have well-developed error correction, eliminating the need to verify backup copies but not the need to test stored media. Storage conditions must be climate controlled and free from electromagnetic interference to avoid degradation of media. Agencies may opt to outsource storage to cold sites. A **cold site** is a commercial service that provides storage for backup materials or the capacity to handle the disaster-stricken facility's computer equipment (Wold and Vick 2003). Often backup materials are found on a combination of different media. Materials are shipped from the institution to the cold site, where backups from multiple organizations are kept in protected vaults under controlled conditions. Agency personnel are responsible for backup, dating, and labeling materials for storage. Cold sites should be located in areas free from floods and tornadoes and at least 5 miles away from the agency to avoid disaster conditions. Commercial cold sites provide environmental controls and possibly communication links and uninterrupted power sources. They are relatively inexpensive but cannot be tested as a backup facility unless equipment is shipped there and communication links are installed.

Traditional backup dumps data to a storage medium such as CDs, DVDs, cartridges, or tape for transfer to another site for storage and, if needed, system restoration. While tape is still used, higher-capacity forms are now preferred and are often used in combination with other methods such as flexible disk arrays to reduce the possibility of operating errors. Tape dumps for off-site storage start off with a gap between creation and pickup/delivery time. Data may be lost in this gap and recovery from tapes is unreliable and time consuming (Apicella 2003; Vaulting provides 2001).

Storage media differ but should permit permanent or semipermanent record keeping. Magnetic tape remains a popular, and relatively inexpensive, storage medium. Optical disks are another storage option with a longer shelf-life and a higher cost. Electronic transfer over high-speed telephone lines to another site is a faster, more reliable means of backup that eliminates transportation concerns. When electronic transmission is not an option, a second set of backup media should be made and transported separately to ensure against accidental loss or destruction. Archived data must be inspected regularly to ensure that it can be processed and that the medium has not deteriorated or become outdated in light of current backup systems.

Personal and Notebook Computers Although the primary focus for IS disaster plans is on the major systems, large amounts of information important for daily operations are also found on PCs and notebook computers. This is particularly true as mobile workers and telecommuters comprise a greater percentage of the workforce (McKilroy 2003). Mobile workers spend at least 50% of their time at a location outside of the main institution using notebooks or PDAs. Homecare staff exemplify one such group of mobile workers. Another population of health care professionals telecommute using the Internet and remote connections to access and transmit information. Telecommuters face information system threats that do not affect internal employees such as firewall maintenance and denial of service attacks, and lost productivity when network connections are not available. For these reasons, IS disaster plans need to include notebook computers, PDAs, mobile devices, and remote users. Routine maintenance prevents many problems. Box 14–2 lists tasks suggested for maintenance. Agencies cannot assume that users know how to perform these chores or perform them regularly. Instruction and assistance should be provided. For example, computer support personnel should perform periodic backups. This has the added benefit of standardizing backup procedures and media.

Box 14–2 **Recommended PC/Notebook Maintenance**

- Create several DOS boot diskettes. Boot diskettes allow the PC to start even if the hard drive will not work. Keep at least one copy with backup tapes/diskettes.
- Keep original software handy in the event that it must be reinstalled.
- Print out copies of SYSTEM.INI, AUTOEXEC.BAT, CONFIG.SYS, and WIN.INI files, update them every time new software is added, and keep the printouts in an accessible area.
- Establish a secure place for backup diskettes or CDs away from the PC, preferably in a fire proof safe or file cabinet. Backup media stored under poor conditions or kept in the same area as the PC are vulnerable to the same threats.
- Do an incremental backup daily, a full backup weekly, and a full system backup monthly and backup/store files on network drives whenever possible.
- Test backup CDs/diskettes to ensure that they are good. Establish a policy for routine replacement of backup media.
- Periodically delete files from the hard drive that are no longer needed.
- Defragment all hard drives monthly.
- Maintain air flow around the PC/notebook to allow cooling.
- Keep diskettes away from magnetic fields, including electronic devices.
- Periodically clean PCs/notebooks.
- Run virus protection software regularly and obtain updated versions as available.

MANUAL VERSUS AUTOMATED ALTERNATIVES

The decision to use manual alternatives when the system is down has implications for the delivery of care, the cost of care given, record management, and employee system training. A backup alternative is a different means to accomplish a common task than what is ordinarily used. An example of a manual backup alternative is when staff must complete requests for laboratory tests via paper forms that must then be delivered to the laboratory, instead of selecting the ordered test from a menu option on a computer screen. Implementation of a backup alternative may delay delivery of services for several reasons. First, personnel are less familiar with the alternative procedure and will take longer to accomplish their work. Results reporting and processing requests for services will be delayed. Manual forms may no longer exist or may not be current in listing available tests or test names. Because automation eliminated personnel who supported the manual process, there may be few people available who know the manual alternative. Automated backup alternatives may also be available. For example, staff may be able to access information through a different screen than the one they generally use. Despite these problems, implementation of backup alternatives permits ongoing delivery of care, even if it is at a slower pace.

Calculation of backup costs goes beyond initial setup costs and ongoing expenditures. One-time recovery costs can be high because they include costs of hiring IS personnel and training staff to use backup alternatives; additional user costs for dual entry; costs for cleanup, repair, or replacement of computer equipment; and payment for backup computing or recovery services. Another cost is the impact on the quality of services rendered during the downtime.

The expense for manual versus automated alternatives varies according to the length of time that the system is down, backup alternatives employed, and the resources they require. Because implementing a backup alternative is costly, administrators must decide if the anticipated downtime merits initiating the alternative. Extremely short down periods are usually not worth the additional time and trouble. Costs include additional labor for IS and other personnel, increased potential for error, and space requirements. Data entry into the system following a manual backup requires additional personnel and a place for them to work. For example, laboratory tests that were requested but not completed before downtime must be requested by nursing again manually. During downtime, laboratory staff must try to match manual requisitions against those that were entered but not processed before downtime. When the system goes live, laboratory tests that were ordered and completed during downtime, along with results, must be entered so that the client record is not fragmented.

Staff Training The successful implementation of a manual alternatives plan hinges on the cooperation and support of everyone in the institution, from top management down. One way to ensure this success is through training. Detailed instruction on every aspect of the system, the plan, and implementation of manual alternatives may be incorporated into initial computer training. However, this approach requires a longer training period, and recall of manual procedures is often poor when long periods of time elapse between instruction and implementation. A more effective strategy entails posting plans in conspicuous places, yearly review of contingency plans, mock disasters, and the provision of step-by-step reference guides to help staff implement manual alternatives. Other measures to increase disaster awareness and ensure successful recovery efforts are listed in Box 14–3.

When it is not possible to maintain IS continuity, recovery is the next option. It sounds simple, but it is not. Few institutions have actually reconstructed IS from backups. And few information technology staff are well equipped to deal with data recovery (Margeson 2003). Even when it would appear that equipment and storage media are damaged, no assumptions should be made that data are permanently lost, nor should persons unacquainted with salvage measures attempt to restore equipment or storage media (Olson 2002). For these reasons, it is best to call in recovery specialists when significant data loss has occurred. Successful recovery requires stabilization of the affected system and good problem-solving skills,

Box 14–3	Ways to Ensure Business Continuity and Successful Recovery

- Display contingency plans in conspicuous places, and post revised versions as soon as they are available.
- List key contact people responsible for implementing contingency and recovery plans.
- Review staff responsibilities periodically.
- Provide clear step-by-step reference aids for staff to guide them through continuity and recovery options including manual alternatives.
- Emphasize the importance of disaster preparedness by incorporating mock disaster situations into training.
- Review the contingency and recovery plans at least yearly along with other mandated programs, such as safe lifting, fire safety, and the materials safety data sheets.
- Schedule at least two mock disasters per year—one of which is community wide.
- Test backups periodically.
- Label backup materials and include explicit directions with them.
- Provide up-to-date hot and cold site information to persons responsible for recovery.
- Include 24-hour telephone numbers, contracts, and payment authorization numbers.
- Emphasize the need for emergency care arrangements for dependents and pets to personnel involved in disaster and recovery plan implementation.

staff preparedness, and good backups. Recovery is complicated when backups are not verified, delaying the detection of problems until restoration is attempted. Also, large institutions have information located in several areas: the mainframe, networks, PCs, laptops, PDAs, and paper documents. Last, most institutions use a combination of backup formats and programs.

Restoration of system operation may result from one of several techniques. First, materials stored at a cold site can be shipped back to the institution and reloaded onto the system. Second, information may be restored from RBSs or electronic vaulting. A third option is the use of hot sites. Commercial hot sites are fully equipped with uninterrupted power supplies, computers, telecommunication capabilities, security, and environmental equipment. Hot sites may accept transmission of backup copies of computer data, allowing restoration of operations using backup media (Wold and Vick 2003). This is accomplished at another location served by a different power grid and central telephone office to avoid the effects of the disaster that affected the health care enterprise. The organization may develop its own hot site or outsource for services. When possible, hot sites should be close enough for practical employee travel, with sufficient space, power, cabling, parking, and satellite dish accommodations to support IS function.

A dedicated hot site usually sits idle when not needed but is available in the event of an emergency and is compatible with agency systems for ease of system restoration and updates. The creation of redundant computer capabilities and the acquisition of a dedicated hot site are costly. At one time, it was common to share the center with other health care alliance partners. A tenant would have to agree to relinquish the site in the event of a disaster. Sharing a site presumes that it is unlikely that two or more partners at separate locations would have a disaster at the same time. Shared arrangements are no longer practical because most systems now have extensive online processing. Hot sites may not be adequate to process critical applications or be able to provide for special equipment needs such as unique laser printers and forms handling equipment. Mobile hot sites are also available. Another option is the creation of a backup facility on-site in another building owned by the organization. This option reduces real estate costs but still requires system redundancy. Internal hot sites can continue to provide processing for critical business functions, although typically this occurs at a reduced level of service. When not in use as a hot site, it can be used for other processing, eliminating fees.

Commercial hot site services charge monthly reservation fees in addition to restoration charges but are less costly than establishing an independent site. There is a risk of being bumped by another client who requires services at the same time. Commercial vendors should be able to offer the assurance of a proven track record for mainframe recovery. Unfortunately, the uniqueness of most client–server environments made commercial recovery services unprofitable and unavailable until recently, forcing institutions to develop their own internal recovery options.

Vendor Equipment Vendors may offer processing capability through their equipment. This solution may work for a select few applications but does not address the needs of an entire organization. There are also issues related to costs, software versions and customizations, availability, and testing.

An alternative to system restoration is distributed processing. Distributed processing uses a group of independent processors that contain the same information, but these may be at different sites. In the event that one processor is knocked out, information is not lost because remaining processors can continue IS operation with little or no interruption. Distributed processing is more expensive upfront but eliminates downtime. Rapid replacement of equipment is yet another recovery strategy, but it is not always feasible because it is costly to maintain extra hardware.

Salvaging Damaged Records

Once alternative arrangements have been made to maintain business options, restoration of the facility and secondary records becomes a focus. Few IS staff possess the skills necessary to salvage damaged records and equipment, but internal staff should know how to act quickly and effectively to

Box 14-4 **General Salvage Rules**

- Stabilize the site.
- Pump any standing water out of the facility.
- Decrease the temperature to minimize mold and mildew growth and damage.
- Vent the area.
- Do not restore power to wet equipment.
- Open cabinet doors, remove side panels and covers, and pull out chassis to permit water to exit equipment.
- Absorb excess water in equipment with cotton, using care not to damage pins and cables.
- Call in professional decontamination specialists when hazardous chemicals or wastes are present.
- Initiate salvage options within 48 hours.

contain damage and to obtain outside help. In small, localized disasters, knowledge of recovery techniques and being able to complete simple recovery steps may be all that is required to save the records, information, or equipment (Rike 2003). Whether the computing center was without climate control or was physically damaged by an event that exposed it to heat, humidity, and/or smoke damage, there are guidelines to follow to salvage materials; Box 14-4 lists some of these. The first rule is to stabilize the site. In most scenarios, internal staff do not participate in the actual recovery process. Many processes require the use of hazardous and dangerous chemicals or knowledge of detailed salvage methods.

Disaster recovery experts can best ensure data recovery from damaged media, particularly from magnetic media. Fires, heat, and floods leave behind residues that damage electronic equipment and storage media. Additional damage may occur when media are improperly stored and handled after the disaster and with the passage of time. Degradation of media also impedes recovery efforts. Data integrity is compromised when storage media are damaged. Recovery specialists must verify data bit by bit and reconstruct files before data can be recorded onto new media. Having written agreements with restoration companies is particularly crucial in times of widespread disasters, such as earthquakes or floods, when many organizations will be seeking help at the same time. Box 14-5 lists some recovery measures.

Recovery Costs The cost for recovery is frequently overlooked (Winkler 2002). It should not be. It can be an extremely expensive process, involving the following factors:

- Lost consumer confidence
- Lost profits

Box 14–5 **Recommended Storage Media Recovery Techniques**

General efforts recovery methods for paper-based materials:

- Have record salvage professionals on retainer. Initiate recovery within 48 hours of the disaster for best results.

- Consult recovery specialists before attempting any record salvage!

- Separate coated papers such as ECG tracing and ultrasound records to prevent them from permanently fusing together.

- Remove noncoated documents from file cabinets or shelves in blocks—do not pull each page apart, as this increases mold growth.

- Store paper documents in a diesel-powered freezer trailer until proper drying arrangements can be finalized.

- Remove excess mud and dirt before freezing documents.

- Pack wet files or books in a box with a plastic trash liner and allow room for circulation of air.

- Place files with open edges facing up and books with spines down.

- Label all boxes precisely and create a master inventory.

- Freeze-dry priority documents and sterilize and use fungicide as needed.

General magnetic media recovery techniques:

- Open and dry water-damaged floppy disks with isopropyl alcohol, place in empty jackets, and copy files to new disks.

- Clean soot-damaged floppy disks manually. Use recovery software to recover and copy information to new disks.

- Freeze-dry tape cartridges, then use recovery software to recover and copy information to new tape cartridges.

- Dry reel-to-reel tapes on a tape-cleaning machine, using warm air to evaporate moisture. Use recovery software to recover and copy information to new storage media.

- Temporary computer services, including space rental, equipment, furniture, extra telephone lines, and temporary personnel
- Shipping and installation costs
- Post-disaster replacement of equipment
- Post-disaster repairs and bringing the building up to new codes
- Recovery and possible decontamination
- Overtime hours for staff during the disaster for the implementation of manual alternatives, and after the disaster for entering data into the system that was generated during system downtime
- Reconstruction of lost data

Insurance coverage is recommended as a means to help pay for IS disasters. Table 14–2 lists types of available coverage. One person should be designated to interact with the insurance company and a mechanism should be identified for how disaster-related costs will be documented.

Restarting Systems

System restarts after downtime must be planned carefully. All critical data for client management and agency administration should be targeted for restoration first. For example, client admission systems are needed before client-related entries can be made. Therefore, it is logical to make the admissions and discharge functions one of the first areas restored. Users can help identify critical functions. Usage tends to be heavy once the system is live again as users try to catch up on their work. Communication is critical at this point. IS personnel must provide users with a sense of confidence, prevent system overload, and bring the system back online slowly to prevent further problems. Economic factors should also be considered. For instance, if charges are calculated with the documentation of a medication, or intravenous fluid, this process must be restored as soon as possible. Nonessential functions and reports should be deferred until the system is fully operational to prevent additional downtime.

Decisions Regarding the Extent of Data Reentry Health care administrators must determine how they will handle late entries and documenta-

Table 14–2	Recommended Insurance Coverage
Coverage	**Purpose**
Business interruption	Provides replacement of lost profits as a result of a covered loss. Must be certain that insurance covers the same period as the event.
Extra expense	Provides financial recovery for out-of-the-ordinary expenses such as a temporary office or center of operations, and additional costs for rent, staff, and rental of equipment and furniture while regular facilities cannot be used.
Code compliance	Often overlooked. Insurance will normally reimburse only for expenses associated with repair or replacement of a damaged building, but not additional costs associated with building code changes implemented since the building was built. This coverage provides for those additional costs.
Electronic data processing	Replaces damaged or lost equipment and media from a covered incident such as storm damage not covered in normal property insurance. May also include coverage for business interruption and extra expenses.

Source: Adapted from Cox, L. P. (1996). Disaster recovery: How do you pay for it? *Disaster Recovery Journal, 9*(2), 19–20.

tion that occurs during system downtimes. One factor that frequently goes unconsidered is the cost for entering information gathered manually into the system once normal operations have resumed. This is a labor-intensive process. The importance of data for inclusion in the automated record and the possible legal ramifications for data stored only on paper must be weighed. For example, is it necessary to include all vital signs and intake and output in the automated record, particularly if these have been within normal limits? A mechanism must be developed that indicates the availability of additional record information in paper form. Additional considerations include whether the entry of information collected manually and entered into the automated record later might be more prone to error and how the original paper record should be dealt with.

PLANNING PITFALLS

Contingency plans are subject to the following pitfalls:

- *Few information technology budgets have sufficient funding for business continuity efforts.* Contingency plan budgets need to be spread across the organization.

- *Lack of access to the plan.* If the plan is available online, measures must be taken to ensure that the computers that house the plan are accessible. All employees responsible for implementing any part of the plan should have a copy at home, at work, and in their briefcase. These copies may be on paper, PDAs, and/or notebooks. CD-ROM may also be an acceptable distribution method. Everyone should be aware of their roles and responsibilities (Alvord and Fuqua 2002; Stephens 2003).

- *Failure to include all information and devices in the plan.* Businesses evolve and institute new processes. Many plans lag behind the technology in use. An increasing amount of important information is found on laptops and desktop PCs, and even in paper format. Many plans fail to consider the importance of e-mail, enterprise resource planning (ERP) systems, and Web-based transactions to daily operations. Many health care providers also have separate databases for various populations. Information services may not be aware of these separate databases until problems arise. There are also applications supported by application service providers (ASPs). One such example might include a renal database for dialysis patients. Contingency plans must consider how services will be provided in the event that the vendor's database is unavailable due to failure on their end or inability to access the database due to downed Internet or telephone connections (Bannan 2002). Another example might include the failure to consider the multivendor environment seen in most health care systems today. Data are frequently housed on several computers.

- *Failure to incorporate data growth into the plan.* Unprecedented data growth threatens recovery plans. Organizations need to focus on critical data to ensure business continuity and reduce recovery time. This can be done by separating inactive from active data as a means to keep operating databases at a manageable size and improve application availability (Lee 2003).

- *Failure to update the plan.* The contingency plan is a fluid document that is subject to change as operations and personnel come and go and determinations are made that some portions of the plan do not work well. The planning committee should control the change process printing review and revision dates on each page. A change manual can be used to note changes, the date, and reason for each change (Smalley and Glenn 2003).

- *Failure to test the plan.* A significant percentage of organizations that have contingency and disaster recovery plans never test them or do not know if they have been tested (Rike 2003; Saran 2003). Some businesses do not even have a comprehensive disaster recovery plan in place.

- *Failure to consider the human component* (Jackson and Dec 2003; Lewis 2003, Rike 2003). Preservation of human life is the top priority in any disaster, followed by preservation of critical functions. Even so, loss of personnel is a distinct possibility. In times of disaster, the institution should be prepared to assist employees and their families, including communication links to check on employees and providing such amenities as transportation to work and possibly temporary housing. Restoration of peace of mind for employees and families is just as important as recovering data from a computer and maintaining business continuity. This includes reestablishing user confidence once normal operations are restored and addressing the emotional impact that the disaster had on employees.

USING POST-DISASTER FEEDBACK TO IMPROVE PLANNING

Post-disaster feedback is invaluable to revising disaster plans for future use. Personnel input after mock disasters or prolonged downtime should be used to identify what worked and what did not. Systems and organizations change. Plans that looked good before a disaster may not look good after one. Recovery expenses usually exceed anticipated costs, leading to a change in recovery strategies for future use. Figure 14–2 depicts a checklist to evaluate the success of a disaster and recovery plan.

Another option for the development, revision, and management of contingency plans for resource-strapped organizations is the use of a managed service provider (Midgley 2002). Managed service providers offer continuous data backup safeguarding against data loss while allowing for im-

Checklist Item	Yes	No
Are backup(s) available? tested?	❑	❑
Are disaster/recovery plan copies available/accessible?	❑	❑
Are duplicate processors or storage options in place?	❑	❑
Are hot-site contract copies available/accessible?	❑	❑
Do key personnel have emergency care arrangements for dependents? pets?	❑	❑
Is home-site staffing coverage adequate?	❑	❑
Are the hot-site locations and access procedures known?	❑	❑
Are the cold-site storage sites and procedures for retrieval of backups known/arranged?	❑	❑
Is travel to the cold and hot sites feasible?	❑	❑
Has authorization for recovery-related expenses been confirmed?	❑	❑
Are contracts with record salvage services in place?	❑	❑
Is shipping information accurate for backup tapes from cold to hot sites and back again?	❑	❑
Is documentation accurate for tape restoration available with starting and ending tape numbers?	❑	❑
Are backup media labeled accurately?	❑	❑
Have network/communications persons been sent to the hot site?	❑	❑
Do restoration procedures agree with current software?	❑	❑
Have previous arrangements been made to have persons stay after hours at the remote site?	❑	❑
Are communications links for backup confirmed, appropriate, and available?	❑	❑
Are phone numbers available for all vendors and services?	❑	❑
Are stored supplies intact/usable?	❑	❑
Is a timeline for anticipated restoration of operations identified and appropriate?	❑	❑
Are packing materials and labels available to ship media from cold to hot sites and back again?	❑	❑
Is an extra container for reports among supplies?	❑	❑
Are human needs for food and rest adequately included in the plan?	❑	❑

FIGURE 14–2 • Checklist for successful implementation of an IS disaster and recovery plan

mediate recovery and restoration of services in the event of a disaster. Organizations using managed service providers retain control of data processing operations while the managed care provider provides the resources. Customers can manage their data processing through a personalized Web management interface that allows them to initiate recovery from any location

Challenges for the future include (1) finding ways to protect the growing amount of information, no matter where it is stored or used, and

(2) finding ways to make sure people can stay connected to their data, no matter what the disruption. Without addressing and linking these two elements, a plan may fall far short of its goals.

LEGAL AND ACCREDITATION REQUIREMENTS

The HIPAA security rule requires contingency planning and disaster recovery processes (Averell 2003; Bogen 2002; Miller and Lehman 2002; Zawada 2003). All health care organizations must have a data backup plan, a recovery plan, an emergency mode of operation plan, and testing and evaluation procedures. Although HIPAA does not specify the exact processes or procedures for compliance, it does demand safeguards for the security of protected health information while operating in both normal and emergency modes. These safeguards encompass the creation, access, storage, and destruction of manual records. The final contingency planning component of the HIPAA regulations requires compliance by April 2005 for most entities. Smaller providers have until April 2006 to achieve compliance.

JCAHO set disaster preparedness standards as a requirement for hospital accreditation more than 30 years ago (Cutlip 2002; JCAHO urges 2001). Until 2000, standards focused on disasters and accidents such as power plant failures and chemical spills. In 2001, JCAHO introduced new emergency management standards for hospitals, long-term care facilities, and behavioral health and ambulatory care that focus on the concept of community involvement in the management process. These guidelines address information security, disaster preparedness, and recovery planning. JCAHO has since added bioterrorism to the list of events that organizations must consider in their plans (McGowan 2002).

JCAHO suggests that organizations conduct at least two emergency drills per year with one community-wide drill. Accreditation standards mandate that health care organizations have an emergency plan that identifies potential hazards, their impact on services, and measures to handle and recover from emergencies. Accredited organizations must demonstrate a command structure, emergency preparedness training for staff, a mechanism to enact an emergency plan, and identify their role in community-wide emergencies.

Together JCAHO and HIPAA require that health care providers perform a business impact analysis, crisis management, conduct employee training, implement ongoing contingency plan reviews, plan for information technology disasters and recovery, and audit their contingency plan processes (Zawada 2003). Several other accrediting bodies require disaster plans though their focus is personal safety rather than information safety. There are other groups that demonstrate varying levels of interest in business contingency management; these include the Food and Drug Administration (FDA), the Federal Emergency Management Agency (FEMA), the National Institute of Standards and Technology (NIST), the Disaster Recovery Institute International, the Bioterrorism Task Force of the Association for Professionals in Infection Control and Epidemiology, and the Bioterrorism Working Group of the Centers for Disease Control and Prevention. Recommendations from these other groups provide voluntary guidelines for better business continuity management that help contingency planners to achieve HIPAA and JCAHO compliance.

CASE STUDY EXERCISES

As the clinical representative for your unit on the Disaster Planning Committee, you are charged with identifying all forms in your area that require completion of a physical vital records inventory sheet. What forms would you list and why?

· · ·

Work crews at Wilmington Hospital inadvertently cut the cable connecting all terminals at the hospital with the computer center. As the on-duty nursing supervisor, what should you tell your employees and why? Who would you contact for further information? How do you determine whether to initiate manual alternatives?

· · ·

An early morning train wreck near St. Luke's Hospital derailed seven freight cars carrying chemicals that can emit toxic fumes. The accident took out power lines for the neighborhood and for St. Luke's. Emergency crews evacuated a seven-block area, stopping just outside of the hospital's main entrance. Power has already been out for 12 hours and restoration is not expected for at least another 12 to 24 hours. You are on an executive administrative committee charged with determining what information will be brought online first and what will remain in paper form. What would you restore first? What records, if any, would you not restore? Explain your rationale. How would you document, for record management purposes, that part of the record is automated and part is manual?

· · ·

As IS project manager, you are responsible for helping the Renal Department select a new database. One of the top vendors must cancel its Web-based demonstration because its server was stolen. What types of questions should this situation raise for disaster planning with the use of vendor-supported applications?

· · ·

You recently learned that the information services network engineer responsible for conducting backups on the server for the tumor registry database failed to ensure that regular backups occurred properly. This was discovered when the database was found to be corrupt. Approximately 20,000 entries were lost as a result. As the liaison between the tumor registry and the IS department, how would you ensure that this would not happen again?

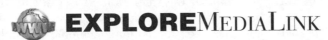

Muliple choice review questions, case studies, and other interactive resources for this chapter can be found on the Web site at *http://www.prenhall.com/hebda*. Click on "Chapter 14" to select the activities for this chapter.

SUMMARY

- Contingency planning is the process of ensuring the continuation of critical business services regardless of any event that may occur. It includes information technology disaster planning.

- Contingency planning consists of several steps. The first step requires business impact analysis and a determination of vital organization functions and information.

- The second step in contingency planning is the development of the plan itself. This step determines the probabilities of all types of disasters, their impact on critical functions, and factors necessary for restoration of services.

- The third step in contingency planning is the implementation of the strategies identified to maintain business continuity, delivery of patient services, and restoration of lost or damaged data. This includes policies and procedures and contracts with vendors and various service providers.

- The fourth step in contingency planning is evaluation.

- Disasters that threaten information systems operation may be natural or man-made. Contingency plans help to ensure uninterrupted operation or speedy resumption of services when a catastrophic event occurs.

- The identification of information vital to daily operation is best determined through interviewing system users. The purpose, flow, recipients, need for timeliness, and implications of information unavailability must be considered in this process.

- Not all information used in daily operations is automated. A vital records inventory should be conducted to identify additional information that requires protection.

- Documentation is essential to the development and successful implementation of a disaster plan. Plans must be detailed, current, and readily available to be useful.

- Careful attention to backup and storage helps ensure that information may be retrieved, or restored, later. Backup may be handled internally or outsourced. Commercial backup services provide transport or electronic transmission of backup media and special storage conditions until materials are needed.

- Manual alternatives to information systems ensure ongoing delivery of services, although it is at a slower rate. Staff must receive instruction and support as they resort to manual methods.

- Restoration of information services post-disaster is not simple because backup media may be faulty and some information kept on other media is lost forever.

- System restoration may reload backup media stored at cold sites or resort to remote backup service or hot sites. Distributed processing and rapid replacement of equipment are other alternatives.

- Restoration is costly because it generally requires outside professional services, additional equipment, and extra hours from support staff. Expenses may be partially recouped through insurance coverage.

- Salvage of damaged records is an important aspect of recovery that is best handled by experts.

- System restarts require planning to avoid system overload as users try to catch up on work. Administrators must consider what functions should be restored first and how to integrate backup paper records with automated records.

- Post-disaster feedback is key to the design and implementation of a better plan for future use.

- Contingency planning needs to consider legal and regulatory requirements.

REFERENCES

Alvord, C., and Fuqua, J. (2002). Maximizing Internet use for business continuity. *Disaster Recovery Journal*, *15*(4). Available online at http://www.drj.com/articles/win03/1601-14p.html. Accessed January 7, 2004.

Apicella, M. (February 17, 2003). Disaster recovery finds prominence: More IT leaders are fortifying their business recovery strategies with thoughtful design and advanced storage technologies. *InfoWorld*, *25*(7), 29.

Averell, H. (June 1, 2003). Disaster recovery, HIPAA style. *ADVANCE for Health Information Executives*. Available online at http://www.advanceforhie.com/. Accessed January 27, 2004.

Bannan, K. J. (January 29, 2002). Building your safety net—Every company needs a disaster recovery plan, but e-businesses have some special needs to guarantee they're running around-the-clock. *PC Magazine*, *21*(1), 2.

Bell, J. (2003). Why some recovery plans won't work. *Disaster Recovery Journal*, *16*(2). Available online at www.drj.com/articles/spr03/1602=03;html. Accessed January 7, 2004.

Bogen, J. (2002). Implications of HIPAA on business continuity and disaster recovery practices in healthcare organizations. *Healthcare Review*, *15*(5), 14.

Chandler R. C., and Wallace, J. D. (2002). What disaster recovery experts were thinking just before the attacks. *Disaster Recovery Journal, 15*(1). Available online at http://www.drj.com/articles/win02/1501-03p.html. Accessed April 23, 2004.

Cope, J. (July 15, 2002). Put your IT eggs in different baskets: Distributing IT resources across multiple locations could make it easier to recover from a disaster. *Computerworld, 36*(29), 38.

Cutlip, K. (2002). Strengthening the system: Joint commission standards and building on what we know. *Hospital Topics, 80*(1), 24.

Davies, T. (2003). Do your homework before you start building a backup data center. *Disaster Recovery Journal, 16*(1). Available online at http://www.drj.com/articles/win03/1601-05p.html. Accessed January 20, 2004.

Desmond, P. (May 27, 2002). Disaster-proofing storage systems. From remote copy to synchronous mirroring, these techniques bring resiliency to storage systems. *Network World,* 10.

Disaster resource guide. (2003). Business continuity planning: All the right moves. Available online at http://www.disaster-resource.com/articles/02p_045.shtml. Accessed January 7, 2004.

Herbig, J. (2003). Understanding and communicating risk assessment. *Disaster Recovery Journal, 16*(3). Available online at www.drj.com/articles/sum03/1603-16p.html. Accessed January 20, 2004.

Hickman, T. (2003). Protecting documents shouldn't stop at server. *Disaster Recovery Journal, 16*(1). Available online at http://www.drj.com/articles/win03/1601-09p.html. Accessed January 20, 2004.

Iverson, J. (summer 2003). Multi-terabyte data recovery in a few clicks. *Disaster Recovery Journal, 16*(3). Available online at www.drj.com/articles/sum03/1603-18p.html. Accessed January 7, 2004.

Jackson, J. A. and Dec, D. A. (2003). A new look at planning for disasters. *Disaster Recovery Journal, 16*(1). Available online at http://www.drj.com/articles/win03/1601-13p.html. Accessed January 20, 2004.

JCAHO organizations must focus on emergency planning. (2002). *Behavioral Health Accreditation & Accountability Alert, 7*(1), 6.

JCAHO urges immediate congressional action on developing effective bioterrorism response. (October 10, 2001). *US Newswire,* p1008283n0745.

Kirchner, T. A., and Ziegenfuss, D. E. (2003). Audit's role in the business continuity process. *Disaster Recovery Journal, 16*(2). Available online at http://www.drj.com/articles/spr03/1602-11.html. Accessed January 7, 2004.

Lee, J. (2003). Effective strategy for meeting disaster recovery SLAs for mission-critical applications. *Disaster Recovery Journal, 16*(2). Available online at http://www.drj.com/articles/spr03/1602-15p.html. Accessed January 20, 2004.

Lewis, G. (2003). The human(e) side: Recovering human technology. *Disaster Recovery Journal, 16*(3). Available online at http://www.drj.com/articles/sum03/1603-12p.html. Accessed January 7, 2004.

Marcella, A. J. (2004). CYBERcrime: Is your company a potential target? Are you prepared? *Disaster Recovery Journal, 17*(1). Available online at http://www.drj.com/articles/win04/1701-04p.html. Accessed April 23, 2004.

Margeson, B. (2003). The human side of data loss. *Disaster Recovery Journal, 16*(2). Available online at http://www.drj.com/articles/spr03/1602-08p.html. Accessed January 20, 2004.

McCormick, J. (2003). Picking up the pieces: To prepare for a disaster, whether natural or man-made, you will need both backup and recovery applications—and a plan. *Government Computer News, 22*(5), 42.

McDaniel, L. D. D. (1996). First steps to take after a fire. *Communication News, 33*(3), 26.

McGowan, B. (2002). The board's role related to disaster preparedness. *Healthcare Review, 15*(2), 15.

McKilroy, A. A. (2003). Connecting the islands: Disaster recovery planning for teleworking environments. *Disaster Recovery Journal, 16*(1). Available online at http://www.drj.com/articles/win03/1601-07p.html. Accessed Janaury 20, 2004.

Miano, B. (fall 2003). Key considerations for proactive planning. *Disaster Recovery Journal, 16*(4). Available online at http://www.drj.com/articles/fall03/1604-04p.html. Accessed January 20, 2004.

Midgley, C. (2002). Protecting your data, protecting your business. *Disaster Recovery Journal, 15*(3). Available online at http://www.drj.com/articles/sum02/1503-09p.html. Accessed January 20, 2004.

Miller, V., and Lehman, K. (2002). Assessment of HIPAA security requirements on disaster recovery planning. *Disaster Recovery Journal, 15*(1), 62–64.

Moore, P. (March/April 1996). Records recovery necessities. *Contingency Planning & Management*, 25–29.

Morgenthal, J. P., and Walmsley, P. (February 2000). Mining for metadata. *Software Magazine*. Available online at http://www.findarticles.com/cf_0/m0SMG/1_20/61298805/print.jhtml. Accessed January 27, 2004.

Olson, G. (2002). Recovering data in a snap. *Disaster Recovery Journal, 15*(4). Available online at http://www.drj.com/articles/fall02/1504-12p.html. Accessed January 20, 2004.

Pelant, B. F. (2003). Business impact analysis. *Disaster Recovery Journal, 16*(1). Available online at http://www.drj.com/articles/win03/1601-03p.html. Accessed January 4, 2004.

Price, E. S. (summer 2003). Application-aware solutions: The building blocks of business continuity. *Disaster Recovery Journal, 16*(3). Available online at www.drj.com/articles/sum03/1603-20p.html. Accessed January 20, 2004.

Puttagunta, N. (2002). Database availability and recovery solutions. *Disaster Recovery Journal, 15*(3). Available online at http://www.drj.com/articles/sum02/1503-14p.html. Accessed January 20, 2004.

Regard, E. (2003). Business continuity via satellite communications. *Disaster Recovery Journal, 16*(3). Available online at http://www.drj.com/articles/sum03/1603-19p.html. Accessed January 20, 2004.

Reshaur, L. M., and Luongo, R. P. (2000). Lessons in business continuity planning: One hospital's response to a disaster. *Disaster Recovery*

Journal, 13(2), 12–13. Available online at http://www.drj.com/articles/spring00/1302-01.html. Accessed January 20, 2004.

Rike, B. (May–June 2003). Prepared or not . . . that is the vital question: When unplanned events or full-blown disasters strike, RIM professionals must have a strategy to ensure survival and at a cost that organizations can afford. *Information Management Journal, 37*(3), 25.

Saran, C. (October 14, 2003). Disaster recovery; CIOs fail to put a price on data loss. *Computer Weekly,* 32.

Smalley, T. M., and Glenn, J. (2003). Security vs. need-to-know. *Disaster Recovery Journal, 16*(2). Available online at http://www.drj.com/articles/spr03/1602-07p.html. Accessed January 20, 2004.

Spath, P. (September 2002). Treatment is priority, but plan to safeguard info. Available online at http://www.findarticles.com/cf_0/m0HKF/9_2-/012-6010/print.jhtml. Accessed December 27, 2003.

Stephens, D. O. (January–February 2003). Protecting records in the face of chaos, calamity, and cataclysm: Even organizations that do not think they are prime targets for terrorists do not have the luxury of considering themselves exempt from disaster planning. *Information Management Journal, 37*(1), 33.

Sussman, S. (2002). Securing windows workstations in real time. *Disaster Recovery Journal, 15*(4). Available online at http://www.drj.com/articles/fall02/1504-15p.html. Accessed January 21, 2004.

Vaulting provides disaster relief. (July 2001). *Communications News, 38*(7), 48.

Wiles, J. (2004). Auditing your disaster recovery plan: A closer look at high tech crime. Will this be your most likely disaster in the 21st century? Available online at http://www.disaster-resource.com/cgi-bin/article_search.cgi?id='93'. Accessed January 8, 2004.

Wilson, B., Corcoran, P., and Eckles, J. (fall 2003). Vendors provide inside look into power outages. *Disaster Recovery Journal, 16*(4), 24, 26, 28.

Winkler, C. (December 9, 2002). Recovery on the cheap: How to cut costs while still safeguarding mission-critical data in the event of a disaster. *Computerworld, (36)*50, 52.

Wold, G. H., and Vick, T. L. (2003). Comparing & selecting recovery strategies. *Disaster Recovery Journal, 16*(2). Available online at www.drj.com/articles/spr03/1602-05p.html. Accessed January 4, 2004.

Zalewski, S. (2003). Online data replication . . . provides new opportunities for business continuity. *Disaster Resource Guide.* Available online at http://www.disaster-resource.com/articles/03p_062.shtml. Accessed February 5, 2004.

Zawada, B. J. (2003). Regulatory pressure on technology for business continuity. *Risk Management, 50*(7), 20.

Zein, M., Cohn, S., and Broadway, T. (2002). Business continuity: Planning is a process not a project. Available online at http://www.disaster-resource.com/articles/02p_036.shtml. Accessed January 7, 2004.

Three

Specialty Applications

15

Using the Computer to Support Health Care Education

After completing this chapter, you should be able to:

- Identify specific ways that computer technology may be used to support education.

- List benefits associated with *computer-assisted instruction (CAI)*, *distance education*, and *Web-based instruction (WBI)*.

- Compare and contrast *e-learning* with other educational uses of computers.

- Provide examples of how computer technology may support education in each of the following settings: formal nursing programs, continuing education, and client or consumer education.

- Describe factors that contribute to the successful use of an instructional computer lab.

- Review options for the individual interested in learning more about nursing informatics.

 MEDIALINK

Additional resources for this content can be found on the Companion Website at *www.prenhall.com/hebda*. Click on "Chapter 15" to select the activities for this chapter.

Companion Website

- Glossary
- Multiple Choice
- Discussion Points
- Case Study: Meeting Educational Needs
- Case Study: Instructional Applications of Computer Technology
- Case Study: How Computers Support Education
- MediaLink Application: Computers in the Clinical Setting
- Web Hunt: On-line Education
- Links to Resources
- Crossword Puzzle

Educational applications of computer technology can enhance the presentation of content, ease the burdens associated with course management for faculty, erase geographic boundaries for students, make learning opportunities available 24 hours a day, tailor instruction to individual learning needs, improve learning outcomes, provide a safe learning environment, and reduce the challenge of acquiring, maintaining, and expanding skill sets—helping to keep the present workforce competent (Bradley 2003). Proponents see its potential to revolutionize education for health care professionals and consumers and promote critical thinking skills. The realization of this potential requires good planning, design, use, and evaluation by educators and administrators. Technology is increasingly prevalent in today's society and workplaces. It should be a part of the education process but only when there is a match with the objectives of the curriculum, it is well used, and it facilitates the learning process. Educators must become adept in the evaluation and use of technology that they plan to use. Students and health care consumers need to investigate the quality of technology-mediated courses and programs prior to enrollment.

INSTRUCTIONAL APPLICATIONS OF COMPUTER TECHNOLOGY

Computer related technology may be used in a variety of ways to support or provide instruction. These often include:

- Word-processing software to prepare presentations and examinations.
- Slide presentation software to create presentations and audio-visual aids.
- Spreadsheets or course management tools to maintain attendance records and grades.
- Course management tools to administer and score examinations and evaluation tools.
- Communication tools such as instant messaging, e-mail, Web blogs, threaded discussions, chats and Web postings to answer student questions and provide feedback to students on their progress.
- Online literature searches to research content prior to developing or revising a presentation. These may be accomplished directly through databases available through libraries or through Web sites such as Sigma Theta Tau's Virginia Henderson Library and the National Library of Medicine. Abstracts and some full text articles can be retrieved online.

Other instructional applications of computer technology include computer-assisted instruction (CAI), competency-based training, teleconferencing, multimedia presentations, simulation, virtual reality, distance

Box 15–1   Applications of Computers in Health Care Education

Formal opportunities

- Continuing education
- Distance education
- Online journals
- Client education

Information opportunities

- E-mail
- Listservs and usenet news groups
- Support groups
- Online literature searches and databases
- Chats or instant messaging
- Blogs

Administrative support

- Webcasts
- Preparation of presentations, handouts, slides
- Record keeping
- Course management tools inclusive of test administration scoring and statistical analysis

---

education, Web-based instruction, and computer learning labs. Box 15–1 lists some ways that computers may be used to facilitate education.

Computer-Assisted Instruction

Computer-assisted instruction (CAI) is the use of the computer to organize and present instructional materials for use by an individual learner. CAI aids learning by actively involving the learner as a participant. In addition, CAI offers 24-hour availability, the ability to proceed at a comfortable pace, and consistency in instructional approach. Many individuals believe that CAI laid the groundwork for modern distance education (Kozlowski 2002). In CAI, the computer teaches a subject (other than computing) to the student through interactive software. Advocates of CAI allege that it enhances computer literacy, facilitates decision making, reduces computer anxiety, and positively affects student achievement (Gleydura, Michelman, and Wilson 1995). Although originally designed to promote individualized learning, CAI can enhance group learning as well (Calderone 1994). Numerous studies have been done comparing the efficacy of CAI to traditional instruction. The general finding is that CAI is at least as effective as traditional instruction although some critics find the methodology of many of these studies faulty—calling for more research (Wang and Sleeman 1993a, 1993b; Rouse 2000). It has been suggested that CAI may provide a means to introduce technology into the curriculum and even to pave the way for distance education (Greco and O'Connor 2000; Kozlowski 2002). CAI is often used to supplement classroom instruction (Myles 2000).

CAI offers the following advantages (Glover and Kruse 1995):

- *Improved reading habits.* Learners can proceed at a pace conducive to comprehension.
- *Convenience.* CAI can be offered at any site that has computer access. Programs may be available for single users on freestanding PCs or via network connections.
- *Reduced learning time.* Because learners can proceed at their own pace, they can skim through familiar content and focus on weak areas.
- *Increased retention.* The active nature of the media requires learner participation, which improves retention.
- *Twenty-four-hour access.* CAI is available at any time of the day or night so that learners can use it at times convenient to them.
- *Consistent instruction in a safe environment.* CAI allows learners to practice new skills without fear of harm to themselves or others.

Three major variables influence CAI effectiveness: quality of the software, the environment of computer use, and characteristics of the learner. Some factors that can lead to negative attitudes toward CAI include the following design issues (Gleydura et al. 1995; Khoiny 1995):

- *Poor design.* Many CAI applications do nothing more than automate page turning.
- *Lack of feedback on incorrect answers.* This is frustrating to learners who want to know why their selections were wrong.
- *Lack of control.* Control encompasses the ability to advance, repeat, or review portions of the program, or to quit at any point.
- *Lack of intellectual stimulation.* Programs that fail to maintain interest may cause learners to feel that they wasted their time.

Drug calculation programs are a common CAI application in most nursing schools. These programs are popular because drug calculation is a basic skill needed by all nurses, and, as such, drug calculation programs fit well into the curriculum, while programs on other content areas may not match curriculum objectives. An example is the case of a CAI program that addresses the care of the critically ill client. Concepts from such an offering may be too complex for junior level students in some schools but not others.

Competency-Based Training

Competency-based training and testing are particularly important in the clinical setting as institutions need to demonstrate that staff are able to perform skills safely (Bradley 2003; O'Gara 2003). Simulation technology allows users to learn and then demonstrate their skills or test different scenarios without negative consequences. Initial research indicates highly positive effects of simulation on skill and knowledge acquisition (Ravert 2002). Computer-based competency training and testing have the potential to free instructor time, streamline instruction and testing, and eliminate costs associated with employee travel.

Multimedia

Nursing education has always used multimedia whether that media included chalkboard diagrams, overheads, slide presentations, video, skill demonstrations, computer-based instruction, interactive video disk (IVD), CD-ROM, DVD, or streaming video (Batscha 2002; Billings 1995; Calderone 1994; Gleydura et al. 1995; Simpson 2002; Smith-Stoner and Willer 2003; Sternberger and Meyer 2001). Now it is possible to add virtual reality to the list of examples. Quite simply, multimedia refers to presentations that combine text, voice or sound, images, and video, or hardware and software that can support the same. Tools change with technological advances. Multimedia is an excellent approach for nurses because they must learn and communicate complex issues to clients. Research has shown that learning retention is facilitated with an approach that incorporates seeing, hearing, doing, and interactivity. Multimedia has been found to be at least as effective as traditional instruction and offers greater satisfaction (Maag 2004). Group-paced instruction with multimedia decreases costs associated with individual instruction, increases comfort with computers, and improves learning as long as the environment is conducive to group use. Nurse educators need to select and use multimedia well and creatively to realize its benefits (Cuellar 2002; Ross and Tuovinen 2001). Multimedia can be incorporated into tests as well (Rossignol and Scollin 2001). Virtual reality is a form of multimedia that fully envelops learners in an environment. It is already used to help medical students, surgeons, and other health care professionals with procedural skills such as physical assessment and the insertion of intravenous needles. It offers the next best option to performing the skill on a real person but without any risks to the learner or the client.

Changing technology now makes tailored multimedia presentations feasible via the use of compact discs (CDs), digital video discs (DVDs), and videoclips on the Web (Calderone 1994; Gleydura et al. 1995; Goodman and Blake 1996; Smith-Stoner and Willer 2003). The tools to produce streaming video are increasingly available. Streaming video can be uploaded to Web pages or course management tools such as Blackboard and WebCT. It may also be reproduced and distributed on CDs. Video is converted to a digital format for use on the Web or CD. Quality multimedia should reduce labor costs for instructor and participant time, improve overall instructional effectiveness, and foster productivity through user satisfaction and enjoyment. CD and DVD drives are now standard equipment on PCs. Multimedia can enhance CAI by using the interactivity, information management, and decision-making capabilities of computers (Billings 1994; Cambre and Castner 1993; Goodman and Blake 1996).

Authoring tools allow program design to match learning objectives and foster higher cognitive development. Authoring tools are software applications designed to allow persons with little or no programming expertise to create instructional programs. These tools require time for mastery: As many as 50 to 200 hours may be needed to prepare 1 hour of instruction and work out the program bugs. Educators can exercise creativity in the design of multimedia. It is possible to use slide presentation software to prepare and customize programs for student learning (Batscha 2002; Smith-Stoner and Willer 2003). Slide presentation software is easily learned, is adaptable, allows the insertion of simple programming commands, and is easily revised. It can also be used to house streaming video presentations. Faculty who are comfortable with the various forms of multimedia usually do a better job of integrating it into their instruction for optimal student benefit. Figure 15–1 depicts an online tutorial on arterial blood gases that was developed by a faculty member.

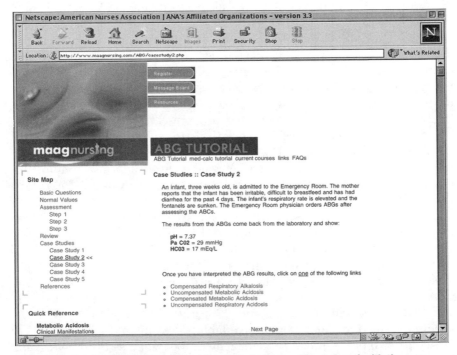

FIGURE 15–1 • An example of online educational offering (Reproduced with the permission of the author Dr. Margaret Maag.)

Teleconferencing

Teleconferencing is the use of computers, audio and video equipment, and high-grade dedicated telephone lines to provide interactive communication between two or more persons at two or more sites. Recent developments make teleconferencing capability possible from desktop computers. Teleconferencing is particularly useful for graduate and doctoral students and staff nurses because it brings educational opportunities to areas that may not otherwise offer courses or programs. In teleconferencing, learners at one site view and interact with an instructor and other learners at separate locations. Participants can pool resources to establish collaborative programs, thus maximizing resources through shared classes and conferences. Teleconferencing requires start-up funds and an investment in equipment and transmission media. Classes may be offered entirely online along with assignments and feedback. Content may be clinically oriented or focus on nursing informatics. This approach extends the reach of educational programs and continuing education courses by accommodating students who would otherwise be unable to attend programs because of their distance from offered programs.

Distance Education

Distance education is the use of print, audio, video, computer, teleconferencing capability, or the World Wide Web to connect faculty and students who are located at a minimum of two different locations. Print media is inexpensive and low technology and can be developed quickly. Audio conferences take place over the telephone. Video and teleconferencing have been popular in recent years. Video signals may be one-way or two-way transmissions over telephone lines, cable, satellite, or network connections. Improved Internet capabilities, telephone use, and teleconferencing have virtually eliminated the barriers faced by nurses in remote locations who wish to further their education via formal study or through continuing education programs, or who require additional job training (Corwin 2000; Kozlowski 2002). Distance education may occur in real, or synchronous, time or via a delay. In real time all parties participate in the activity at the same time; this may include a classroom session or chat. With the delayed, or asynchronous, approach, the learner reviews material at a convenient time. Asynchronous learning can be enhanced with the incorporation of ongoing electronic discussion to aid the clarification of ideas, promote retention, and aid critical thinking (Cartwright 2000; Harden 2003). Synchrony influences instructional design, delivery, and interaction. Distance education requires additional course preparation and organization by faculty and a concerted effort on the part of students to remain active participants. The transition from traditional classroom to online learning is not easy. It can, however, be an effective means of instruction.

There is a strong push among institutions of higher learning to offer distance education as a means to improve student access, meet student demands, extend geographic boundaries, remain viable, and keep students on the cutting edge of technology (Bentley, Cook, Davis, Murphy, and Berding 2003; Charp 2003; Cuellar 2002). However, good market research and planning remain key to the success of distance education courses and programs (Wong, Greenhalgh, Russell, Boynton, and Toon 2003). Careful consideration must be given to the market, course objectives, choice of software platform, staff training, design of active learning, quality, technical and administrative issues, finances, and the fit with the overall institution. Distance education has rapidly become an acceptable mode of nursing education, with more than one-half of all schools of nursing surveyed by the American Association of Colleges of Nursing demonstrating some involvement in distance education (Faison 2003; Sapnas et al. 2002). As more institutions and faculty move toward Internet-based distance education, The Institute for Higher Education Policy prepared a report sponsored by the National Education Association and Blackboard Inc., an Internet education company, that identified 24 benchmarks deemed essential to ensure excellence in Internet-based distance education (IHEP 2000). These benchmarks are broken down into seven categories and are summarized here:

Institutional Support Benchmarks

- Documented technology plan that includes security measures such as password protection, encryption, and back-up systems
- Reliable technology delivery system
- Centralized support system for building and maintaining the distance education infrastructure

Course Development Benchmarks

- Guidelines that specify minimum standards for course development, design, and delivery
- Periodic review of instructional materials for compliance with program standards
- Course and program requirements call for students to use analysis, synthesis, and evaluation

Teaching/Learning Benchmarks

- Students interact with faculty and other students as a part of instruction; communication facilitated through voice and/or e-mail
- Timely and constructive faculty feedback to students on questions and assignments
- Instruction on the methods of effective research and evaluation of resources for students

Course Structure Benchmarks

- Counseling for students on online instruction before starting a course or program to determine if they meet the technology and commitment requirements
- Supplemental course materials that address course objectives, concepts, and learning outcomes
- Access for students to sufficient library resources
- Agreement by faculty and students on course expectations

Student Support Benchmarks

- Students receive program information inclusive of admission requirements, tuition and fees, and technical and proctoring requirements
- Hands-on training is provided to help students access electronic databases, interlibrary loans, government archives, news services, and other pertinent resources
- Technical assistance is available at all times
- Student services answer questions accurately and quickly and have a mechanism to handle complaints

Faculty Support Benchmarks

- Technical assistance is available to faculty
- Assistance is available to help faculty make the transition from traditional to online teaching
- Instructor training and assistance, including peer mentoring, are available all through online courses
- Faculty have written guidelines to help students with issues related to the use of electronically accessed data

Evaluation and Assessment Benchmarks

- Evaluation processes use several methods and specific standards to determine educational effectiveness
- Enrollment data, costs, and applications of technology are used to evaluate program effectiveness
- Learning outcomes are regularly reviewed for clarity, utility and appropriateness

Faculty must acquire new skills and teaching methodologies for distance education (Geibert 2000; Im and Lee 2003; Kozlowski 2004; McKenna and Samarawickrema 2003). Communication and flexibility are essential qualities. Students may feel isolated, particularly if they experience difficulties in getting online. For this reason technical assistance must be readily available and faculty must maintain frequent communication with students. This communication may take place through postings to the class as well as e-mail to individual students. Students come to distance education with varying levels of technical skills. Students must be enrolled in the course and the electronic roster for access to the distance education offering. Late course registration, down servers, and poor computer skills can frustrate students; they must have Internet access. Time spent on e-mail may seem excessive but actually frees up time otherwise spent in group meetings addressing concerns (VandeVusse and Hanson 2000). All assignments should be clear. Course requirements need to stipulate file formats for paper submission. Faculty must realize that students may experience difficulty with firewalls, file transfer, and occasional Internet problems. Faculty need to design assignments that help students to develop a sense of community. Online collaboration may be accomplished via the use of e-mail, videoconferences, group projects, instant messaging, threaded discussions, and bulletin board postings. Thurmond (2003) states that developing interaction opportunities are a core element of online courses. Learners must engage with course content, other learners, the instructor and technology. Learner-content interaction occurs when students examine content and participate in class activities. Print media is less likely to engage a learner than are hyperlinks, interactive software, and discussions. Reciprocal action aids learning. Learner-learner interactions provide an opportunity to share ideas and benefit from the experiences of others. Collaborative projects facilitate this interaction through the creation of a community. Learner-instructor interactions occur with prompt feedback and meetings. Frequent communication through postings, e-mail, and online discussion facilitates this process. The fourth type of interaction described in discussions of distance education is learner-interface. Learner-interface interaction is facilitated when students are successful in getting online and accessing course materials. Faculty and students must avoid slang and use unambiguous language because participants can come from any part of the globe.

Distance education offers many advantages, but it also requires student commitment. Distance learners must assume responsibility for active learning, thus becoming more independent and self-disciplined (Theile 2003). Box 15–2 lists key points for the participant in distance education. Distance education broadens educational opportunities and eliminates long commutes. For this reason it may serve as a recruitment and retention mechanism for schools of nursing and health care agencies. It can provide access to experts and cut costs by paying faculty to teach at one site rather than multiple sites. Despite these advantages, distance education often faces budget constraints as well as slow planning and decision making.

The growth of distance education programs has implications for library services as well (Gandhi 2003). Academic libraries must demonstrate the ability to provide equivalent resources and services electronically or through some other means to both on-campus and distance learners to meet accreditation requirements. Some institutions have distance education librarians who work closely with faculty teaching distance education courses to meet student needs. This may be done through digitizing reserve materials

Box 15–2
Key Points for Students Involved in Distance Learning

- Reception sites may be in students' homes or workplaces.
- Increases educational opportunities by eliminating long commutes.
- Class rosters with phone numbers and addresses are generally distributed to all class members (pending individual approval) as a means to encourage interaction among students.
- Faculty can hold office hours online and provide feedback by telephone, electronic posting, chats, and e-mail as well as during class time.
- Students may remain online after class to ask questions.
- The sponsoring agency notifies students of information pertaining to hardware and software requirements reception sites, parking, and technical support.
- Additional effort is required from both students and faculty to maintain interactive aspects of the education process.
- Some modifications may be required in the use of audiovisual aids. Additional attention must be given to how well audiovisual aids transmit and whether they are visible to persons at other sites.
- Successful offerings are the result of a team effort that involves instructional designers, graphic artists, computing services, faculty training, and technical support.

and placing them on electronic reserves accessible only to students enrolled in the course. Restricted access, along with a prominent display of copyright notices on all readings help to ensure compliance with copyright and fair use laws. Permission should be obtained from the copyright holder for each item used. Reserve lists must be submitted in sufficient time to allow librarians time to secure permissions and scan materials.

As more schools of nursing move to distance education, there are concerns over the ability to socialize students to the profession. Obviously, this aspect of education requires careful attention in any setting. It is even more critical when there are no regular, face-to-face meetings between faculty and student. Studies indicate that it can take place in distance education, although additional research into this area is suggested (Faison 2003). Hirumi (2002) notes that technological advances are happening faster than research can keep up on the effectiveness of these advances. There are also issues related to faculty workload and class size, and intellectual property rights for electronic courses (Bentley et al. 2003).

Web-Based Instruction (WBI)

Web-based instruction (WBI) uses the attributes and resources of the World Wide Web, such as hypertext links and multimedia, for educational purposes. WBI may be offered as a stand-alone course or as a complement to traditional classes. Independent WBI provides access to most or all class materials, resources, and interaction via Internet technology. This is in contrast to Web-supported courses that rely on physical meetings of students and teachers but integrate assignments, readings, computer-mediated communications, and/or links to sites into the course activities. Some synonyms for WBI include Web-based training (WBT), Web-assisted instruction (WAI), Internet-based training (IBT), Web-based learning (WBL), Web interactive training (WIT), and online courses.

WBI is a popular educational use of computers (Cragg, Edwards, Yue, Xin, and Hui 2003; Cragg, Humbert, and Douchette 2004; Geibert 2000). It shares many of the advantages associated with CAI, such as self-paced learning, 24-hour availability, prompt feedback, and interactivity. Web-based instruction also supports multimedia, a high level of learner interactivity, and hyertext links, which enable learner-centered control over information and learning (Vogt, Kumrow, and Kazlauskas 2001). WBI is free from geographic constraints and can be revised as needed. The Web provides a user-friendly format along with access to multimedia in a fairly consistent manner. Most WBI sites provide basic course information, such as syllabus, schedule, announcements, and reading lists. Many other sites include synchronous or asynchronous communication, online testing, discussion groups, conferences, whiteboards, streaming audio and video, and, in some cases, online help. WBI can be used as a stand-alone course for distance education or as a complement to traditional courses. Teleconferencing capability is sometimes included. There is debate as to whether WBI is actually cost effective when development and support costs are considered. In the case of course materials, printing costs are shifted from the institution to the student.

It is important to consider a number of issues before Web-based instruction is offered (Bruckley 2003; Chen 2003; Choi 2003; Gould III 2003; Rose, Frisby, Hamlin, and Jones 2000; Sakraida and Draus 2003). These include the following:

- *Institutional commitment of resources.* WBI requires human and material resources. It is labor intensive to develop and manage. It requires administrative support for needed equipment, technical staff, and help for faculty interested in using this medium. Good design requires input from software specialists, service technicians, learning specialists, and possibly psychologists.

- *The technology infrastructure.* Networking and technical support staff should be consulted to determine server and network specifications, technical standards, bandwidth, and software requirements for Web-based instruction. Requirements to support and receive instruction must be identified. When teleconferencing is used, it is important to look at room layout in relationship to equipment capabilities.

- *Web course management tools and online peer collaboration tools.* This type of software provides the infrastructure, or shell, for faculty to present content, documents, and media (Kropf 2002; Mills 2000). Common features include tracking, threaded discussions, chat capability, a whiteboard, e-mail, the ability to post information, scheduling capability, templates, the ability to share files, grading components, exam and evaluation capability, and administrative and security features that limit access to authorized users. Some examples include Blackboard, WebCT, FirstClass, TopClass, LearningSpace, LearnLinc I-Net, and Centra Software's Symposium. Course management tools may be used to supplement traditional instruction or to supplant it. Some course management tools are fairly intuitive while others require a higher learning curve for faculty use. Typically colleges and universities make the software available and provide instruction and support to faculty and students seeking to use it (Sakraida and Draus 2003).

- *Adaptation of course materials and delivery for online instruction.* Successful WBI makes use of the hypertext capabilities of the Web; this includes links to other sites of potential interest. It represents a deviation from traditional class structures and acknowledges that the locus of control for learning lies with the learner. For this reason, activities that require active involvement on the part of the learner such as structured or threaded discussions and group projects are recommended.

- *Faculty commitment.* Web-based instruction is time consuming to create and maintain. Students require more feedback than might be needed in a traditional setting. Faculty must learn the tools and the teaching methodologies and keep materials and links up-to-date.

- *Practice time before the actual start of instruction.* One cannot assume that faculty or students come to Web-based instruction with an intuitive grasp of the technology. For this reason it is important to practice using the tool before the start of a course. Preparatory tutorials ensure that instructional time is not squandered on technical assistance for a few. Faculty must consider that Web-based courses generally have a slow start because Web-based learning is still a new learning environment for many students. They must exercise patience and ensure that technical support is available until all students demonstrate the basic skills required to navigate the course. Support may be available via orientation sessions, written and online materials, and telephone support.

- *Develop and communicate a contingency plan.* While the advantages of WBI include 24-hour availability from any location, there may be instances when access cannot be accomplished. This may be related to an individual's PC or Internet service provider, power outages, or problems with the organization's infrastructure. It is of particular concern when classes are synchronous. Identify alternative means of communicating assignments early in the class.

Box 15–3 includes a few suggestions for faculty who are developing Web-based instruction or considering its use.

Box 15-3	Do's and Don'ts for Teaching a Web-Based Course

Do's

- *Humanize the course.* Encourage students to provide background information about themselves and their goals at the onset of the course.
- *Post materials prior to class and discussions.* This provides reinforcement and promotes active listening when WBI is used as an adjunct to traditional classes.
- *Provide mechanisms for student feedback.* Use threaded discussions, chats, e-mail, blogs, and whiteboard capability.
- *Keep lessons short and modular.* Long documents online do not facilitate learning.
- *Use methods to factor interaction.* Include situations and ask participants to identify how they would respond. Encourage discussion among classmates. Assign group projects.
- *Incorporate a mechanism to access library resources.* Provide reserve lists to the library well in advance to allow time for signing.
- *Use formative feedback.* This will allow faculty to modify the course as needed to benefit students.
- *Provide information related to resources for technical support.*
- *Be flexible.* Not all students have the same level of computer skills.

Don'ts

- *Don't assume preexisting knowledge.* Provide a tutorial prior to class or as part of the first class to familiarize students with the technology.
- *Don't assume that everyone has the latest versions of software or fastest processor.* Students who cannot access all documents or portions of the class will become frustrated.
- *Avoid items that take a long time to download.* People will not wait. Large files also place a heavy demand on the server and network.
- *Avoid "plug-ins."* These programs can change the way the user's computer processes tasks as well as place additional demands on the processor.

WBI requires time for planning, implementation, and maintenance. Course design needs to incorporate learning activities that encourage collaborative efforts. As with distance education in general there are changes for faculty and student roles as a shift occurs from content-driven, or teacher-centered, to a student-centered approach. Faculty must move into the role of facilitator as they help students to organize information and use critical thinking (Kozlowski 2002). WBI increases access to educational offerings but learners still need access to computers and the Internet and basic computer skills.

E-learning

E-learning is the delivery of content and stimulation of learning primarily through the use of telecommunication technologies such as e-mail, bulletin board systems, electronic whiteboards, inter-relay chat, desktop video conferencing, and the World Wide Web (Hirumi 2002). It may also occur as the result of a satellite broadcast, audio/video tape, interactive TV, and/or CD-ROM. The basic premise behind e-learning is that it encourages more effective learning. The term is often used to refer to corporate training. It offers flexibility, self-paced instruction, and the ability to focus on needed content or skills. E-learning may or may not incorporate the opportunity to interact with faculty or other students.

Computer Labs

Computer labs have become an important instructional tool and a feature that students look at when they choose an educational facility. Box 15–4 identifies some features for students to consider when they have the opportunity to evaluate computer labs. There are three types of instructional computer labs: public access, limited access, and computer classrooms. Public access facilities provide a collection of general-purpose software and are open to all members of the institution on a first-come, first-served basis. Limited access labs are usually located within a particular department and are open only to people associated with that department. Limited-access lab software is determined by subject need. Computer classrooms are used as an instructional tool by faculty who conduct classes in the lab. This arrangement calls for one computer per learner. Computer classrooms may be used as public or limited access facilities when not in use as a classroom. Lab purpose determines the type and amount of hardware and software needed and has implications for size, the number of hours that it is accessible for use, and how it is staffed. Most computer labs rely on local area networks (LANs) instead of freestanding PCs because LANs are easier to administer, offer lower support costs, and permit sharing of resources, including software, printers, and information.

A successful computer lab requires careful planning and commitment to its ongoing support. Unfortunately there are few published guidelines for the setup of an instructional lab. Childs (2002) examined this issue with nursing labs that are also referred to as *clinical resource centers*. Typically, this type of facility is found within health sciences schools and contains a mixture of equipment, models, and computers that can be used for hands-on learning and simulation. Clinical resource centers should provide an orientation for users and be located at a convenient site with hours convenient to users. Equipment and software must be current. Staff should have a working knowledge of PCs and/or networks, software, and peripheral devices to provide user support. In addition to taking care of equipment and assisting users, computer lab staff maintain security, create and monitor user accounts, track system use, and back up software to prevent accidental damage. Faculty contribute to computer lab success by encouraging its use and through the selection of high-quality instructional software. Given the range of computer-enhanced learning tools, the clinical

Box 15–4 **Evaluation Criteria for a Computer Lab**

Lighting

- Windows, if present, are high up on the walls with shades, blinds, and/or curtains to control glare.
- Lighting for the room and at each computer is adjustable to accommodate the use of overheads, reading, note-taking, and computer work, while avoiding fatigue and headaches.

Heating/Ventilation/Air Conditioning

- Room temperature ranges between 70° and 72° F.

Acoustics

- Outside noise that can decrease concentration is minimal or nonexistent.

Furniture

- Chairs are comfortable and adjustable in height, with good lumbar support, wheels, and armrests that fit under tables to minimize restlessness and fatigue.
- Large tables support writing, training materials, and computer equipment while providing knee room.
- Surfaces are free from glare.
- Furniture has rounded corners to decrease risk of injury.
- A separate, portable master workstation with room for a PC, mouse pad, and projector provides a place for faculty to demonstrate program features.

Color

- The room is a cheerful medium to light color.

Power/Cabling/Phone Jacks

- There are sufficient electrical outlets and phone jacks to accommodate each workstation.
- Cables are properly secured and out of the way, so as not to pose a safety hazard.

SOURCE: Adapted from "Planning a computer lab: Considerations to ensure success," 1994, *IALL Journal of Language Learning Technologies,* 27(1), 55–59

resource lab will undoubtedly receive greater attention in the future. Many institutions use their facilities for students from several health care disciplines and even competency testing for graduates.

One source of frustration for students using computer labs is when they cannot access or use a particular software program. Careful lab management should limit this problem. Inability to access software may result when installation is improper, when a program is designed for use by one user, or when the number of users permitted by the lab's site license has been met. Site licenses are an agreement between the computer lab and the software publisher on the terms of use. For example, the site license for a network version of a word processing package may allow up to 25 users at one time. Additional individuals cannot access the software until another user has logged off. Institutions and lab administrators must estimate software use to negotiate site licenses that meet their needs. Lab users should exit applications and log off of the system so that others may access the software. Publishers may offer special site license agreements for the computer lab market, particularly if a need for special agreements is demonstrated (Happer 1995).

AUDIENCES FOR COMPUTER-ENHANCED EDUCATION

Educational applications of computers adapt well to a diversity of settings and learners. The very flexibility of educational applications of computer technology make it suitable for use in formal health care education programs, as well as continuing education and consumer education.

Formal Nursing Education

Advocates of computer-enhanced education note that its applications in health care are limited only by imagination (Bloom and Hough 2003; Charp 2003; Greco and O'Connor 2000). Critics of nursing education claim that computers and the Internet only promise to revolutionize the way that nursing is taught as instruction moves away from the traditional classroom lecture and clinical instruction to modalities that better accomodate the learning needs of individual students, promote the development of critical thinking skills, and foster skills needed in the work place (Bentley et al. 2003; Choi 2003; Cragg et al. 2003). The activities that can accomplish this may include simulations, virtual reality, CAI as a supplement to classroom instruction, slide presentations, Internet searches, collaborative learning, computerized testing, and the availability of reference materials online and on PDAs (Bloom and Hough 2003; Myles 2000). These activities may replace, or supplement, the traditional lecture format, which supports passive rather than active learning. Institutions are also responding to consumer demands for new models and methods for instructional delivery. Computer-enhanced communication and education can increase student access to experts and educational programs through the removal of geographical boundaries. The inclusion of computers in education is vital to the development of basic computer skills needed in the work place. Many programs suggest, and some require, that students purchase and use PDAs in the classroom and clinical settings to access reference materials and take notes. Computers are used in the clinical setting to document client care on hospital information systems. As a result of this expanding use of computers, most nursing programs have institutional academic computer plans, policies, and facilities. This reflects expectations that nursing graduates possess basic computer literacy skills (AACN 1998; ANA 2001). Nursing education programs are a logical place to introduce or expand basic computer skills such as word processing, Internet access, e-mail, and to introduce electronic searches, and spreadsheet and database applications. These computer literacy skills are important in the everyday workplace serving to increase access to information, facilitate the teaching/learning process, decrease anxiety associated with computer use, and enhance job skills. Basic computer literacy provides a framework for the development of another skill set expected of new graduates, namely rudimentary information management. For these reasons most basic nursing programs require that students take an introductory computer course.

Many nursing students are exposed to National Council Licensure Examination for Registered Nurses (NCLEX-RN) review programs while in school. This is important because all nurses in the United States take their licensure examination via computer. The NCLEX-RN examination uses computer-adaptive testing (CAT) with the goal of determining candidate ability based on the difficulty of questions answered correctly, not the number (Wendt 2003). When a question is missed, the candidate is given an easier item to answer. If the candidate is able to answer the easier item correctly the next item is more difficult. The NCLEX-RN uses an established minimum number of questions that must be answered but the total number of questions will vary by candidate. CAT offers several advantages over paper and pencil examinations. It saves time by matching items to individual ability, examinations are tailored to the individual, results may be available immediately, and it supports a variety of different reports (Latu and Chapman 2002; Van Horn 2003). NCLEX-RN preparation programs vary in quality, ranging from simple drill and practice to those that provide rationale for answers. Educators and nursing students need to be discriminating consumers. One question to consider is the approach and intended purpose of the program. For example, some provide a means to decrease anxiety over the NCLEX-RN examination through practice under similar conditions. They may also attempt to simulate the examination experience. Other programs claim to predict student success on the NCLEX-RN examination. Box 15–5 lists some criteria to consider when selecting NCLEX-RN preparation software.

The benefits associated with computer-supported learning have led to an increased availability of courses and educational software related to nursing and health care topics. It is important to evaluate the quality of these applications and to use them in an effective manner. The nurse educator is responsible for evaluating the merits of available tools prior to their implementation. It is not necessary to be a software expert to do this. Faculty should use the same criteria to evaluate computer uses in education that they apply to any other instructional medium. Box 15–6 lists criteria that may be used to evaluate the quality of instructional software.

Administrative computer applications improve record keeping for program attendance, performance, and evaluation and can save time for the construction, administration, and scoring and statistical analysis of test results. Although most evaluative tools focus on testing, computers and PDAs lend themselves nicely to notes and anecdotal accounts of clinical learning that can be used to evaluate individuals and the quality of specific learning experiences as well as support curriculum changes (Meyer, Sedlmeyer, Carlson, and Modlin 2003). An increasing number of faculty are turning towards software applications and technology to make the clinical evaluation process less ar-

Box 15–5 **Features to Look for in NCLEX-RN Preparation Programs**

- Ease of use
- Good feedback for answers. For example, does it provide rationale and scores?
- Effective screen design and keyboard use. If the goal of the program is to simulate the examination, then screen design and keyboard use must be the same as the NCLEX-RN.
- Questions that are high quality and clear, and in adequate numbers.
- Questions presented in a randomized fashion, as in the actual examination
- A match between the preparation program content and NCLEX-RN examination content
- A bookmark feature that allows students to mark the spot where they quit, exit the program, and return to that spot later
- Clear instructions
- Adequate technical support
- A warranty
- An upgrade policy
- Acceptable system requirements (type of computer, memory requirements, etc.)

SOURCE: Adapted from "Computerized NCLEX-RN preparation programs: A comparative review," by D. Billings et al., 1996, *Computers in Nursing,* 14(5), 262–263, 266.

Box 15–6 **Evaluation Criteria for Instructional Software**

- Does it support the overall course objectives?
- Is the material presented clearly?
- Is content accurate?
- What is the quality of the design? Does it maintain learner interest and provide the ability to customize learning to individual needs?
- Is information presented in a logical order?
- Does it provide appropriate and immediate feedback?
- Does it make good use of graphics, design, and multimedia?

duous. In some cases Web-based tools accept input from both faculty and students tabulating results and providing information for curriculum decisions.

Hospital Information Systems Connectivity with real hospital information systems (HIS) is another important use of computers in nursing education. The incorporation of hospital and nursing information systems into nursing school curricula promotes professional socialization, helps students see the effects of their decision making with care plans or maps, and decreases orientation time for new graduates. Computer-generated care plans or maps allow students to devote to analysis of data the time once spent writing care plans, and allow staff more time to mentor students. This use of information systems ensures that graduates have exposure to computers and possess marketable job skills, and helps students to see the whole clinical picture. Students may receive live training sessions in system use by faculty or by hospital-based trainers or use computer-based training (CBT). Training may occur at the school or healthcare facility. Students can retrieve information for use in preparing for client assignments, but should not be able to make changes or add information to the actual client record from remote sites.

Access to hospital information systems as a learning tool in schools of nursing offers the following benefits (Doorley, Renner, and Corron 1994; Kennedy 2003; Poirrier, Wills, Broussard, and Payne 1996):

- Provides time to analyze clinical information
- Provides the student with adequate time to compose care plans or review critical pathways
- Allows students to review their plans with faculty or hospital nursing staff prior to entry into the system
- Increases students' knowledge and proficiency when they enter the actual clinical setting

HIS connectivity may be provided at schools of nursing. This requires negotiation with the vendor for permission. Other considerations include increased demands upon the information system and concerns related to confidentiality of client information. HIS connectivity allows students to be more familiar with their assigned clients and poses fewer interruptions for staff from students requesting information. Incorporation of hospital and nursing information systems at schools of nursing also facilitates role transition from student to graduate nurse, makes graduates more attractive to prospective employers, and allows hospitals to cut orientation time for graduates with prior HIS training.

Continuing Education

Nationwide budget cuts caused many institutions and employers to reduce or eliminate continuing education program offerings provided by traditional classes, conferences, and workshops. There is now an increased reliance on outside agencies and technology to meet this need. The traditional approach to this problem has been home study offered through professional journals and organizations. Readers review articles, answer related questions, send in their test form and fee, and wait to find out whether they received credit. The journal approach offers little, if any, interaction with peers. Mandatory education requirements such as fire safety were often met through the review of video or paper self-learning modules. Another approach is the use of the Internet for continuing education courses. This approach offers several benefits. It is available without a subscription 24 hours a day to a large population. Furthermore, it can provide instant feedback and highly individualized instruction, since the incorporation of links allows users to skip familiar content or seek additional information as required. It allows staff to attend mandatory programs at convenient times without interruption to client services and decreases expenses for travel between sites and instructor hours (Harrington and Walker 2003). Internet continuing education programs may be found through professional publications and organizations, as well as Web searches. Unfortunately, this option requires access to a computer.

Computers can also be used for administrative support of continuing education (Cragg et al. 2004). For example, computerized records can be searched rapidly to determine if and when a particular student attended a program such as fire safety or cardiopulmonary resuscitation (CPR). It is also possible to administer and score proficiency examinations and evaluation tools. Other tracking features can show individuals who started, but did not complete, an educational unit or the number of attempts needed to achieve successful completion. Improved records also help to determine program costs and demonstrate staff development or continuing education staff productivity.

E-Learning has been suggested as an alternative delivery method for mandatory educational programs as well as other programs that provide employees with opportunities to improve or maintain skill sets (Hequet 2004; Hirumi 2002; Joch 2003). The rationale for this approach is that e-learning allows employees to learn at their own pace and to skip material that they already know. There are no costs associated with travel, lodging, or meals. It also helps to meet deadlines for mandatory education programs. Training is available upon demand and course materials and tests are online. Institutions using E-learning to meet mandatory educational programs should choose a product that easily allows customization as regulations change and programs need revised. e-Learning can support synchronous or asynchronous communications but asynchronous communications are more common and are often mediated by technology. Appraisal of the effectiveness of e-learning may be done through participant evaluation as well as a review of technical support logs.

Client Education

Although many computer applications directly benefit nurses and other health care professionals, consumers derive much of their health care information from the Internet and educational software and e-mail. Some sites allow consumers to pose questions and then provide an answer within 24 hours. Home pages on the World Wide Web provide information on a variety of topics, including preparation for diagnostic tests. They may even show film clips. Web-based client education materials must be designed with the following factors in mind: purpose, target population, expected clinical and learning outcomes, educational framework, design principles, and ongoing site evaluation for readability and ease of navigation (Smith, Cha, Puno, Magee, Bingham, and Van Gorp 2002). Effective instructional websites should also incorporate different learning modalities (Vogt et al. 2001). Client education materials and discharge instructions can be generated by hospital information systems as well. An example of this application may be seen with a client who had heart bypass surgery. Instructions should include the following: when to schedule a follow-up visit with the cardiac surgeon and the primary physician, wound care, signs or symptoms that should be reported to the physician, and discharge medications. Computer generation of discharge instructions can tailor instructions to the individual client and the physician authorizing the discharge, and offers the following advantages:

- Consistent instruction despite the fact that different nurses provide teaching
- Improved quality and detail
- Speed
- Clarity and legibility
- Eliminates repetition. Nurses no longer need to write the same instructions over and over again.
- Compliance with physician recommendations.

ISSUES RELATED TO COMPUTER-ENHANCED EDUCATION

The mere presence and use of computers for education do not ensure successful learning. Consideration of the following factors and guidelines will enhance the effectiveness of using computers for education:

- *Institutional planning.* Computer-enhanced education must be a part of an overall plan that makes provisions for infrastructure, as well as financial and technical support.
- *Hardware and software must be accessible.* This includes technical support, servers, and all software that the learner is expected to use. Problems with access and poor service immediately set a negative tone.
- *User comfort with the technology.* Not all learners are familiar with computers or know how to use them. This lack of knowledge and skills may lead to anxiety. For this reason computer literacy should be a prerequisite, and a basic introduction provided before the introduction of any new technology. This applies to faculty and students. Short, highly interactive training sessions that cover small amounts of information at one time are recommended. Once the learner is comfortable with the technology other learning needs can be met (Chen 2003; Scollin 2001).
- *Opportunities to ask about material not understood.* Although the computer is an invaluable instructional aid, the ability to question and discuss information presented must also be available.
- *Instruction is well designed and well matched to course objectives.* High-quality Web-based instruction and computer programs for education must maintain learner interest and provide the appropriate information (Bloom and Hough 2003).

- *Evaluation criteria are identified to monitor the effectiveness of the computer as a tool.* These may include increased use of e-mail, increased job satisfaction, and improved student achievement. Online course evaluations may also be used.

There are a number of issues that must be addressed for faculty that are either interested in developing online courses and other means of computer-enhanced instruction, or who feel that they are under pressure from their respective institutions to teach online courses. These include:

- *Faculty workload, or hours, for the development and presentation of computer-enhanced instruction.* Administrative support of faculty who develop and present online courses, computer tutorials, and other applications that support education must include release time and/or financial rewards.

- *Promotion and tenure policies.* The design, development, and ongoing support of computer-enhanced or online instruction are time-consuming and labor-intensive yet these activities rarely receive the same level of recognition as professional presentations and publications when faculty are considered for promotion in rank and tenure. As more institutions adopt computer-enhanced instruction this area must be addressed.

- *Intellectual ownership.* Many faculty remain unclear on questions of intellectual ownership for computer-enhanced learning activities and online courses that they develop or materials that they post online as part of a course. Institutional policy needs to address this. Most faculty feel that they "own" a course that they developed and that no one else should be given that course to teach without their permission.

Educational Opportunities in Nursing Informatics

Until recent years the opportunities for nurses and other health care professionals to learn more about informatics were largely limited to programs sponsored by special-interest groups. Only a handful of undergraduate and graduate nursing programs offered introductory nursing informatics courses. This situation is changing rapidly now as nursing informatics has become a popular topic. An increasing number of schools offer a graduate degree or a certificate with a nursing informatics focus. Some of these programs use distance or Web-based education, while others use the traditional classroom setting. Doctoral programs are still limited. There are also a number of programs with a focus on health information management or health informatics.

CASE STUDY EXERCISES

You are on the education committee at your small community hospital. Your staff development department was eliminated several years ago.

You and your colleagues are charged with developing strategies to meet the educational needs of agency registered and licensed practical nurses. Limited capital and the isolated location of your community make this a difficult assignment. Your institution does have Internet and World Wide Web access in the medical library, as well as teleconferencing capability. Develop a proposal to meet your charge using available resources. Be prepared to defend your proposal to an administration loathe to part with monies beyond those already budgeted.

• • •

You are the client educator at a medical center in the Pacific Northwest. Your clientele are drawn from a 150-mile radius and beyond. For this reason it is difficult to have clients complete diabetic education or other classes. You have been told to improve client completion of classes or face elimination of your department. The medical center has both teleconferencing capability, presently used for consults, and an established Web page that provides basic information about the institution. How might you use these resources to develop alternative strategies for client education? Address budget considerations, necessary resources, target populations that might be better served, and how you propose to link distant clients with instructional offerings.

• • •

You recently joined the faculty at a small, private rural college. Because you express an interest in computers and are slightly more knowledgeable about computers than are your faculty colleagues, you have been asked to establish a computer lab for the nursing department and to incorporate computer use in all of the nursing courses. Current resources are quite limited. Provide a detailed plan of how you would accomplish this charge from start to finish. Identify potential stumbling blocks and ways that you would address them.

 EXPLOREMediaLink

Multiple choice, review questions, case studies, and other interactive resources for this chapter can be found on the Web site at *http://www.prenhall.com/hebda*. Click on "Chapter 15" to select the activities for this chapter.

SUMMARY

- Computer technology can help revolutionize education in formal nursing programs, continuing education, and consumer education. It also provides informal opportunities for networking among professionals via e-mail and discussion groups.

- Successful use of computers for education requires careful planning, orientation to the technology, convenient access, opportunities to question what is not understood, and good instructional design.

- Formal nursing education is a logical place to introduce or expand basic computer skills, such as word processing, Internet access, e-mail, and online literature searches.

- Educational software should be subject to the same review criteria applied to other instructional materials before their adoption.

- Computer instruction should match curriculum level and objectives.

- NCLEX-RN preparation programs are a popular use of computerized test programs in basic nursing programs.

- Connectivity to hospital information systems from schools of nursing allows students more opportunity to analyze client information before scheduled clinical experiences and facilitates professional socialization.

- Computers provide invaluable assistance in the preparation of educational materials and presentations, the delivery of instruction, examinations, and evaluations, and the maintenance of educational records.

- Computer-assisted instruction is the use of a computer to teach a subject other than computing via direct interaction of the student with the computer. It offers the following advantages: convenience, decreased learning time, and increased retention.

- Teleconferencing is the use of computers, audio and video equipment, and high-grade dedicated telephone lines, cable, and satellite to provide interactive communication between two or more persons at two or more sites.

- Distance education is the use of print, audio, video, computer, or teleconference capability to connect faculty and students located at a minimum of two different sites. Distance education may take place in real time or on a delayed basis. It expands educational opportunities without the need for a long commute.

- Web-based instruction uses the attributes and resources of the Internet to deliver and support education. It may be used as a stand-alone course or to supplement traditional classes.

- E-learning uses electronic media to present instruction. It is often suggested for corporate training because it is considered to be efficient. It allows users to skip material that they already know.

- Multimedia refers to the ability to deliver presentations that combine text, voice or sound, images, and video. Multimedia presentations tend to improve learning by actively engaging the senses.

- Computer labs are an asset to educational facilities. Most use local area network technology to share information, software, and other resources.

- Educational opportunities in nursing informatics range from the informal to the formal. There are numerous introductory courses on undergraduate and graduate levels. Some institutions offer areas of specialization within a degree on the graduate level or certificate programs. Opportunities for doctoral work in nursing informatics are limited.

REFERENCES

American Association of Colleges of Nursing (AACN). (1998). *Essentials of baccalaureate education for professional nursing practice.* Washington, DC: AACN.

American Nurses Association (ANA). (2001). *Scope and standards of nursing informatics practice.* Washington, DC: American Nurses Publishing.

Batscha, C. (2002). The pharmacology game. *CIN Plus, 5*(3), 1, 3–6.

Bentley, G. W., Cook, P. P., Davis, K., Murphy, M. J., and Berding, C. B. (2003). RN to BSN program: Transition from traditional to online delivery. *Nurse Educator, 28*(3), 121–126.

Billings, D. M. (1994). Effects of BSN student preferences for studying alone or in groups on performance and attitude when using interactive videodisc instruction. *Journal of Nursing Education, 33*(7), 322–324.

Billings, D. M. (1995). Preparing nursing faculty for information age teaching and learning. *Computers in Nursing, 13*(6), 264, 268–270.

Bloom, K. C., and Hough, M. C. (2003). Student satisfaction with technology-enhanced learning. *CIN: Computers, Informatics, Nursing, 21*(5), 241–246.

Bradley, C. (2003). Technology as a catalyst to transforming nursing care. *Nursing Outlook, 51*(3), S14–S15.

Bruckley, K. M. (2003). Evaluation of classroom-based, web-enhanced, and web-based distance learning nutrition courses for undergraduate nursing. *Journal of Nursing Education, 42*(8), 367–370.

Calderone, A. B. (1994). Computer-assisted instruction: Learning, attitude, and modes of instruction. *Computers in Nursing, 12*(3), 164–170.

Cambre, M., and Castner, L. J. (March 1993). The status of interactive video in nursing education environments. Presented at FITNE: Get in Touch with Multimedia, Atlanta, GA.

Cartwright, J. (2000). Lessons learned: Using asynchronous computer-mediated conferencing to facilitate group discussion. *Journal of Nursing Education, 39*(2), 87–90.

Charp, S. (2003). Technology for all students. *T.H.E. Journal, 30*(9), 8.

Chen, T. (2003). Recommendations for creating and maintaining effective networked learning communities. *International Journal of Instructional Media, 30*(1), 35.

Childs, J. C. (2002). Clinical resource centers in nursing programs. *Nurse Educator, 27*(5), 232–235.

Choi, H. (2003). A problem-based learning trail on the Internet involving undergraduate nursing students. *Journal of Nursing Education, 42*(8), 359–363.

Corwin, E. J. (2000). Distance education: An ongoing initiative to reach rural family nurse practitioner students. *Nurse Educator, 25*(3), 114–115.

Cragg, C. E., Edwards, N., Yue, Z., Xin, S. L., and Hui, Z. D. (2003). Integrating web-based technology into distance education for nurses in China. *CIN: Computers, Informatics, Nursing, 21*(5), 265–274.

Cragg, C. E., Humbert, J., and Douchette, S. (2004). A toolbox of technical supports for nurses new to web learning. *CIN: Computers, Informatics, Nursing, 22*(1), 19–23.

Cuellar, N. (2002). Tips to increase success for teaching online: Communication! *CIN Plus, 5*(1), 1, 3–6.

Doorley, J. E., Renner, A. L., and Corron, J. (1994). Creating care plans via modems: Using a hospital information system in nursing education. *Computers in Nursing, 12*(3), 160–163.

Faison, K. A. (2003). Professionalization in a distance learning setting. *The ABNF Journal: Official Journal of the Association of Black Nursing Faculty in Higher Education, 14*(4), 83–85.

Gandhi, S. (2003). Academic librarians and distance education: Challenges and opportunities. *Reference & User Services Quarterly, 43*(2), 138.

Geibert, R. C. (2000). Integrating web-based instruction into a graduate nursing program taught via videoconferencing: Challenges and solutions. *Computers in Nursing, 18*(1), 26–34.

Gleydura, A. J., Michelman, J. E., and Wilson, C. N. (1995). Multimedia training in nursing education. *Computers in Nursing, 13*(4), 169–175.

Glover, S. M., and Kruse, M. (1995). Making the most of computer-assisted instruction. *Nursing 95, 25*(9), 32N.

Goodman, J., and Blake, J. (1996). Multimedia courseware: Transforming the classroom. *Computers in Nursing, 14*(5), 287–296.

Gould J. W., III (2003). Program planning of asynchronous online courses design complexities and ethics. *Acquisition Review Quarterly, 10*(1), 63.

Greco, J. F., and O'Connor, D. J. (2000). A role for computer-assisted instruction in the beginning undergraduate course. *Financial Practice & Education, 10*(1), 239–244.

Happer, S. K. (1995). Software, copyright, and site license agreements: Publishers' perspective of library practice. Thesis. Kent, OH: Kent State University.

Harden, J. K. (2003). Faculty and student experiences with web-based discussion groups in a large lecture setting. *Nurse Educator, 28*(1), 26–30.

Hardy, J. L., Lindqvist, R., Kristofferzon, M. L., and Dahlberg, O. (1997). The current status of nursing informatics in undergraduate nursing programs: Comparative case studies between Sweden and Australia. *Studies Health Technology and Informatics, 46*, 132.

Harrington, S. S., and Walker, B. L. (2003). Is computer-based instruction an effective way to present fire safety training to long-term care staff? *Journal for Nurses in Staff Development, 19*(3), 147–154.

Henderson, R., and Deane, F. (1995). Assessment of satisfaction with computer training in a healthcare setting. *Journal of Nursing Staff Development, 11*(5), 255–260.

Hequet, M. (2004). Training no one wants: Restive, rebellious, reluctant—Sometimes you're faced with employees who just don't want to be trained. What should you do? *Training, 41*(1), 22 (6p).

Higa, D., and McNatt, B. (2003). Automation impact. *ADVANCE for Health Information Executives, 7*(2), 66–74.

Hirumi, A. (2002). The design and sequencing of e-learning interactions: A grounded approach. *International Journal on E-Learning, 1*(1), 19–27.

Im, Y., and Lee, O. (2003). Pedagogical implications of online discussion for preservice teacher training. *Journal of Research on Technology in Education, 36*(2), 155.

Institute for Higher Education Policy (IHEP). (2000). *Quality on the line: Benchmarks for success in Internet-based distance education.* Available at http://www.ihep.com/Pubs/PDF/Quality.pdf. Accessed February 19, 2004.

Joch, A. (2003). Sites for sore eyes. *Healthcare Informatics, 20*(4), 31–33.

Kennedy, R. (2003). The nursing shortage and the role of technology. *Nursing Outlook, 51*(3), S33–S34.

Khoiny, F. E. (1995). Factors that contribute to computer-assisted instruction effectiveness. *Computers in Nursing, 13*(4), 165–168.

Kozlowski, D. (2002). Using online learning in a traditional face-to-face environment. *Computers in Nursing, 20*(1), 23–30.

Kozlowski, D. (2004). Factors for consideration in the development and implementation of an online RN-BSN course: Faculty and student perceptions, *CIN: Computers, Informatics, Nursing, 22*(1), 34–43.

Kropf, R. (2002). How shall we meet online? Choosing between videoconferencing and online meetings. *Journal of Healthcare Information Management, 16*(4), 68–72.

Latu, E., and Chapman, E. (2002). Computerised adaptive testing. *British Journal of Educational Technology, 33*(5), 619.

Maag, M. (2004). The effectiveness of an interactive multimedial learning tool on nursing students' math knowledge and self-efficacy. *CIN: Computers, Informatics, Nursing, 22*(1), 26–33.

McKenna, L. G., and Samarawickrema, R. G. (2003). Crossing cultural boundaries: Flexible approaches and nurse education. *CIN: Computers, Informatics, Nursing, 21*(5), 259–264.

Meyer, L., Sedlmeyer, R., Carlson, C., and Modlin, S. (2003). A web application for recording and analyzing the clinical experiences of nursing students. *CIN: Computers, Informatics, Nursing, 21*(4), 186–195.

Mills, A. C. (2000). Creating web-based, multimedia, and interactive courses for distance learning. *Computers in Nursing, 18*(3), 125–131.

Myles, J. (November 27, 2000). The Internet advances nursing education. *Healthcare Review, 13*(10), 4. Available at http://www.findarticles.com/cf–0/m-HSV/10_13/82393991/print.jhtml. Accessed January 21, 2004.

O'Gara, N., and American Academy of Nursing. (2003). Recommendations of the American Academy of Nursing Conference participants. *Nursing Outlook, 51*(3), S39–S41.

Planning a computer lab: Considerations to ensure success. (1994). *IALL Journal of Language Learning Technologies, 27*(1), 55–59.

Poirrier, G. P., Wills, E. M., Broussard, P. C., and Payne, R. L. (1996). Nursing information systems: Applications in nursing curricula. *Nurse Educator, 21*(1), 18–22.

Ravert, P. (2002). An integrative review of computer-based simulation in the education process. *CIN: Computers, Informatics, Nursing, 20*(5), 203–208.

Ring, D. M., and Vander Meer, P. F. (Summer 1994). Designing a computerized instructional training room for the library. *Special Libraries,* 154–160.

Rose, M. A., Frisby, A. J., Hamlin, M. D., and Jones, S. S. (2000). Evaluation of the effectiveness of a web-based graduate epidemiology course. *Computers in Nursing, 18(4),* 162–167.

Ross, G. D., and Tuovinen, J. E. (2001). Deep versus surface learning with multimedia in nursing education. *Computers in Nursing, 19*(5), 213–223.

Rossignol, M., and Scollin, P. (2001). Piloting use of computerized practice tests. *Computers in Nursing, 19*(5), 206–212.

Rouse, D. P. (2000). The effectiveness of computer-assisted instruction in teaching nursing students about congenital heart disease. *Computers in Nursing, 18*(6), 282–287.

Sakraida, T. J., and Draus, P. J. (2003). Transition to a web-supported curriculum. *CIN: Computers, Informatics, Nursing, 21*(6), 309–315.

Sapnas, K. G., Walsh, S. M., Vilberg, W., Livingstone, P., Asher, M. E., Dlugasch, L. and Villanueva, N. E. (2002). Using web technology in graduate and undergraduate nursing education. *CIN Plus, 5*(2), 1, 33–37.

Scollin, P. (2001). A study of factors related to the use of online resources by nurse educators. *Computers in Nursing, 19*(6), 249–256.

Simpson, R. L. (2002). Virtual reality revolution: Technology changes nursing education. *Nursing Management, 33*(9), 14–15.

Smith, C. E., Cha, J., Puno, F., Magee, J. D., Bingham, J., and Van Gorp, M. (2002). Quality assurance processes for designing patient education web sites. *CIN: Computers, Informatics, Nursing, 20*(5), 191–200.

Smith-Stoner, M., and Willer, A. (2003). Video streaming in nursing education. *Nurse Educator, 28*(2), 66–70.

Sternberger, C., and Meyer, L. (2001). Hypermedia-assisted instruction: Authoring with learning guidelines. *Computers in Nursing, 19*(2), 69–74.

Theile, J. E. (2003). Learning patterns of online students. *Journal of Nursing Education, 42*(8), 364–366.

Thurmond, V. A. (2003). Defining interaction and strategies to enhance interactions in web-based courses. *Nurse Educator, 28*(5), 237–241.

VandeVusse, L., and Hanson, L. (2000). Evaluation of online course discussions: Faculty facilitation of active student learning. *Computers in Nursing, 18*(4), 181–188.

Van Horn, R. (2003). Technology: Computer adaptive tests and computer-based tests. *Phi Delta Kappan, 84*(8), 567.

Vogt, C., Kumrow, D., and Kazlauskas, E. (2001). The design elements in developing effective learning and instructional web-sites. *Academic Exchange Quarterly, 5*(4), 40.

Wang, S., and Sleeman, P. J. (1993a). A comparison of the relative effectiveness of computer-assisted instruction and conventional methods for teaching an operations management course in a school of business. *International Journal of Instructional Media, 20*(3), 225–235.

Wang, S., and Sleeman, P. J. (1993b). Computer-assisted instruction effectiveness: A brief review of the research. *International Journal of Instructional Media, 20*(4), 333–348.

Wendt, A. (2003). Frequently asked questions about computer-adaptive testing. *Computers, Informatics, Nursing: CIN Plus, 21*(1), 46–48.

Wong, G., Greenhalgh, T., Russell, J., Boynton, P., and Toon, P. (2003). Putting your course on the web: Lessons from a case study and systematic literature review. *Medical Education, 37*(11), 1020–1023.

16

Telehealth

After completing this chapter, you should be able to:

- Define the term *telehealth*.
- List the advantages of telehealth.
- Identify equipment and technology needed to sustain telehealth.
- Discuss present and proposed telehealth applications.
- Describe legal and practice issues that affect telehealth.

- Review the implications of telehealth for nursing and other allied health professions.
- Identify several telenursing applications.
- Discuss some issues pertaining to the practice of telenursing.

 MEDIALINK

Additional resources for this content can be found on the Companion Website at *www. prenhall.com/hebda*. Click on "Chapter 16" to select the activities for this chapter.

Companion Website

- Glossary
- Multiple Choice
- Discussion Points
- Case Study: Productive Teleconferencing
- Case Study: Telecommunication Breakdown
- MediaLink Application: Future Implications of Video Nursing
- Web Hunt: Telehealth
- Links to Resources
- Crossword Puzzle

Telehealth is the use of telecommunication technologies and computers to exchange health care information and to provide services to clients at another location. This was once known as telemedicine, but applications are now widely used by other members of the health care community. The American Nurses Association (1996) prefers the term *telehealth* as a more inclusive and accurate description of the services provided. Telehealth services include health promotion, disease prevention, diagnosis, consultation, education, and therapy. Teleconferences and videoconferences are tools used to deliver these services. Electronic, visual, and audio signals sent during these conferences provide information to consultants from remote sites. Many common medical devices have been adapted for use with telemedicine technology. Distant practitioners and clients benefit from the skills and knowledge of the consultants without the need to travel to regional referral centers. Telehealth is a tool that allows health care professionals to do the following (DiCianni and Kobza 2002; Harrison 2002; Marcin, Ellis, Mawis, Nagrampa, Nesbitt, and Dimand 2004, Waldo 2003):

- Consult with colleagues
- Conduct interviews
- Assess and monitor clients
- View diagnostic images
- Review slides and laboratory reports
- Extend scarce health care resources
- Decrease the number of hospital visits for patients with chronic conditions
- Decrease health care costs
- Improve the quality of client care
- Improve the overall quality of the client's record

Telehealth-related terms describing these capabilities have proliferated (see Box 16–1 for a partial listing).

TERMS RELATED TO TELEHEALTH

Initially *telemedicine* was the predominant term for the delivery of health care education and services via the use of telecommunication technologies and computers. It has since largely been replaced by the term *telehealth*. Telehealth encompasses telemedicine but is a broader term that emphasizes both the delivery of services and the provision of information and education to health care providers and consumers. For example, federal agencies use the Internet to provide health care professionals, consumers, and their families with medical information. The Public Health Service's Agency for Health Care Policy and Research (AHCPR) places clinical

Box 16-1 Some Common Telehealth Terms

- *E-care.* The provision of health information, products, and services online as well as the automation of administrative and clinical aspects of care delivery.

- *E-health.* A broad term often used interchangeably with the term telehealth to refer to the provision of health information, products, and services online.

- *E-medicine.* The use of telecommunication and computer technology for the delivery of medical care.

- *Telecardiology.* Transmission of cardiac catheterization studies, echocardiograms, and other diagnostic tests in conjunction with electronic stethoscope examinations for second opinions by cardiologists at another site.

- *Teleconsultation.* Videoconferencing between two health care professionals or a health care professional and a client.

- *Telehomecare.* The use of telecommunication and computer technologies to monitor and render services and support to home care clients.

- *Telementoring.* Real-time advice is offered during a procedure to a practitioner in a remote site via a telecommunication system.

- *Telenursing.* The use of telecommunication and computer technology for the delivery of nursing care.

- *Telepathology.* Transmission of high-resolution still images, often via a robotic microscope, for interpretation by a pathologist at a remote site.

- *Teleprevention.* The use of telecommunication technology to provide health.

- *Telepsychiatry.* Variant of teleconsultation that allows observation and interviews of clients at one site by a psychiatrist at another site.

- *Telerehabilitation.* The use of interactive technology to facilitate exercise and rehabilitation activities.

- *Teleradiology.* Transmission of high-resolution still images for interpretation by a radiologist at a distant location.

- *Telesurgery.* Surgeons at a remote site can collaborate with experts at a referral center on techniques.

- *Teletherapy.* The use of interactive videoconferencing to provide therapy and counseling.

- *Teleultrasound.* Transmission of ultrasound images for interpretation at a remote site.

---

practice guidelines online. The U.S. National Library of Medicine provides information on health, various medical conditions and procedures, clinical trials, and the capability to conduct searches of several databases on its Web site. There also are a number of professional journals and articles available online. Some require subscription; some do not. One example of an online journal is The National Cancer Institute's *JNCI Cancer Spectrum*. This publication incorporates a wide range of cancer information from respected sources. It allows readers to browse by topic, and does require a subscription. As a consequence of the information explosion, health care professionals and clients gain access to the most current treatment options at essentially the same time. No matter what term is used, the basic premise of telehealth is that it can provide services to underserved communities. Another frequently used term is *e-health*, which is often used interchangeably with the term *telehealth*. **Telenursing** is the use of telecommunications and computer technology for the delivery of nursing care.

Teleconferencing

Teleconferencing implies that people at different locations have audio, and possibly video, contact, which is used to carry out telehealth applications. The terms *teleconference* and *videoconference* may be used synonymously, because both use telecommunications and computer technology.

Videoconferencing

Videoconferencing implies that people meet face-to-face and view the same images through the use of telecommunications and computer technology even though they are not in the same location. It saves travel time and costs, which actually encourages people to meet more frequently. Videoconferencing is an appealing concept that can be used for many applications, especially distance learning and telehealth (although some applications may require high resolution and audio quality and high-speed transmission). For example, videoconferences provide a means to improve quality and access to care in Alaska, where clinics are connected. Live conferences are used to view critically ill clients, and specially adapted medical equipment is used to collect and send assessment data digitally. Communities benefit by saving travel time and costs for this arrangement, and appropriate care can be initiated in a timely fashion (Smith 2004).

Desktop Videoconferencing

Desktop videoconferencing (DTV) is a synchronous, or real-time, encounter that uses a specially equipped personal computer with telephone line hookup to allow people to meet face-to-face and/or view papers and images simultaneously. DTV is less expensive than custom-designed videoconference systems, but it may not be acceptable for telehealth applications that require high-resolution or high-speed transmission, such as interpretation of diagnostic images where slower frame rates produce a jerky image or lengthy transmission times.

HISTORICAL BACKGROUND

Telehealth began with the use of telephone consults and has become more sophisticated with each advance in technology (Brantley, Laney-Cummings, and Spivack 2004; McGee and Tangalos 1994; Perednia 1995;

Perednia and Allen 1995). During the past four decades the U.S. government played a major role in the development and promotion of telehealth through various agencies. Interest waned as funding slowed to a trickle in the 1980s but subsequent technological advancements made telehealth attractive again. Federal monies and the Agriculture Department's 1991 Rural Development Act laid the groundwork to bring the information superhighway to rural areas for education and telehealth purposes.

The most aggressive development of telehealth in the United States has been by NASA and the military (Brown 2002). NASA provided international telehealth consults for Armenian earthquake victims in 1989. The military has also had several projects to feed medical images from the battlefield to physicians in hospitals and on robotics equipment for telesurgery for improved treatment of casualties.

Until recently, one of the single largest U.S. projects has been at the University of Texas at Galveston, where the medical branch provides care to inmates across the state (Brown 2002). Other states also use telehealth to treat prisoners avoiding the costs and danger of transporting prisoners.

One major barrier to telehealth was removed with the passage of the Telecommunications Act of 1996, which allowed vendors of cable and telephone services to compete in each others' markets (Schneider 1996). This event helped to open the door to create the information superhighway needed to provide the framework to support telehealth. The Snowe–Rockefeller Amendment required telecommunications carriers to offer services to rural health providers at rates comparable to those charged in urban areas so that affordable health care may be available to rural residents.

Grant monies to fund the development of telehealth applications and studies are available through several sources (Brantley, Laney-Cummings, and Spivack 2004; Galblum 2004). The majority of these sources are federal and state agencies; these include the U.S. Departments of Defense, Commerce, Agriculture, Education, Justice, Health and Human Services, and Veterans Affairs. The Department of Homeland Defense is a recent addition to this list. There are also private, nonprofit groups such as the Center of Excellence for Remote and Medically-Underserved Areas (CERMUSA) and the Acumen Fund. The majority of private parties providing funds focus on specific applications, often to promote a particular product. Additional research is needed. Questions remain about the evidence of the efficacy and cost-benefits of telehealth applications. These questions arise not so much because there have been a lack of projects so much as a lack of a coordinated approach to the development, research, testing, and evaluation of applications. The Lewin Group (2000) noted that despite an earlier call by the IOM (1996) to evaluate telemedicine applications in terms of quality of care, outcomes, access to care, health care costs, and the perceptions of clients and clinicians, methodology problems remain. These include small sample sizes and a lack of control groups (AHRQ 2001). There also is a lack of long-term data (Waldo 2003). AHRQ recommends that projects involving chronic conditions that use the bulk of resources or have the greatest barriers to care receive the highest priority for telemedicine research. The National Institute of Nursing Research has solicited grant applications to study telehealth technologies that can improve clinical outcomes. The National Cancer Institute's Center to Reduce Cancer Health Disparities is looking for technology and telehealth applications that can facilitate early detection and screening. Despite the emphasis in this text on U.S. development of telehealth, it is an international phenomenon. The United States may lead in the development of technologies that enable telehealth, but Australia, Canada, Norway, and Sweden are among the current world leaders in the use of telehealth applications (Brehl 2002; Brantley, Laney-Cummings, and Spivack 2004).

DRIVING FORCES

Recent attention to patient safety, cost containment, managed care, shortages of health care providers, and uneven access to health care services make telehealth an attractive tool to improve the quality of health care and save money (Brantley, Laney-Cummings, and Spivack 2004; Coen Buckwalter, Davis, Wakefield, Kienzle, and Murray 2002; DiCianni 2002; Hagland 2003; Lind 2003; Russo 2001; Smith 2004; Taylor 2003).

Savings may be realized via the following measures:

- Improved access to care, which allows clients to be treated earlier when fewer interventions are required.
- Clients may receive treatment in their own community where services cost less.
- Improved quality of care; expert advice is more easily available.
- Extending the services of nurse practitioners and physician assistants through ready accessibility to physician services
- Improved continuity of care through convenient follow-up care
- Improved quality of client records; the addition of digital information such as monitored vital signs and wound images provide better information for treatment decisions and help to decrease errors.
- Time savings; health care professionals can cut down on the amount of time spent in travel and instead spend it in direct client care.

Telehealth is also a marketing tool (Girzadas and Given 2003; Kelly 2002; Kohn 2002). Many institutions post health promotion or quality benchmark information on their Web pages with the hope that it will attract new customers. Large institutions offer links with the understanding that additional services will be rendered at their facilities. For example, imagine that a client with symptoms of coronary artery disease is seen at a community hospital that has no facilities for cardiac surgery. The client is more likely to follow up at the larger institution that has established links to the community hospital, because a rapport has been established with the consulting physician. Telehealth services can eliminate the need for visas for international clients. Some facilities provide scheduling and online claim authorization as convenient services. Telehealth services deemed valuable by physicians can also attract new medical staff. As a result of the above factors, many agencies offer telehealth or plan to do so in the near future. Telehealth services need to be addressed in enterprise-wide strategic plans. Box 16–2 lists some additional benefits associated with telehealth.

APPLICATIONS

Telehealth applications vary greatly. Examples include monitoring activities, diagnostic evaluations, decision support systems, storage and dissemination of records for diagnostic purposes, image compression for efficient storage and retrieval, research, electronic prescriptions, voice recognition for dictation, education of health care professionals and consumers, and support of caregivers (Brown 2002; Brantley et al. 2004). Sophisticated equipment is not always necessary. Some applications are "high tech," whereas others are relatively "low tech." Real-time videoconferencing between physicians or health care professionals and clients and the transmission of diagnostic images and biometric data are examples of high-tech applications. An example of a low-tech application is a home glucose-monitoring program that uses a touch-tone telephone to report glucose results. Desktop PCs outfitted with video cameras can provide telehealth opportunities for applications that do

---

Box 16–2 **Telehealth Benefits**

- *Continuity of care.* Clients can stay in the community and use their regular health care providers.

- *Centralized health records.* Clients remain in the same health care system.

- *Incorporation of the health care consumer as an active member of the health team.* The client is an active participant in videoconferences.

- *Collaboration among health care professionals.* Cooperation is fostered among interdisciplinary members of the health care team.

- *Improved decision making.* Experts are readily available.

- *Education of health care consumers and professionals.* Offerings are readily available.

- *Higher quality of care.* Access to care and access to specialists is improved.

- *Removes geographic barriers to care.* Clients living away from major population centers or in economically disadvantaged areas can access care more readily.

- *May result in lower costs for health care.* Eliminates travel costs. Clients are seen earlier when they are not as ill. Treatment may take place in local hospitals, which are less costly.

- *Improved quality of health record.* The record contains digitalized records of diagnostic tests, biometric measures, photographs and communication.

not require high resolution. Current telehealth technologies can be grouped into at least nine broad categories, although for general discussion purposes, there are two types: store-and-forward and interactive conferencing. Store-and-forward is used to transfer digital images and data from one location to another. It is appropriate for nonemergent situations. It is commonly used for teleradiology and telephathology. Interactive conferencing primarily refers to video conferencing and is used in place of face-to-face consultation. Telehealth is not a technology so much as it is a technique for the delivery of services. Increasingly it is perceived as a framework for a comprehensive health system integrating various applications, as well as the management of information, education, and administrative services. Box 16–3 lists some other actual and proposed applications.

Online Databases and Tools

Online resources can include the following:

- *Standards of care.* These may include recommended guidelines for care for a particular diagnosis.
- *Critical pathways and client outcomes.* A critical pathway is a suggested blueprint for the care of a client with a particular diagnosis such as pneumonia. The pathway outlines recommended multidisciplinary interventions and outcomes for the expected length of stay.
- *Computerized medical diagnosis.* This database assists the physician to match symptoms against suspected diagnoses.
- *Drug information.* One important application is the determination of the most effective, least expensive antibiotic for a particular infection.
- *Electronic prescriptions.* This permits the physician to "write" a prescription that is sent automatically to the pharmacy. It decreases errors associated with poor handwriting and sound-alike drugs (Hagland 2003). When integration exists among health care systems, physicians, and pharmacies, there is no need to enter patient history, allergies, demographic, and insurance information more than once. Electronic prescribing is being adopted in more systems as part of patient safety initiatives.
- *Abstracts and full-text retrieval of literature.* These can be retrieved easily at any time of the day.
- *Research data.* This information is available via literature searches and Web access.
- *Bulletin boards, reference files, and discussion groups on various specialty subjects.*

Ready access to information improves care delivery and decreases related costs. For example, the incorporation of national standards of care and drug information eliminates redundant efforts by individual institutions to

Box 16–3   **Current and Proposed Telehealth Applications**

- *Cardiology.* ECG strips can be transmitted for interpretation by experts at a regional referral center, and pacemakers can be reset from a remote location.

- *Counselling.* Clients may be seen at home or in outpatient settings by a counselor at another site.

- *Data mining.* Research may be conducted on large databases for educational, diagnostic, and cost/benefit analysis.

- *Dermatology.* Primary physicians may ask specialists to see a client without the client waiting for an appointment with the specialist and travelling to a distant site.

- *Diabetes management.* Clients may report blood glucose readings by using the touch-tone telephone.

- *Mobile unit postdisaster care.* Emergency medical technicians (EMTs) and nurses at the site of a disaster can consult with physicians about the health needs of victims.

- *Education.* Health care professionals in geographically remote areas can attend seminars to update their knowledge without extensive travel, expense, or time away from home.

- *Emergency care.* Community hospitals can share information with trauma centers so that the centers can better care for clients and prepare them for transport.

- *Fetal monitoring.* Some high-risk antepartum clients can be monitored from home with greater comfort and decreased expense.

- *Gariatrics.* Videoconference equipment in the home permits home monitoring of medication administration for the client with memory deficits who is otherwise able to stay at home.

- *Home care.* Once equipment is in the client's home, nurses and physicians may evaluate the client at home without leaving their offices.

- *Military.* Physicians at remote sites can evaluate injured soldiers in the field via the medic's equipment.

- *Pharmacy.* Data can be accessed at a centralized location.

- *Pathology.* The transmission of slide and tissue samples to other sites makes it easier to obtain a second opinion on biopsy findings.

- *Psychiatry.* Specialists at major medical centers can evaluate clients in outlying emergency departments, hospitals, and clinics via teleconferences.

- *Radiology.* Radiologists can take calls from home that receive images from the hospital on equipment they have in place. Rural hospitals do not need to have a radiologist on site.

- *School clinics.* School nurses, particularly in remote areas, can quickly consult with other professionals about problems observed.

- *Social work.* Social workers can augment services with telehealth home visits.

- *Speech–language pathology.* More efficient use can be made of scarce speech–language pathologists.

prepare their own standards and formularies. It also decreases malpractice claims through adherence to standards of care. Standards of care reflect best practices based on research findings. Online research databases facilitate research through the systematic collection of information on large populations, with potential for data mining at a later time. Further benefits from online resources will be accrued as more projects are implemented to develop common terms to facilitate sharing of data, such as the National Library of Medicine's Unified Medical Language System.

Education

Telehealth affords opportunities to educate health care consumers and professionals through increased information accessibility via online resources, including the World Wide Web, distance learning, and clinical instruction. Grand rounds and continuing education are two of the most touted applications for education.

Grand rounds are a traditional teaching tool for health professionals in training (Ellis and Mayrose 2003; Sargeant, Allen, O'Brien, and MacDougall 2003). As the name indicates, a group of practitioners review a client's case history and present condition, at which time they mutually determine the best treatment options. Grand rounds help to maintain clinical knowledge and expertise but are not always available in smaller institutions. Telehealth facilities allow the incorporation of diagnostic images, client interviews, and biometric measurements from outlying hospitals into medical center grand rounds, thereby allowing practitioners from two or more sites to participate. Videoconferencing allows more practitioners to attend this educational offering than might otherwise be possible. In like fashion, consultations and images from major teaching centers may be made available to remote facilities to enhance the practice of professionals in outlying areas.

Continuing Education

Telehealth offers direct access to traditional continuing education and extemporaneous teaching opportunities with every teleconsultation and distance education offering. Training costs for continuing education may be decreased by bringing people together from many distant sites without travel or lodging expenses or extended time away from their responsibilities.

Home Health Care

Telecommunication technology can reduce home health care costs while increasing the frequency and availability of services (Brennan 1996; Brown 2002; Coen Buckwalter et al. 2002; DiCianni and Kobza 2002; Joch 2003; McCarty and Clancy 2002; Mitchell 2003; Russo 2001; Schurenberg 2003). It also supports automatic collection of data and allows clinicians to handle more clients than via traditional care models. For example, use of a home monitoring system in Japan provides 24-hour contact and medical response for clients as needed in addition to regularly scheduled visits. Biometric measurements such as heart rate and pattern, blood pressure, respiratory rate, and fetal heart rate can be monitored at another site, with electronic or actual house calls provided as needed. Women with high-risk pregnancies, diabetics, and cardiac and postoperative clients can be monitored at home. Clients who require wound care comprise another population that can be managed well at home through telehealth applications. Nurses can also transmit digital photographs of wounds to certified wound ostomy continence nurses (WCONs). Photographs are stored in the database. The WCON can make recommendations and follow more clients through the use of telehealth than would otherwise be possible. Internet access for home health clients and their families also provides convenient access to support groups, treatment information, and electronic communication with their health care providers, while decreasing feelings of isolation. The REACH (Resources for Enhancing Alzheimer's Caregiver Health) initiative sponsored by the National Institutes for Health exemplifies a support program for caregivers that encourages them to engage in relaxation exercises. As the number of elderly grows, televisits eliminate the discomfort and inconvenience of travel and long waits to be seen. Equipment required is dictated by the nature of the monitoring. For example, telemetry requires continuous monitoring, necessitating a dedicated telephone line as well as the monitoring devices supplied by the home health care agency. Other clients may require less-expensive, low-technology monitoring, while another group requires equipment with videoconference and monitoring capability. A Web-based solution for care coordination can integrate information from biometric measures and diagnostic tests and automatically alert the clinician of panic values. The benefits of telehealth technology allow clinicians to cut travel time without decreasing client contact and help to improve the organization of the health record with automatic collection of data and better coordination of care among clinicians. Figure 16–1 depicts a teleconference that connects a home health care client, a nurse, and a physician. The use of sensors to detect falls and whether the refrigerator has been opened and closed has also been suggested as a means to alert nurses to problems in the homes of elderly and frail patients (Harrison 2002). These devices could help keep clients in their own homes rather than long-term care. Some providers of advanced home telemonitoring services have formed partnerships with home care companies that make the technology available to providers. This arrangement eliminates the need for home health care companies to invest in the equipment needed to support telehealth (Strategic Partnership 2003).

Disease Management

The bulk of U.S. health care costs result from chronic conditions (Coen Buckwalter et al. 2002; Denbar 2003). For this reason it is essential to find better ways to manage the health of individuals with chronic medical

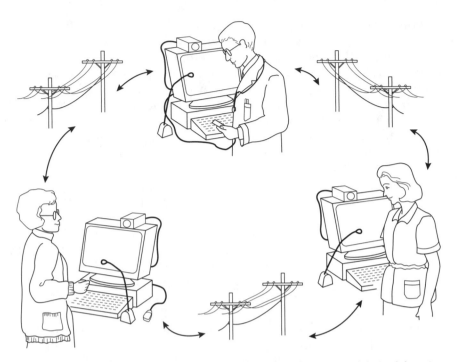

FIGURE 16–1 • Diagram of a teleconference involving client, nurse, and physician at separate sites

conditions. Telehealth applications can help. The U.S. Department of Veteran Affairs is launching the largest telemedicine initiative in the United States to this date. Plans call for the use of computer and telephone-based medicine in the homes of 25,000 chronically ill veterans by the end of 2004. Technology ranges from automated reminders to take medications and handheld vital sign monitors to two-way video computers that are equipped with everything from a stethoscope to an electrocardiograph. Participation will be voluntary and clients have the option to continue traditional care. Technology costs may be as high as $7500 per client plus an additional $1200 per year in operating costs. Similar initiatives are under way at home care agencies and through private medical centers throughout the country. Examples of other programs include Resource Link of Iowa (RLI), the Diabetes Education and Telemedicine Project (IDEATel), and the use of Health Buddy.

Resource Link of Iowa (RLI) uses two-way interactive video to manage the care of chronically ill patients in their homes throughout Iowa (Coen Buckwalter et al. 2002). Criteria for enrollment included a high utilization of care, clinical indications that more aggressive monitoring could reduce use of services, and a willingness to use technology. The technology has been well received and a reduction in the number of face-to-face visits noted. The Diabetes Education and Telemedicine Project (IDEATel) began

February 2000 as a 4-year clinical trial to maximize clients' control of their diabetes by providing them with a computer link to their caregivers for input of glucose and vital signs. Eligibility requirements included a high utilization of care, clinical indications that aggressive monitoring could reduce the use of services, and an expressed willingness to use technology. Caregivers receive alerts with critical values. Health Buddy is an in-home communication device that has been used to provide heart failure disease management (Telehealth Program Suitable 2004). Findings suggest that Health Buddy may be as effective as telephone follow-up and home visits. Telehealth can also be used to remind clients to take their medications helping to reduce unnecessary complications and the number of hospital visits.

LEGAL AND PRIVACY ISSUES

Reimbursement and licensure issues remain two of the major barriers to the growth and practice of telehealth (Brantley et al. 2004; Brown 2002; Hutcherson 2001; Meyers 2003; Sarkar 2004; Weil 2004). There are also concerns about the impact of telehealth on record privacy, particularly with the implementation of the Health Insurance Portability and Accountability Act (HIPAA).

HIPAA, Referral, and Payment

Brantley et al. (2004) concluded that federal, state, and private sector policies have impeded the advance of telehealth and that an entirely new framework is necessary to determine reimbursement for telehealth services. The Balanced Budget Act of 1997 first authorized Medicare reimbursement for some services that did not traditionally require a face-to-face meeting between client and practitioner such as radiology or electrocardiogram interpretation (Hutcherson 2001; Lauderdale, Lacsamama, and Palsbo 2003; McCarty and Clancy 2002; Puskin 2001; Thede 2001). Almost 2 years passed before any reimbursement occurred. There were limitations on who could receive services, what services were covered, who got paid, and how services were reimbursed. Only clients in federally designated rural areas deemed as having a shortage of health professionals were eligible. Store-and-forward technologies were not covered in some cases. And there were issues related to what practitioners were eligible for reimbursement and how they were paid. Reimbursement rules were loosened with the Medicare, Medicaid, and SCHIP Benefits Improvement and Protection Act of 2000 but not enough to make a significant difference in Medicaid reimbursement or to encourage other third party payors in the United States to pay for telehealth services. As a result, some physicians and other providers who do teleconsultation have not been paid for their services. A temporary procedural (CPT) code for billing developed by the American Medical Association may help to increase physician interest in performing online consultations (Dannenfeldt 2004). Up until now, increased client volume at referral centers has been regarded as a means to make up for lost revenue.

Support Personnel

While the technology behind telehealth should be easy to use, technical support may be required. Support staff should be capable, flexible, and preferably experienced. At the present, questions have not been fully resolved as to who will train health care professionals to participate in telehealth and how compensation will be derived for the additional hours associated with installation, training, and use of telehealth technology. There is also an issue of confidentiality. Technical support staff who are present during the exchange of client information need to be aware of institutional policies as well as laws such as HIPAA that are designed to protect client privacy. These individuals should sign the same sort of statement that clinical personnel sign on the receipt of their information system access codes.

Liability

Telehealth is plagued by a number of liability issues (ANA 1996; Hutcherson 2001; McCarty and Clancy 2002; Sarkar 2004). First, there is the possibility that the client may perceive it as inferior because the consulting professional does not perform a hands-on examination. The ANA cautions that telehealth shows great promise as long as it is used to augment, not replace, existing services. Second, professionals who practice across state lines deal with different practice provisions in each state and may be subject to malpractice lawsuits in multiple jurisdictions, raising questions about how that liability might be distributed or which state's practice standards would apply. Theoretically, clients could choose to file suit in the jurisdiction most likely to award damages. The basic question here is, where did the service occur? Third, how might liability be spread among physicians, other health care professionals, and technical support persons? And fourth, HIPAA legislation added new concerns to the mix. These issues still need sorted out.

Telehealth has the potential to raise or lower malpractice costs. For example, Pennsylvania's HealthNet records teleconferences to provide a complete transcript of the session. Clients receive a videotape for later review and as a means to clarify their comprehension, and the original videotape is kept as part of the client record. The American Nurses Association (1999) also calls for the development of documentation requirements for telehealth services that address treatment recommendations as well as any communication that occurs with other health care providers. This strategy should decrease malpractice claims through better documentation and improved client understanding. On the other hand, liability costs may increase if health care professionals can be sued in more than one jurisdiction.

Major issues for nurses include questions of liability when information provided over the telephone is misinterpreted, when advice is given across state lines without a license in the state where the client resides, or, particularly, when an unintentional diagnosis comes from the use of an Internet chat room. Liability is unclear in these areas. Regulation of telenursing practice by boards of nursing is difficult when practice crosses state lines. Unless nurses are licensed in every state in which they practice telenursing, respective regulatory boards are unaware of their presence. Authority to practice telenursing across state lines provides the following advantages (National Council of State Boards 1996):

- It establishes the nurse's responsibility and accountability to the board of nursing.
- It establishes legitimacy and availability to practice telenursing.
- It provides jurisdictional authority over the discipline of telenursing in the event that unsafe delivery becomes an issue.

Until this issue has been resolved, nurses must also be cautious when providers from other states give them directions. Several state boards of nursing specifically forbid taking instructions from providers not licensed in the current state. Box 16–4 summarizes barriers to the practice of telehealth.

Licensure Issues

In general, current laws require health care professionals to be licensed in the state in which they practice. Application for licensure in additional states can be lengthy and expensive. Telehealth advocates want to remove legal barriers to practice through nationwide licensing or changes in practice acts that permit practitioners from any state to consult with practitioners from another state without the need to be licensed in that second state. The Federation of State Medical Boards drafted legislation to address this issue that calls for the establishment of a registry for telehealth physicians, who would enjoy shorter license application periods and lower fees but have some practice restrictions. Some licensing laws pertaining to

---

Box 16–4

Barriers to the Use of Telehealth Applications

- *Regulatory barriers.* State laws are either unclear or may forbid practice across state lines.
- *Lack of reimbursement for consultative services.* Most third party payors do not provide reimbursement unless the client is seen in person.
- *Costs for equipment, network services, and training time.* Equipment capable of transmitting and receiving diagnostic-grade images is still expensive, although costs are declining.
- *Fear of health care system changes.* Personnel may fear job loss as more clients can be treated at home and hospital units close.
- *Lack of acceptance by health care professionals.* May stem from liability concerns and discomfort over not seeing a client face-to-face.

telehealth have been enacted or are under consideration but no resolution has been achieved as yet. Task forces of the National Council of Nurses suggested multistate licensure as a means to support telenursing. The resulting mutual recognition model holds a nurse licensed to practice in one state accountable to the practice laws and regulations in the state where telehealth services are provided. The American Nurses Association (1998) does not support this proposed model, however, citing concerns related to discipline, revenue for individual state boards of licensure, and knowledge issues related to allowable practice in other states. Until changes are implemented, delivery of services across some state lines via telehealth may be illegal and practitioners must proceed cautiously.

Confidentiality/Privacy

Although telehealth should not create any greater concerns or risks to medical record privacy than any other form of consultation, records that cross state lines are subject to HIPAA regulations and state privacy laws.

OTHER TELEHEALTH ISSUES

There are a number of other important issues related to telehealth. They include the following:

- *Lack of standards.* The lack of plug-and-play interoperability among telehealth devices and point-of-care and other clinical information systems is cited as a major obstacle (Brantley et al. 2004; Waldo 2003). There is a need for a standard interface specification that allows telehealth data to be merged easily with information from other clinical information systems. Work is in process on the development of these standards using HL7 messages constructed with Extensible Markup Language.

- *National Health Information Infrastructure (NHII).* In succinct terms, the NHII is all about the secure exchange of health care information between a requestor and provider (Brantley et al. 2004; Meyers 2003; Palmer 2004). The NHII is at present a vision, not a reality. It requires an identity management system that can be trusted on a national scale that will give information providers a means to validate the electronic identity of a requestor. Similar work is presently under way with the U.S. government. Rules are still needed to create electronic IDs for the NHII. The Department of Health and Human Services, the American Telemedicine Association (ATA), and the Rand Corporation, among other entities, have been discussing the NHII.

- *Homeland security.* The homeland security community has not given significant consideration to telehealth technology when assessing its needs, strategies, and desired outcomes (Brantley et al. 2004). It can make use of various surveillance systems to analyze symptoms on a large scale for possible biological and chemical attacks.

- *Mainstream acceptance.* Despite its advocates, many health care professionals continue to have reservations about its use (Thede 2001). These include the perception that telehealth offers few benefits to them, concerns over privacy and legalities, and fears that telehealth applications will reduce the number of health care professionals needed.

- *Accreditation and regulatory requirements.* The Joint Commission on Accreditation of Healthcare Organizations first identified medical staff standards for credentialing and privileging for the practice of telemedicine in 2001 and approved revisions in 2003. Practitioners are required to be credentialed and have privileges at the site where the client is located. Credentialing information from the distant site may be used by the originating site to establish privileges if the distant site is JCAHO accredited. The Food and Drug Administration (FDA) has several guidelines for the use of telehealth-related devices.

- *Patient safety.* The majority of discussions that address patient safety emphasize the potential of telehealth to enhance patient safety through applications such as e-prescribing. Some literature makes mention of threats to patient safety when telehealth applications fail to render the same level of care as hands-on care or when problems occur with the use of electrical devices.

ESTABLISHING A TELEHEALTH LINK

Successful establishment and use of a telehealth link require strategic planning as well as consideration of the following factors: necessary infrastructure, costs and reimbursement, human factors, equipment, and technology issues.

Formulating a Telehealth Plan

Any plans for the use of telehealth applications should be in concert with the overall strategic plan of the organization. A telehealth plan minimizes duplicate effort and helps to ensure success. Goals should address the following:

- Current services and deficits
- Telehealth objectives
- Compliance with standards
- Reimbursement policies that favor desired outcomes rather than specific processes
- Periodic review of goals and accomplishments in light of changing technology and needs
- How telecommunication breakdowns will be handled: Will backup be provided? What happens when a power outage in the home severs a link?

The people who will use the system need to be involved in its design from the very beginning. It is wise to start small and expand offerings. Most

Box 16–5 | **Strategies to Ensure Successful Teleconferences**

- Select a videoconferencing system to fit your needs, such as a desktop or mobile system or customized room.
- Locate videoconferencing facilities near where they will be used, yet in a quiet, low-traffic area.
- Schedule sessions in advance to avoid time conflicts. Start on time.
- Establish a working knowledge of interactive conferencing features.
- Provide an agenda to keep the conference on track.
- Introduce all participants.
- Set time limits.
- Send materials needed in advance to maintain focus and involve participants.
- Summarize major points at the conclusion.
- Start by asking all participants if they have a good audio and video feed.
- Participate in a conference call as if it were a face-to-face meeting. Enunciate clearly.
- Minimize background noise or use the mute feature.
- Promote interactivity through questions and answers.
- Have technical support available to resolve any problems that might arise.

institutions begin with continuing education and later expand capability. Educational teleconferences require larger rooms that are not suitable for client examinations. Selection of equipment should be based on transmission speed, image resolution, storage capacity, mobility, and ease of use. Higher bandwidth generally improves performance. Equipment should match defined telehealth goals. Box 16–5 lists some strategies to ensure successful teleconferences.

Building the Supporting Framework

Other considerations in telehealth are who will build the infrastructure to support telehealth and what role the federal government should take. Federal and state governments already commit considerable resources to telehealth and related technology. The Department of Commerce, HCFA, Office of Rural Health Policy, and Department of Defense are some federal agencies that have conducted telehealth research and demo programs. Most states have projects in process. The NIIT is a consortium of corporations, universities, and government agencies that views the development of a national information infrastructure as a means to create jobs, promote prosperity, and improve health care by reducing redundant procedures and creating an electronic record repository. In their discussion of the infrastructure needed to support telehealth, Nevins and Otley (2002) estimate that an investment of about $20 to $30 billion is needed.

Telehealth transmissions can be supported by satellite or microwave, telephone lines, or the Internet. The cost and speed of the service are inter-related. Satellite and microwave transmission is not feasible for most users. **Asynchronous transfer mode (ATM)** service is a high-speed data trans-mission link that can carry large amounts of data quickly. Speeds range from 0.45 megabits per second (Mbps) to 2.48 gigabits per second (Gbps). ATM works well when large sets of data, such as MRIs, need to be exchanged and discussed. Present ATM use is limited for reasons of cost, availability, and lack of standards. Another option for data transmission is switched multimegabit data service (SMDS), better known as a T1 line. **T1 lines** are high-speed telephone lines that may be used to transmit high-quality, full-motion video at speeds up to 1.544 Mbps. T1 services are leased monthly at a fixed charge independent of use. Next in descending order of speed are DSL (digital subscriber lines) and integrated service digital network (ISDN) lines. DSL uses existing copper telephone wires to transfer high bandwidth data. DSL availability has traditionally been limited by distance from the central telephone office. Variants of DSL technology can rival T1 lines for speed of data transmission. ISDN lines carry 128 kilobits per second (kbps), although lines can be bundled for faster speeds. Each ISDN line costs ap-proximately $30 per month plus costs for calls. ISDN lines support medical imaging, database sharing, desktop videoconferencing, and access to the In-ternet. Telehealth's identification of 384 kbps as its practical minimum bandwidth renders plain old telephone service (POTS) unsuitable for most applications. Faster access speeds are required for continuing medical edu-cation, telemetry, remote consults, and network-based services.

The Internet already carries e-mail for many health care professionals and is a powerful tool for obtaining and publishing information. Security and access issues will determine the extent to which client-specific informa-tion is interchanged on the Internet. The American Medical Association has published guidelines for e-mail correspondance for clients on its Web site.

Cable TV also has the potential to bring high-resolution x-ray images to on-call radiologists at home via its broadband capabilities.

Human Factors

On-site support and commitment from administrators and health care pro-fessionals are necessary for successful telehealth. Acceptance is frequently more difficult to obtain from health care providers than it is from clients. Overall, satisfaction is high, particularly when clients perceive that care is easier to obtain or otherwise more convenient (Coen Buckwalter et al. 2002; Marcin et al. 2004). Health care professionals should provide input about the type of telehealth applications that they would like to see to their professional organizations and health care providers. One application, con-tinuing education distance learning programs, is well received and serves to introduce other applications. Adequate training time is needed to learn how to use equipment, and support staff must be available. Telehealth, and all of its applications, is new to most people and time is needed to get accustomed to it. An example of this may be seen in teleradiology, where radiologists must learn how to interpret images using a monitor.

Equipment

Equipment must be reliable, accurate, and flexible enough to meet varying needs. One example of this principle may be seen when equipment purchased for continuing education also supports high-resolution images needed for diagnostic images. However, it is not necessary to have all the latest, most expensive technology to start telehealth. Desktop videoconferencing uses specially adapted personal computers to operate over telephone lines. These PCs may be merged with existing diagnostic imaging systems and other information systems. While it usually lacks broadcast picture quality, DTV provides an opportunity to practice some telehealth applications at a fairly low cost. Consulting parties may be able to see each other and diagnostic images by splitting the PC screen into segments. Box 16–6 lists components needed to support DTV.

Telehealth Costs

Estimates for setting up videoconferencing vary greatly, depending on the type of system and applications chosen. Desktop systems are fairly inexpensive. Better resolution increases costs. Costs include equipment purchase, operation, and maintenance; network services; and time to learn a new skills. Time needed to learn how to use telehealth applications is often underestimated. Installation of DTV in physicians' offices and ambulatory care settings is now feasible.

Technology Issues

Many of the early technical problems associated with telehealth have been largely resolved. Present issues include resolution, frame rate,

---

Box 16–6	Basic DTV Components for Telehealth Applications

- PC
- PC adapter cards
- Camera
- Microphones
- Video overlay cards
- External speakers on existing PCs with broadband switches
- Special adapative tools, such as an electronic stethoscope

standards, and record storage and location. Resolution is the sharpness or clarity of an image. The resolution needed for interpretation of diagnostic images requires a broad bandwidth that is at least 384 kilobits and 30 frames per second (FPS). Video systems work by rapidly displaying a series of still images referred to as *frames.* Frames per second (FPS), or the frame rate, refers to the number of these images that are captured, transmitted, and displayed in one second. The higher the FPS, the smoother the picture. Broadcast quality transmission is 30 FPS. Lower FPS rates produce marginally acceptable video that may be suitable for purposes other than interpretation of diagnostic images. Many DTV systems do not offer broadcast quality at this time. Bandwidth, the efficiency of compression, and hardware and software limitations all determine videoconference frame rates. Another issue related to frame rate is the delay that is noted for one videoconferencing party to respond to another. Although this period is only a few seconds long, it must be factored into teleconferences. Another issue related to resolution is the need to digitize x-rays for transmission and storage. For these reasons, teleradiology applications require more costly equipment and telecommunication services.

Health care personnel need to shape the development of technological standards by determining the minimal acceptable standards to ensure quality at the lowest possible costs. Acceptance of international standard H.320 for passing audio and video data streams across networks allowed videoconferencing systems from different manufacturers to communicate. H.320 is a standard for the connection and transfer of multimedia data that allows the transmission and reception of image and sound. It supports a wide range of transmission rates. Prior to the adoption of H.320, only systems produced by the same vendor could communicate. Work continues in this area so that continued improvements can be expected. Other important standards for telehealth include the Digital Image Communication in Medicine (DICOM) standard and the Joint Photographic Experts Group (JPEG) compression standard for digital images. DICOM seeks to promote the communication, storage, and integration of digital image information with other hospital information systems, while JPEG is used to compress images as a means to decrease transmission time and storage requirements. Work is under way for the development of plug-and-play standards to integrate and exchange information captured with telehealth technology with that housed in clinical information systems.

Most discussions of telehealth include the electronic health record (EHR) as a means to make client data readily available and store diagnostic images. **Picture archiving communications systems (PACS)** are storage systems that permit remote access to diagnostic images at a time convenient to the physician. While PACS technology has been available for a number of years, its early history was troubled. Recent technological improvements make PACS feasible.

TELENURSING

At one time the number of references noted in the literature relative to tele-nursing was limited even though telenursing has been in existence for decades, using available technology to serve its purposes. For example, the telephone has long been used as a communication tool between nurses and health care consumers as well as other professionals. As new technology be-came available, it was also adapted to educate consumers and peers, main-tain professional contacts, and provide care to clients at other sites. As a result, nurses currently use telephones, faxes, computers, teleconferences, and the Internet in the practice of telenursing. Potential applications are varied, but common uses are telephone triage, follow-up calls, and checking biometric measurements. Other examples include education, pro-fessional consultations, obtaining test results, and taking physician instruc-tions over the phone. Interactive television or teleconferences enable home health nurses to make electronic house calls to clients in their homes; thus nurses can see more clients per day than would be possible via on-site vis-its. Another instance of telenursing is the Telenurse project in Europe, which seeks to standardize the mechanism for describing and communi-cating nursing care as a means to enable comparisons of nursing practice from one site to another without regard to region or country.

The International TeleNurses Association (ITNA) was founded in 1995 to promote and support nursing involvement in telehealth and serve as a resource for nurses. This group maintains an active listserv. The American Nurses As-sociation (1999) published their Core Principles on Telehealth in 1999. These guidelines are intended to help nurses to protect client privacy during the de-livery of telehealth services. Other health care providers have also developed policy statements or standards of practice and special interest groups.

Future Development

Many providers expect that telehealth will change the way that health care is delivered and carve out new roles for health care providers (AMA 2003; ANA 1996; Brehl 2002; Galblum 2004; Lind 2003; Marcin et al. 2004; Russo 2001). Changes have already started. Telehealth offers new means to locate health information and communicate with practitioners through e-mail and interactive chats or videoconferences. It provides new ways to monitor clients and cuts down on the need to travel and miss work to seek care. Web-based disease management programs encourage clients to assume greater responsibility for their own care. The migration of applications developed for the military are available for emergency treatment in some communities. Remote monitoring and use of global positioning systems (GPSs) to direct ambulances to the closest, or best, treatment centers are available now. Mobile technology such as PDAs and point-of-care systems capture data quickly and efficiently facilitate its transmission for analysis and use by administrators when they need it, not months or years later. The growth of telehealth has been stymied in the United States primarily due to a lack of reimbursement. Demands for quality, patient safety, and more care options will help change the reimbursement picture, opening the door for more telehealth applications. Brantley et al. (2004) note that better coordination of planning, policy-making, and allocation of resources is needed.

The Federal Communications Commission (FCC) along with the National Rural Health Association and the Healthcare Information and Management Systems Society have been working together to help rural providers take better advantage of a telemedicine grant program (Bazzoli 2004). The FCC's telemedicine program has not been well utilized. In 2003, new rules were announced designed to improve access for rural healthcare programs. The program enables rural providers to obtain access to modern telecommunication technologies through discounts to telecommunication services charges. These changes are expected to encourage the adoption of more telehealth applications.

CASE STUDY EXERCISES

You are the nurse practitioner in St. Theresa's emergency department. A client is brought in with obvious psychiatric problems. You have no psychiatrist available and the nearest psychiatric facility is a 1-hour drive away. St. Theresa is a Tri-State Health Care Alliance Member. Tri-State has telehealth links with the regional hospital, where a psychiatrist is in the emergency department. What steps would you take to initiate a productive teleconference? Justify your response.

• • •

Erin O'Shell, home health nurse, just set up teleconference equipment for Dr. Bobby to evaluate Mr. Richard Goldstein for possible hospitalization for congestive heart failure. Dr. Bobby and the hospital are a 1-hour drive away. Just as the teleconference started, but before Dr. Bobby could listen to Mr. Goldstein's lungs or complete other key portions of the examination, a power outage severed the teleconference link. How should Ms. O'Shell handle this situation? Provide your rationale.

 EXPLOREMediaLink

Multiple choice review questions, case studies, and other interactive resources for this chapter can be found on the Web site at *http://www.prenhall.com/hebda*. Click on "Chapter 16" to select the activities for this chapter.

SUMMARY

- Telehealth is the use of telecommunication technologies and computers to provide health care information and services to clients at another location.

- Telehealth is a broad term that encompasses telemedicine but includes the provision of care and the distribution of information to health care providers and consumers.

- Efforts to contain costs and improve the delivery of care to all segments of the population make telehealth an attractive tool. Telehealth can help health care providers treat clients earlier when they are not as ill and care costs less, provide services in the local community where it is less expensive, improve follow-up care, improve client access to services, and improve the quality of the client's record.

- Telehealth applications vary greatly and include client monitoring, diagnostic evaluation, decision support and expert systems, storage and dissemination of records, and education of health care professionals.

- Teleconferencing and videoconferencing are tools that facilitate the delivery of telehealth services.

- Desktop videoconferencing (DTV) is an important development that enables the expansion of telehealth applications into new areas. DTV uses specially adapted personal computers to link persons at two or more sites.

- Telenursing uses telecommunications and computer technology for the delivery of nursing care and services to clients at other sites.

- Neither telemedicine nor telenursing are new. Applications include education of health care consumers and professionals as well as the provision of care. In addition to the use of the telephone for triage and information, clients may be monitored at home via telephone or teleconferences. Telehealth is a tool that helps health care providers to work more efficiently.

- Major issues associated with the practice of telehealth and telenursing include a lack of reimbursement, infrastructure, plug-and-play standards, licensure and liability issues, and concerns related to client privacy and confidentiality.

- The successful use of telehealth and telenursing is best ensured through the development and implementation of a plan that addresses current services and deficits, goals, technical requirements, compliance with standards and laws, reimbursement, and strategies to handle telecommunication breakdowns.

- Telehealth and telenursing applications are expected to become more commonplace once reimbursement and licensure barriers are removed and technical standards for the exchange of information between telehealth devices and clinical information systems established.

• Telehealth has the capacity to revolutionize the delivery of health care and has already started to do so.

REFERENCES

Agency for Healthcare Research and Quality (AHRQ). (February 2001). *Telemedicine for the Medicare Population. Summary, Evidence Report/Technology Assessment: Number 24.* AHRQ Publication Number 01-E011. Available at http://www.ahrq.gov/clinic/epcsums/ telemedsum.htm. Accessed on February 27, 2004.

American Medical Association. (May 16, 2003). Guidelines for physician-patient electronic communications. Available at http://www.ama-assn. org/ama/pub/category/print/2386.html. Accessed February 28, 2004.

American Nurses Association. (October 9, 1996). Telehealth—Issues for nursing. Available at http://nursingworld.org/readroom/tele2.htm. Accessed February 25, 2004.

American Nurses Association. (June 24, 1998). Multistate regulation of nurses. Available at http://nursingworld.org/gova/multibg.htm. Accessed February 25, 2004.

American Nurses Association. (1999). Core principles on telehealth. Washington, DC: American Nurses Publishing.

Bazzoli, F. (January 2004). Telemedicine gets FCC boost. *Healthcare IT News, 1*(1), 11.

Brantley, D., Laney-Cummings, K., and Spivack, R. (February 2004). *Innovation, Demand and Investment in Teleheatlh.* A report of the Technology Administration, U.S. Department of Commerce Office of Technology Policy. Available at http://www.technology.gov/reports/ TechPolicy/Telehealth/2004Report.pdf. Accessed February 28, 2004.

Brehl, R. (2002). The cutting edge: Canada is fast becoming a world leader in telehealth, which joins high tech to health care. *Time International, 160*(13).

Brennan, P. (October 1996). Nursing informatics: Technology in the service of patient care. Paper presented at the meeting of Alpha Rho Chapter of Sigma Theta Tau, Morgantown, WV.

Brown, N. (2002). Telemedicine coming of age. Available online through the Telemedicine Research Center at http://trc.telemed.org/telemedicine/ primer.asp. Accessed February 29, 2004.

Coen Buckwalter, K., Davis, L. L., Wakefield, B. J., Kienzle, M. G., and Murray, M. A. (2002). Telehealth for elders and their caregivers in rural communities. *Family and Community Health, 25*(3), 31–40.

Dannenfeldt, D. (February 2004). Temporary AMA code may increase online conultations. *Healthcare IT News, 1*(2), 23–24.

Denbar, A. (September 23, 2003). Keeping patients connected. The Boston Globe. Available at http://www.boston.com/bnews/nation/ articles2003/09/23/keeping patients_connected?mode. Accessed February 29, 2004.

DiCianni, M. (2002). Telehealth monitoring turns field nurses into wound-care experts. *Healthcare Review*, *15*(1), 9.

DiCianni, M., and Kobza, L. (2002). A chance to heal: Home health agencies can improve patient care and increase profits with telehealth wound consulting. *Health Management Technology*, *23*(4), 22–24.

Ellis, D. G., and Mayrose, J. (2003). The success of emergency telemedicine at the State University of New York at Buffalo. *Telemedicine Journal and e-Health*, *9*(1):73–79.

Galblum, A. (February 29, 2004). Handheld computers for health workers in Africa. *Health Systems Trust*. Available at http://new.hst.org/za/news/index.php/20021043/. Accessed February 29, 2004.

Girzadas, J., and Given, R. (2003). Distinguish yourself with e-health. *Healthcare Informatics*, *20*(3), 39–40.

Hagland, M. (2003). Reduced errors ahead. *Healthcare Informatics*, *20*(8), 31–38.

Harrison, S. (2002). Telehealth skills hailed as answer to discharge delays: Costs of high-tech monitoring systems compare favourably with long-term care. *Nursing Standard*, *17*(12), 7.

Hutcherson, C. M. (2001). Legal considerations for nurses practicing in a telehealth setting. *Online Journal of Issues in Nursing*, *6*(3). Available at http://www.nursworld.org/ofin/topic16/tpc16_3.htm. Accessed February 25, 2004.

Institute of Medicine (IOM). (1996). *Telemedicine: A guide to assess telecommunications in health care*. Available at http://books.nap.edu/books/0309055318/html/2.html. Accessed March 2, 2004.

Joch, A. (2003). Wired for home care. *Healthcare Informatics*, *20*(9), 66.

Joint Commision for the Accreditation of Healthcare Organizations (JCAHO). (February 2003). Existing requirements for telemedicine practitioners explained. *Joint Commission Perspectives*. Available at http://www.atmeda.org/news/JCP-2003-February2.pdf. Accessed March 2, 2004.

Kelly, B. (2002). Telemedicine begins to make progress. *Health Data Management*, *10*(1), 72–78.

Kohn, D. (2002). E-health initiatives for today's information systems. *ADVANCE for Health Information Executives*, *6*(12), 17–22, 96.

Lauderdale, D., Lacsamama, C., and Palsbo, S. E. (September 2003). Telemedicine issue summary: Medicaid and telemedicine in 2002. Available at http://tie.telemed.org/legal/medic/medicaid2002.asp. Accessed February 26, 2004.

The Lewin Group, Inc. (December 2000). *Assessment of approaches to evaluating telemedicine*. Final report prepared for Office of the Assistant Secretary for Planning and Evaluation, Department of Health and Human Services. Available at http://www.aspe.hhs.gov/health/reports/AAET/aaet.htm. Accessed February 27, 2004.

Lind, J. (September 1, 2003). Mobile technology saves lives and resources in the emergency ward. Available at http://www.itsweden.com/main.aspx?pageid=170&id=13&type=features. Accessed February 29, 2004.

Marcin, J. P., Ellis, J., Mawis, R., Nagrampa, E., Nesbitt, T. S., and Dimand, R. J. (2004). Using telemidicine to provide pediatric subspecialty care to children with special health care needs in an underserved rural community. *Pediatrics, 113*(1pt 1), 1–6.

McCarty, D., and Clancy, C. (2002). Telehealth: Implications for social work practice. *Social Work, 47*(2), 153–161.

McGee, R., and Tangalos, E. G. (1994). Delivery of health care to the underserved. *Mayo Clinic Proceedings, 69*(12), 1131–1136.

Meyers, M. R. (2003). Telemedicine: An emerging health care technology. *Health Care Management, 22*(3), 219–223.

Mitchell, M. (2003). Web-based telemedicine. *ADVANCE for Health Information Executives, 7*(10), 71–74.

National Council of State Boards of Nursing, Inc. (1996). Telenursing: The regulatory implications for multistate regulation. *Issues, 17*(3), 1, 8–9.

Nevins, R., and Otley V. C., III, (2002). Demystifying telehealth. *Health Management Technology, 23*(7), 52, 51.

Palmer, P. (February 2004). Trusted identity management for the NHII. *Healthcae IT News, 1*(2), 15.

Perednia, D. A. (May 9, 1995). Telehealth: Remote access to health services and information. In Bringing health care on-line: The role of information technologies, pp. 1–41. Available at http://www.acl.lanl.gov/sunrise/Medical/ota/09ch5.txt.

Perednia, D. A., and Allen, A. (1995). Telehealth technology and clinical applications. *Journal of the American Medical Association, 273*(6), 483–488.

Puskin, D. S. (2001). Telemedicine: Follow the money. *Online Journal of Issues in Nursing, 6*(3). Available at http://nursing world.org/ojin/topic16/tpc16_1.htm. Accessed February 25, 2004.

Russo, H. (2001). Window of opportunity for home care nurses: Telehealth technologies. *Online Journal of Issues in Nursing, 6*(3). Available at http://nursingworld.org/ojin/topic16/tpc16_4.htm. Accessed February 25, 2004.

Sargeant, J., Allen, M., O'Brien, B., and MacDougall, E. (2003). Videoconferenced grand rounds: Needs assessment for community specialists. *The Journal of Continuing Education in the Health Professions, 23*(2), 116–123.

Sarkar, D. (February 26, 2004). Laws, other hurdles hinder telehealth. *FCW.Com.* Available at http://www.fcw.com/geb/articles/2004/0223/web-telehealth-02-26-04.asp. Accessed February 28, 2004.

Schneider, P. (1996). Washington word: Telecom reform. *Healthcare Informatics, 12*(3), 93.

Schurenberg, B. (2003). Keeping patients at home. *Health Data Management, 11*(7), 56–57.

Smith, E. (2004). Telehealth in the Tundra. *Health Management Technology, 25*(3), 24–26.

Strategic partnership created to make new telehealth services available. (October 20, 2003). *Cardiovascular Week*, 22.

Taylor, C. W. (2003). Bridging the gap: In-home monitoring device reduces cost of treating underserved populations in rural Alabama. *Health Management Technology, 24*(1), 36–38.

Telehealth program suitable for management of heart failure patients. (January 26, 2004). *Cardiovascular Week*, 28.

Telehealth study demonstrates cost savings. (2002). *Journal of Clinical Engineering, 27*(1), 22.

Thede, L. Q. (2001). Overview and summary: Telehealth: Promise or peril? *Online Journal of Issues in Nursing, 6*(3), Available at http://nursing world.org/ojin/topic16/tpc16top.htm. Accessed February 26, 2004.

Waldo, B. (2003). Telehealth and the electronic medical record. *Nursing Economics, 21*(5), 245.

Weil, E. (February 10, 2004). Geared up for health. *Time.* Available at http://www.time.com/time/generations/printout/ 0,88161101040216-588850,00html. Accessed February 29, 2004.

CHAPTER

17

Research

After completing this chapter, you should be able to:

- Describe ways that computers can support all steps of the research process.

- Discuss the advantages of computerized literature searches over manual methods.

- Identify several well-known statistical analysis software programs.

- Relate the significance of computational nursing models for future health care delivery.

- Name several impediments to health care research.

- Discuss the anticipated effects of increased automation and the electronic health record (EHR) on research efforts.

- Explain how students in health care professions may reap the benefits of research tools.

- Discuss the impact of Health Insurance Portability and Accountability Act (HIPAA) legislation on health care research.

 MEDIALINK

Additional resources for this content can be found on the Companion Website at *www. prenhall.com/hebda*. Click on "Chapter 17" to select the activities for this chapter.

Companion Website

- Glossary
- Multiple Choice
- Discussion Points
- Case Study: Using Computers to Support Research
- Case Study: Students Using Computers for Research
- Case Study: Online Data Collection
- MediaLink Application: Online Research
- MediaLink Application: The NURSERES listserv group
- Web Hunt: Database Research
- Links to Resources
- Crossword Puzzle

Ideas for unit 4 paper website

Computer use in nursing research was once limited to data analysis. This situation has changed. Increased access to computers and the availability of software packages in the workplace, schools, and at home now make research feasible for health care professionals in most settings and facilitate the process from start to finish. Fortunately, this phenomenon coincides with a growing need to use research findings to justify actions in health care education, practice, and administration. Research provides data that allow better allocation of scarce resources and support knowledge development, which in turn enhances the theoretical underpinnings of nursing and informatics. Box 17–1 summarizes some ways that computers facilitate the research process.

USING COMPUTERS TO SUPPORT RESEARCH

Computers can assist with every phase of the research process from beginning to end. This is equally true for the student conducting informal research for a class assignment, the staff nurse seeking information about a particular client's diagnosis and treatment, and the nurse researcher embarking on a funded study. All health care professionals should be aware of how computers can support them in their educational endeavors, clinical practice, and research.

Identification of Research Topics

Constant changes in health care and the health care delivery system make it difficult to keep up with the latest findings and identify areas in need of further research. Online discussion groups and communities and publication of research findings help solve this problem. The NURSERES listserv group, at listserv@listserv.kent.edu/archives/nurseres.html, is a discussion list for nurse researchers. There also are discussion groups for specialty practice areas, including education and informatics. Timely and ongoing studies allow health care educators, providers, agencies, and alliances to find trends in information and react to market changes proactively. Box 17–2 lists a few suggested health care informatics topics for research based on reading and discussions with health care professionals.

Literature Searches

The primary databases for searching nursing literature are the Cumulative Index to Nursing and Allied Health Literature (CINAHL), MEDLINE, and PsychINFO. All three are available online in health care libraries, allowing literature searches to be conducted over the Internet. CINAHL also offers individual subscriptions for online and CD-ROM access. MEDLINE incorporates abstracts and references from biomedical journals. It is available free of charge through the National Library of Medicine's Web site. PsychINFO is an

Box 17–1

Computer Applications That Support Health Care

- *Topic identification.* Online literature searches, research reports, e-mail, online communities, and discussion groups can be used to identify areas in need of research.

- *Online and CD-ROM literature searches.* Electronic searches enable the researcher to identify prior research in the area as well as articles pertaining to the theoretical framework for proposed studies.

- *Full text retrieval of articles.* This eliminates the need to physically locate journals and photocopy them.

- *Development of resource files.* Computer files that take the place of index cards and handwritten notes may be searched quickly, allowing researchers to spend valuable time performing research and writing reports instead of performing clerical tasks.

- *Selection or development and revision of a data collection tool.* Online literature searches help researchers locate developed data collection tools. If no suitable tool is found, researchers can develop their own tool using a word processing package and trial it by sending it out via e-mail or the Web.

- *Preparation of the grant/study proposal.* Word processing aids the writing process because revisions can be made quickly.

- *Budget preparation and maintenance.* Spreadsheets and financial planning software assist with this process.

- *Determination of appropriate sample size.* The ability to generalize study findings is related to the size of the sample. Power analysis is the process by which an appropriate sample size may be determined. Software is available for this purpose.

- *Data collection.* Computers aid in the collection of data in several ways. Data may be input into a computer through scanned questionnaires, direct entry of field observations, or the use of an online data collection tool. PDAs and notebook computers aid on-site entry of data eliminating note and paper tools.

- *Database utilization.* Databases allow organization and manipulation of collected data.

- *Statistical analysis/qualitative text analysis.* Statistical analysis software performs complex computations, while qualitative text analysis allows searches for particular words and phrases in text, noting frequency of appearance and context.

- *Preparation of the research findings for report.* Word processing and graphics programs enable researchers to present their findings without the need for clerical assistance or graphic artists.

- *Bibliographic database manager (BDM).* This type of software aids the preparation of research reports by allowing the importation of references from literature databases without the need to rekey and, when used with a word processor, formats citations and reference lists according to the style selected.

- *Electronic dissemination of findings.* Online Journals, Web pages, and e-mail permit researchers to share their findings quickly. This contrasts with the traditional publication of study findings in print media that might take a year or more from the time of submission until distribution.

Box 17–2   **Suggested Health Care Informatics Research Topics**

Attitudes toward computers

- Student/health care provider concepts of health care informatics
- Staff attitudes

Clinical data

- Development and efficacy of acuity and classification systems
- Use of point-of-care
- The impact of informatics on clients' families, and health care providers
- Critical pathway and database development and use, including outcome assessment
- Expert systems, decision trees and support, and artificial intelligence and knowledge engineering
- Client education
- Quality assurance
- Evaluation of SNOMED CT and other standard clinical languages such as NANDA, NIC, and NOC
- Efficacy of telehealth applications
- Tracking resources

Education

- Effectiveness of computer-assisted instruction or Web-based instruction
- Computerized testing

---

electronic database produced by the American Psychological Association that includes the behavioral sciences. It may also be accessed through the American Psychological Association Web site. All three of these databases allow users to enter search subjects and then narrow searches by criteria such as language, journal subset, and/or publication year. For example, MEDLINE users can limit a search to nursing journals and/or research reports. These features allow potential researchers to quickly determine whether research has been conducted in their area of interest and to peruse the reported findings. The user may view article abstracts and, in some cases, retrieve the full text for articles online. Box 17–3 summarizes a few advantages and disadvantages associated with online literature searches. Figure 17–1 depicts an abstract from one of the results obtained from a MEDLINE search for nursing informatics models using the National Library of Medicine's PubMed.

Data Collection Tools

Data collection tools may be located via CD-ROM or online literature searches and discussion lists. There are test references that provide comprehensive information on published tools that are available for purchase

Box 17–3

Pros and Cons of Online Literature Searches

Pros

- Searches may be completed quickly.
- Searches may be done without the aid of a librarian.
- Searches may be limited to specific years, languages, or journal subsets.
- Searches may be general or limited to requesting research reports.
- Online abstracts allow researchers to quickly determine if a particular article suits their purpose.
- When available, full-text retrieval allows the researcher to obtain articles without searching for volumes on a shelf or waiting for copies to arrive from other sites.

Cons

- Searches require a basic level of comfort with computers.
- The person conducting the search must be able to narrow the topic area.
- Search results are directly related to the selection of search terms. Poor selection of terms may falsely indicate no or few articles on a given topic or provide an over number of articles of limited use.
- Researchers may need the services of a librarian to start the programs and for assistance with search terms and limiters.
- Online searches may not entirely eliminate the need to locate volumes and photocopy articles or wait for copies to arrive from other libraries unless full-text retrieval is available.

as well as unpublished instruments that appear in journal articles. The use of an existing data collection tool offers the researcher the benefits of established validity and consistency, and the ability to commence research sooner without spending time to devise and test an instrument. A **data collection tool** is a device that has been created for the purpose of accumulating specific details in an organized fashion. Some examples include a physical assessment form, a graphics record, and opinion questionnaires. Once a suitable tool is found, permission for its use often may be obtained more quickly through e-mail than through traditional mail. In the event that a suitable tool is not located, the construction of a data collection tool via word processing software makes revision easy, while online construction yields immediate feedback.

Once the data collection instrument is constructed, discussion lists and chat rooms may be used to test the instrument, solicit study participants, and even collect data. E-mail interviews and Web-based surveys offer alternative methods to collect research data electronically (Braithwaite, Emery, DeLusignan, and Sutton 2003; Eysenbach and Wyatt 2002; Lenert and Skoczen 2002). E-mail allows varying degrees of structure in the interview process, as well as ease of transcription via downloading without

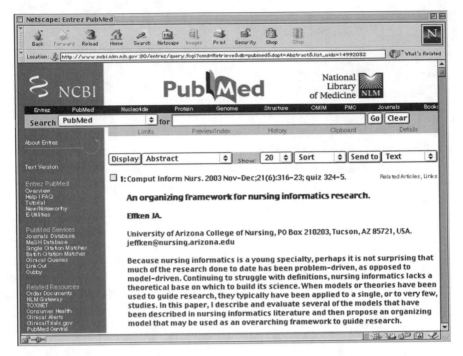

FIGURE 17–1 • Results of a MEDLINE search (Reproduced from a national library of medicine MEDLINE search. Used by permission of Lippincott, Williams C. Wilkins copyright 2003. Abstract depicted Effken, J.A. (2003). Framework for nursing informatics and organizing research. *CIN: Computers, Informatics, Nursing, 21*(6) 316–323.)

interpretation error secondary to pauses and inflection. Data collection via the Internet can offer several advantages. These may include:

- Interactive forms that can be evaluated for completeness and accuracy of data before submission
- Automated data compilation and exportation to other software
- Fast, cost-effective administration of surveys
- Freedom from geographic boundaries
- Ease associated with sending out reminders to complete survey instruments
- Access to previously hidden populations

The Internet population is not representative of the general population, however, because it is not available to all populations. Selection bias is another factor that limits the generalizability of results because the Internet population is nonrepresentative and open surveys conducted via the Web net volunteer participants. Box 17–4 provides some suggestions for the design and administration of Web-based data collection tools. As with traditional research methods, ethical issues must be considered. These issues

Box 17–4	Tips for Design and Administration of Web-Based Data Collection Tools

- Determine the objectives for the tool.
- Write then edit the questions.
- Include the title, introduction, purpose of the tool, and an anonymity statement.
- Critique the tool for reading level.
- Ensure that the tool is visually attractive.
- Limit the amount of information on a page.
- Ask evaluators to rate the tool for readability and time required for completion as well as their suggestions.
- Test the automated data collection process before public posting.
- Pretest the tool before public posting.
- Include a few open-ended questions, and provide a wrap-up.

include informed consent, protection of privacy, and the avoidance of harm. The ability to use cookies to assign a unique identifier to each person viewing a Web-based questionnaire offers the researcher the ability to determine response and participation rates and to filter out multiple responses. Researchers using cookies should publish a privacy policy, state that cookies will be sent, explain their purpose, and set an expiration date based on the date that data collection will end. Researchers must also recognize that there will be occasional problems with online data collection, including programming errors, usability problems, software incompatibilities, and technical problems (Schleyer and Forrest 2000).

Data collection can also be aided through the use of mobile devices such as PDAs and notebook computers at the study site (Bosma, Balen, Davidson, and Jewesson 2003; Kennedy, Charlesworth, and Chen 2003; Meadows 2003). Data can be transmitted, if needed, to another computer for compilation and analysis. This eliminates transcription errors and speeds the data collection and analysis process. Interactive data collection tools offer the advantages of engaging the participant, eliminating redundant data entry, and the time and costs for scrubbing data.

Data Analysis

Data analysis is the processing of data collected during the course of a study to identify trends and patterns of relationships. This task begins with descriptive statistics in quantitative, and some qualitative, studies. Descriptive statistics permit the researcher to organize the data in meaningful ways that facilitate insight by describing what the data show. Theory development and the generation of hypotheses may emerge from descriptive analysis. In addition to descriptive analysis, there are a number of statistical procedures that a researcher must choose when conducting a study. Until recently, researchers embarking on large studies needed the services of statisticians and large computing centers for data analysis. Many practitioners and students in the health care professions thought they were unable to perform meaningful research without these supports. Personal computers now rival larger systems in abilities and can easily link with larger computers, making it easier to conduct research in any setting.

There has been a growing recognition that the huge amounts of data collected within business and health care systems might be tapped and used for a variety of purposes (Allen 2003; Daukantas 2003; Tyagi 2003; The Upside 2003; Versel 2003). The overwhelming volume of data requires computer processing to turn data into useful information. A variety of terms exist to refer to the use and processing of this data. *Knowledge discovery in databases* (KDD) is a term that has been used in other industries (Wilson and Rosen 2003). KDD identifies complex patterns and relationships in collected data. It provides a powerful tool suitable for the analysis of large amounts of data. Commercial packages are available in a range of prices and platforms. KDD may be used to identify risk factors for diseases or efficacy of particular treatment modalities. The confidentiality of individual records may be protected through the use of data perturbation. This technique modifies actual data values to hide confidential information while maintaining underlying aggregate relationships of the database. Further research is needed on the use of data perturbation and its potential to introduce bias. **Data mining** is another term for the use of database applications to look for previously hidden patterns. Its use is growing; it has been investigated for marketing purposes, tracking the factors underlying medication errors, and improving financial performance. Data mining supports sifting through large volumes of data at rapid speeds in ways that were not previously possible due to size or speed limitations (Schuerenberg 2003). This allows real-time access to information for a competitive edge (Reimers 2003). Data mining in conjunction with electronic records can help physicians quickly determine the number of clients in their practice that need examinations and to generate reminders. The use of mined data is contingent on its quality.

Quantitative Analysis The computational abilities of computers readily lend themselves to statistical analysis of qualitative data and render more accurate results than might be available from hand-calculated statistics. Several software packages are available for quantitative analysis; most evolved during the 1960s and 1970s and permit the importation of data from spreadsheet or database software, and sometimes ASCII files. The majority provide versions of their products for a variety of computer platforms. A partial list follows:

- The System for Statistical Analysis (SAS) comprises several products for the management and analysis of data. It is considered an industry standard.

- MINITAB Statistical Software offers an alternative to SAS. Geared to users at every level, it is widely used by high school and college students and incorporates pull-down menus for ease of use.

- BMDP evolved as a biomedical analysis package. It comes in personal and professional editions and offers an easy-to-use interface for data analysis. BMDP also prompts the user until analysis is complete. It offers a comprehensive library of statistical routines.

- SPSS is another well-known software company. SPSS provides products for most computer platforms; it provides statistics, graphics, and data management and reporting capabilities.

- S-Plus is known for its flexibility in allowing users to define and customize functions. It also offers extensive graphics.

- SYSTAT, unlike some of the other packages discussed, was first developed for PC use. It is now available through SPSS.

- DataDesk started as a MacIntosh product, but it now is also available for use with a Windows operating system.

- JMP started as a MacIntosh product and resembles DataDesk. It now is also available for use with Windows operating systems.

Despite the increased use of statistical analysis packages by nurses, some researchers still argue that nurses should work with the traditional users of supercomputers to develop skills needed to use these resources and to access large data archives held by government and private agencies. Supercomputers offer the ability to quickly peruse huge databases. This belief gives rise to a new branch of nursing science, nurmetrics. Nurmetrics uses mathematical form and statistics to test, estimate, and quantify nursing theories and solutions to problems.

Computer Models Computational nursing, a branch of nurmetrics, uses models and simulation for the application of existing theory and numerical methods to new solutions for nursing problems, or the development of new computational methods (Meintz 1994; Van Sell and Kalofissudis 2002). One proposed use of nurmetrics and computational nursing is the formulation and testing of new models for health care delivery by using computers. This application is cost effective and can demonstrate how factors such as education may affect health practices and outcomes over time without the need to first implement the program and wait for results. Nurmetics has not been widely used. Nursing informatics uses computer science and informatics principles to understand how the structure and function of information may be used to solve problems in nursing administration, nursing education, practice, and research. Both graphical user interfaces (GUIs) and global data analysis facilitate modeling and simulation.

Qualitative Analysis Computers also aid the organized storage, tabulation, and retrieval of qualitative data. For example, databases can be used like electronic filing cabinets to store data; software can locate key words or phrases in a database, sort data in a prescribed fashion, code observations or comments for later retrieval, support researcher notes, and help create and represent conceptual schemes. As notes, coding, sorting, and pasting are automated, researchers have more time to analyze data. Despite these benefits, critics cite the following dangers:

- Qualitative research may be molded to fit the computer program.
- Computers tempt researchers to use large populations, thus sacrificing in-depth study for breadth.

Software is available to support qualitative research by allowing researchers to automate clerical tasks, merge data, code, and link data. QSR International provides several products that facilitate qualitative research, including NUD*IST and Nvivo. Ethnograph is another product that supports importation of text-based qualitative data into word processing packages. HyperRESEARCH and TAMS Analyzer represent other examples of qualitative software. AQUAD is a specialized program for users with an advanced knowledge of qualitative research. Text must first be entered or scanned into a word processor and converted into ASCII. AQUAD permits coding on the screen, and researchers may define linkages they wish to explore. Words or phrases in text and their frequency may be noted. There are several listservs that support qualitative research, including QUALRS-L, QUALNET-L, Qual-software, and QUAL-L.

Data Presentation: Graphics

Once data analysis is complete, graphics presentation software helps the researcher put study findings into a form that is easy for the reader to follow in written study reports and for the listener to follow when findings are presented at professional meetings and conferences. Graphics presentation software allows the researcher to design and make slides for use at presentations without the services of a media department. Harvard Graphics and PowerPoint are two well-known commercial packages. PDAs can now be used to store slide presentations. Figure 17–2 shows a bar graph prepared using a graphics application.

Online Access to Databases

The National Institutes of Health (NIH) offers access to several databases useful to nurses interested in research, health policy, and the identification of funded research projects. One of these databases, the Computer Retrieval of Information on Scientific Projects (CRISP), provides information on research grants supported by the Department of Health and Human Services. CRISP lists the following data for each project: title, grant number, abstract, principal investigator, thesaurus terms, and key words. CRISP is updated weekly and is available at *http://crisp.cit. nih.gov/*. Search results may be printed or saved to disk. The Agency for

online databases

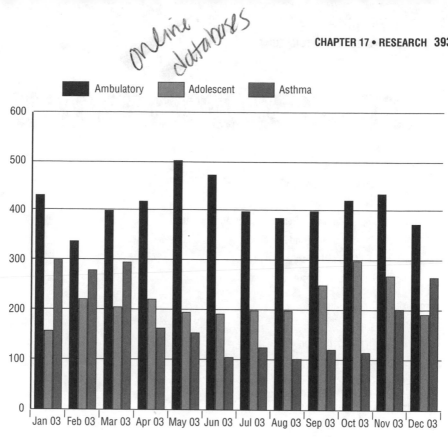

FIGURE 17–2 • Bar graph depicting the number of clinic visits per month for January 2003 Through December 2003

Healthcare Research and Quality (AHRQ) sponsors the National Quality Measures Clearinghouse (NQMC). NQMC is a public repository for evidence-based quality measures and measure sets. NQMC may be accessed through the AHRQ Web site at *http://www.ahrq.gov*. The intent of this database is to provide detailed information on quality measures and to further their use.

Several other agencies provide access to online databases useful to health care researchers, educators, clinicians, and administrators. These include the following:

- The National Library of Medicine (NLM) at *http://www.nlm.nih.gov*.

- Sigma Theta Tau's Virginia Henderson International Nursing Library (INL) at *http://www.stti.iupui.edu/VirginiaHendersonLibrary/*. The INL provides information on grant opportunities, nurse researchers, meeting proceedings, and access to databases that pertain to nursing research.

- The Cochrane Library at *http://www.cochrane.org/reviews/clibintro. htm*. The Cochrane Library consists of a regularly updated collection of evidence-based medicine databases, including the Cochrane Database of Systematic Reviews.

Box 17-5   Possible Funding Sources for Health Care

Government Agencies

- National Institutes of Health
- National Institute of Nursing Research
- National Library of Medicine
- Substance Abuse and Mental Health Services Administration
- Centers for Disease Control and Prevention
- Food and Drug Administration
- Agency for Healthcare Research and Quality

Professional Organizations

- Sigma Theta Tau
- American Nurses Association
- Oncology Nursing Foundation
- Specialty Groups

Foundations and Organizations

- Robert Wood Johnson Foundation
- Skin Cancer Foundation
- Epilepsy Foundation
- Myasthenia Gravis Foundation
- American Cancer Society
- March of Dimes
- Arthritis Foundation

There are a number of other sites that contain links to databases and research-related information. These sites are maintained by government agencies, professional organizations, and publishers, among others. Box 17-5 lists some other sources to consider when seeking research funds. AHRQ is one agency that actively supports research to improve health care, particularly studies that can improve patient safety, access to services, and bioterrorism knowledge and preparedness (Ortiz 2003).

IMPEDIMENTS TO HEALTH CARE RESEARCH

Nursing and health care presently lack information required to deliver more effective health care at a lower cost. The electronic health record (EHR) will help to provide the database needed to accomplish this feat. The EHR will change the way in which information is collected and used and will help to ensure the survival of enterprises that have EHR capability. Unfortunately, the birth to death EHR is not wide spread. In the meantime, automated health care providers can accrue some benefits by tracking information on an ongoing basis and noting emerging patterns. Cost containment may be achieved by decreasing operating expenses, eliminating duplication, and improving quality of care. Client care can be improved by making clinical and financial data available for individual and aggregate profiles and outcome assessments.

Impediments to the realization of the EHR as a source of data to improve health care include competition among health care providers, a lack of common language or data elements, unresolved technical issues, and concerns over the confidentiality of private health information. Hospital mergers and affiliations foster the sharing of data. Competition does not. This presents an obstacle to the creation of large databases required to accurately find trends in health care problems and successful treatment options.

Unified Language Efforts

The lack of a common language to facilitate data collection and decision making was recognized as a problem in nursing several years ago. The Unified Medical Language System project represents an attempt to standardize terms used in health care delivery. The American Nurses Association had a database steering committee working on the Unified Nursing Language System as a means to develop and use other clinical databases to extend nursing knowledge. This committee approved the inclusion of the Nursing Interventions Classification (NIC) and its linkage to the North American Nursing Diagnosis Association (NANDA) diagnoses for inclusion in the Unified Nursing Language System. Despite its name, NANDA and its companion interventions and outcomes are international in their scope and under study across the globe.

At the present, the Uniform Hospital Data Set (UHDS) is the most commonly used data set in the United States, but it does not include data on nursing care and outcomes. The Nursing Minimum Data Set (NMDS) has been defined as a consistent collection of data comprising nursing diagnoses, nursing interventions, nursing outcomes, intensity of care, and demographic and service elements. The NMDS was devised as a means to:

- Collect essential and comparable nursing data across different health care settings
- Describe care
- Demonstrate or project trends for care and allocation of resources
- Stimulate nursing research through links to data existing in hospital information systems

Despite efforts to arrive at a common nursing language, several vocabularies and classification schemes exist. The American Nurses Association established the Nursing Information & Data Set Evaluation Center (NIDSEC) to establish standards for information systems to support the documentation of nursing practice and review systems against these standards (American Nurses Association 2004). The ANA supports the use of multiple vocabularies and classification schemes as a means to support the diversity in nursing practice. NIDSEC also advocates the development of links, or mapping of similar terms, among the different schemes and vocabularies. All schemes must be clinically useful and stated in unambiguous terms and must have an associated unique identifier that leaves a machine-readable audit trail. Box 17–6 lists languages that the ANA recognizes as supporting nursing practice.

In addition to facilitating data collection, uniform languages set the definition of key terms, ensuring that studies can be replicated. Implementation of uniform languages first requires the following:

- Education of staff who are unfamiliar with standardized terms
- Elimination of computer restraints, such as limited characters and lines per field, found with some computer systems
- Database coordination among various clinicians and departments that use terms differently but require access to shared data repositories

Multi-institutional Research

Automation and a uniform language also aid the simultaneous collection of data from multiple sources. At the present, this capability is limited to health care alliances that can, and already do, share data. This feature will become more important once the EHR is realized. Multi-institutional research offers researchers the opportunity to increase the size of their study populations and eliminate idiosyncrasies associated with a particular place as a contributing factor to the findings. In short, multi-institutional research ensures that findings can be applied to a larger population.

Research in Real Time

The potential of hospital information systems to collect large amounts of data almost instantly allows for research in "real time," or essentially as events occur. This ability helps institutions react quickly to changes noted in client populations. Some systems can perform routine work while automatically channeling study information into an appropriate database according to particular study protocols. This is a desirable feature that would eliminate redundant data entry; however, at the present, few information systems are flexible enough to do this. This lack of flexibility creates the need to collect data that are already available on information systems to be gathered and formatted separately each time it is needed for a research study.

Collaborative Research

Collaborative computing and research foster productivity by allowing individuals at dispersed sites to share ideas and information in real time.

Box 17-6 Standardized Languages That Support Nursing Practice

NANDA (North American Nursing Diagnosis Association)	An international effort to develop and classify nursing diagnoses Provides a common language for client problems Gives a diagnostic label, contributing factors, and signs and symptoms Each diagnostic category lists major and minor defining characteristics
Nursing Interventions Classification System (NIC)	Three-level taxonomy of nursing interventions Domains and classes help providers to locate interventions most appropriate for their clients Provides a structure that can be numerically coded for computer use and data manipulation
Home Health Care Classification (HHCC)	Documents the provision of nursing care to patients in their homes Consists of two interrelated taxonomies: HHCC of Nursing Diagnoses and HHCC of Nursing Interventions Developed as a means to predict resource needs and measure outcomes
Omaha System	Model for capturing, sorting, and analyzing client data Used as a component of Nursing Minimum Data Set (NMDS) Problem classification and intervention scheme and problem rating scale for outcomes for community health nursing Provides ability to describe client population and level of service
Nursing Outcomes Classification (NOC)	Classification of patient/client outcomes developed to evaluate the effects of nursing interventions Each outcome consists of a definition, a list of indicators used to evaluate patient status, a target outcome rating, a place to identify the source of data, a five-point Likert scale to measure status, and list of references used to develop the outcome.

(continued)

Collaborative computing may use e-mail, desktop videoconferencing, other telecommunication tools, or shared databases to join persons of like interests. Many health care professionals lack basic competence in research (Byrne and Keefe 2002). This situation has been exacerbated as the requirement for research projects has been shifted from undergraduate and graduate levels to doctoral programs. This discourages many practitioners from applying research findings and from attempting research themselves. Collaboration and mentoring are facilitated through telecommunication technology and should foster the development of research expertise. The American Academy of Nursing (AAN) and the

Box 17–6 **Standardized Languages that Support Nursing Practice—** *continued*

Nursing Management Minimum Data Set (NMMDS)	Supports collection of contextual data to allow comparison of care across like settings Provides data needed by managers for data-based decisions
Patient Care Data Set (PCDS)	Data dictionary of elements for inclusion in clinical information systems Comprised of terms commonly used to describe patient problems, expected outcomes, and care actions in acute care settings
PeriOperative Nursing Data Set (PNDS)	Vocabulary developed to define nursing diagnoses, expected outcomes, interventions, and activities for patients scheduled for invasive or operative procedures
SNOMED CT®	A multidisciplinary terminology intended to provide the underpinnings for an integrated electronic patient record. Consists of concepts, descriptions, and relationships
Nursing Minimum Data Set (NMDS)	Attempt to standardize the collection of essential nursing data Consists of essential elements for nursing care, client demographics, and services, along with a label and conceptual definition for each Developed to allow comparisons of data gathered across different populations, settings, geographic locations, and times
International Classification for Nursing Practice (ICNR®)	Provides a framework to cross map nursing terms, vocabularies and classifications Classifies elements into Nursing Diagnoses/Phenomena, Nursing Actions/Interventions, and Nursing Outcomes
ABC codes (Alternative Billing Concept codes)	Alphanumeric codes used to represent services and supplies for nursing and alternative medicine
Logical Observation Identifiers Names and Codes (LOINC®)	Universal names and codes for laboratory tests and other clinical measures for use in computer databases or electronic transmission

AHRQ sponsor the Senior Nurse Scholar in Residence program as a means to encourage a senior nurse researcher to develop areas of investigation that integrate clinical nursing care questions with issues of quality, costs, and access. Information about this program can be found on the AHRQ Web site.

In addition to the impediments to research already noted, namely the failure to realize the EHR and a lack of standard language across health care, there are impediments to informatics research. Effken (2003) cites the lack of an organizing framework for nursing informatics to guide its direction. Without this framework, there is a tendency to focus on specific problems rather than underlying causative factors. Theory can ensure that study falls within the nursing informatics domain, provide a common language for researchers, and provide a basis for understanding, explaining and predicting outcomes of innovations in nursing informatics.

DISSEMINATION OF RESEARCH FINDINGS

Researchers have a responsibility to share their findings. Research findings may be shared via traditional paper-based journals or online publications. Several weeks may elapse from the time a researcher queries a journal to determine if there is interest in publishing his or her study findings until a reply is received. The process is shortened with electronic publication. Queries, submissions, reviews, and publication can all be done electronically. Results may also be posted without a review either through an established online publication or individually by a researcher. The *Journal of Medical Internet Research* is an example of an online publication with a research focus. Electronic publication has made it possible for more organizations to establish their own journals.

Preparation of the results for publication can be facilitated through the use of a bibliography database manager (BDM) (Nicoll 2003). This software helps to maintain the accuracy of references and properly format in-text citations and the final reference list. BDMs allow the importation of references directly from databases, eliminating the need to rekey and eliminating typographical errors. This process requires an Internet connection to the database, and in some cases an ID and password to access the database. Some examples of available BDMs include EndNote6, Reference Manager 10, and ProCite5.

THE IMPLICATIONS OF HIPAA FOR HEALTH CARE RESEARCH

The passage of HIPAA brought concerns over its implications for health care research. NIH has posted several documents online to clarify information for actual and potential researchers (February 2004, September 2003). HIPAA does have an impact on research. As of April 2003, the Privacy Rule requires many health care providers and insurers to obtain additional documentation from researchers before disclosing health information to them and to scrutinize requests for access to health information more closely. This additional documentation may include written permission from subjects through a special authorization form, or a waiver of the authorization requirement from the institutional review board or privacy board. A signed authorization form for research is valid only to a specific research study, not to future projects. Authorization differs from informed consent in that the authorization allows an entity to use or disclose his or her protected health information (PHI) for a specific purpose such as a study, whereas informed consent constitutes permission to participate in the research. The authorization must specify what PHI will be used or disclosed, who can use or disclose it, the purpose of the use or disclosure, and an expiration date. There must also be statements that address the individual's right to revoke the authorization and how that could be accomplished; whether treatment, payment, enrollment, or eligibility of benefits can be based on authorization; and that the Privacy Rule may no longer apply if PHI is redisclosed by the recipient. The authorization form must be signed and dated. Authorization is not required or may be altered when the covered entity obtains appropriate documentation that an institutional review board or a privacy board has granted a waiver or alteration of authorization requirements. Authorization is not required once information has been de-identified according to Privacy Rule standards.

Researchers are not covered entities unless they are also health care providers or employed by a covered entity or engage in any of the electronic transactions covered under HIPAA. Covered entities include providers that transmit health information electronically for HIPAA transactions, health plans, and clearinghouses. The Privacy Rule allows PHI use or disclosure to researchers to determine if the number and type of study subjects are sufficient to conduct research and if information has been stripped of all or certain identifiers. This second instance is referred to as *limited data.* Covered entities may disclose PHI to researchers to aid in study recruitment. Research started before the enactment of the Privacy Rule may be allowed to continue under a "grandfather" provision. Researchers need to be aware of HIPAA's Privacy Rule because it establishes the conditions under which covered entities can use or disclose PHI. There are implications for the creation and use of databases that contain PHI that may be used at some future point in time. Researchers may be responsible for drafting the authorization form. Not all researchers must comply with the Privacy Rule.

STUDENTS USING COMPUTERS FOR RESEARCH

Students in the health care professions often believe that research has little significance for them, and few carry out the entire research process. This is an unfortunate attitude because students can benefit greatly from information accessed via computers. One of the most obvious applications for student use is the electronic literature search. Despite the availability and merits of this type of search, many students claim that they tried and failed to find anything, when in fact they did not enter search limiters or appropriate terms. Both CD-ROM and online searches yield information that is more current than most of the reference books students use.

A more popular resource is the World Wide Web. It offers a wealth of information for both health care professionals and consumers. It is widely accessible at educational institutions for students who have no home access. It even has sites of particular interest to students in the health care professions. Students might choose to prepare for a community health teaching project by searching for materials on the Web as long as they are attentive to distribution and revision dates.

Students enrolled in research courses may have occasion to use software for statistical analysis, presentation of graphics, and proposal and report preparation. Many texts include software with study questions for mastery of research content.

Despite the fact that computer literacy is an expectation for nursing students, not all students are equally comfortable with computers. For this reason computer skills should be presented early and reinforced as a measure to get students to make good use of computers for research as well as other applications.

CASE STUDY EXERCISES

You are the staff nurse in a busy medical–surgical department at your community hospital. You and several of your colleagues have an idea that client anxiety is decreased in direct proportion to the amount of teaching that they receive preoperatively. Describe how you might use computer applications to look at this issue and prepare a proposal for funding consideration.

• • •

You and your classmates are expected to conduct a health teaching project in a public high school as one of the requirements for your Community Health Nursing course. Identify and discuss resources that you might use to gather material for this project.

• • •

You are working the night shift at your local community hospital. One of your clients was newly diagnosed today with a rare disorder that is unknown to you and your peers. Mrs. Prado is unable to sleep and is asking for more information about her diagnosis. None of the reference books on your unit provide information about her diagnosis. Your unit does, however, have an Internet connection. How might you use resources on hand to meet Mrs. Prado's needs?

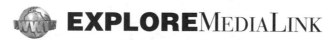

EXPLOREMEDIALINK

Multiple choice review questions, case studies, and other interactive resources for this chapter can be found on the Web site at *http://www.prenhall.com/hebda*. Click on "Chapter 17" to select the activities for this chapter.

SUMMARY

- Research provides data that allows better allocation of scarce resources and supports the development of knowledge.
- Computer applications can aid every facet of nursing research.
- Electronic literature searches, online discussion groups, and research reports all assist the potential researcher to identify topics for further study.
- Both CD-ROM and online literature searches quickly locate articles and provide abstracts. Full-text retrieval is available with some on-line searches.
- Data collection instruments may be located, developed, and even administered online.
- Data analysis is facilitated via the use of software for both qualitative and quantitative analyses.
- Nurmetrics is a branch of nursing science that uses mathematical form and statistics to test solutions to problems. One branch of nurmetrics known as computational nursing uses models and simulations to test solutions and proposed models for care.
- Several organizations maintain databases that contain information useful to nurses conducting research, including CRISP, the National Library of Medicine, the *American Journal of Nursing*, and Sigma Theta Tau.
- The implementation of the electronic health record will provide information required to deliver health care more effectively and at lower costs.
- The lack of a common language to facilitate data collection is a problem in health care. Several projects are under way to address this issue, including the Unified Medical Language System and the Unified Nursing Language System.
- Automation and the implementation of the electronic health record are expected to increase multi-institutional research efforts as well as research in real time and collaborative research.
- Students in the health care professions may reap the benefits of research tools without formally conducting research.
- Researchers need to be aware of relevant legislation such as HIPAA and the requirements that imposes on them in their conduct of research.

REFERENCES

Allen, G. (2003). Data mining technology; hair removal and surgical site infection; cytobrush versus curette sampling; pain wraps. *AORN Journal*, 78(3), 496.

American Nurses Association. (2004). Nursing Information and Data Set Evaluation Center (NIDSECSM). Available at http://www.nursingworld.org/nidsec/. Accessed March 10, 2004.

Bakken S., Warren, J. J., Lundberg, C., Casey, A., Correia, C., Konicek, D., and Zingo, C. (2002). An evaluation of the usefulness of two terminology models for integrating nursing diagnosis concepts into SNOMED Clinical Terms. *International Journal of Medical Informatics, 68*(1–3), 71–77.

Bosma, L., Balen, R. M., Davidson, E., and Jewesson, P. J. (2003). Point of care use of a personal digital assistant for patient consultation management. *CIN: Computers, Informatics, Nursing, 21*(4), 179–185.

Braithwaite, D., Emery, J., De Lusignan, S., and Sutton, S. (2003). Using the Internet to conduct surveys of health professionals: A valid alternative? *Family practice, 20*(5): 545–551.

Byrne, M. W., and Keefe, M. R. (2002). Building research competence in nursing through mentoring. *Journal of Nursing Scholarship, 34*(4), 391–396.

Daukantas, P. (2003). FDA to upgrade its data-mining skills and tools. *Government Computer News, 22*(11), 5.

Effken, J. A. (2003). An organizing framework for nursing informatics research. *CIN: Computers, Informatics, Nursing, 21*(6), 316–323.

Eysenbach, G., and Wyatt, J. (2002). Using the Internet for surveys and health research. *Journal of Medical Internet Research, 4*(2), e13.

Kennedy, C., Charlesworth, A., and Chen J. L. (2003). Interactive data collection: Benefits of integrating new media into pediatric research. *CIN: Computers, Informatics, Nursing, 21*(3): 120–127.

Lenert, L., Skoczen, S. (2002). The Internet as a research tool: Worth the price of admission? *Annals of behavioral medicine: a publication of the Society of Behavioral Medicine, 24*(4): 251–256.

Meadows, B. J. (2003). Eliciting remote data entry system requirements for the collection of cancer clinical trial data. *CIN: Computers, Informatics, Nursing, 21*(5), 234–240.

Meintz, S. L. (1994). High performance computing for nursing research. In S. J. Grobe and E. S. P. Pluyter-Wenting (Eds.), *Nursing informatics: An international overview for nursing in a technological era. Proceedings of the Fifth IMIA International Conference on Nursing Use of Computers and Information Science* (pp. 448–451). New York: Elsevier.

National Institutes of Health. (September 2003). Privacy boards and the HIPAA privacy rule. Available at http://privacyruleandresearch.nih.gov/privacy_boards/hipaa_privacy_rule.asp. Accessed March 10, 2004.

National Institutes of Health. (February 5, 2004). Clinical Research and the HIPAA Privacy Rule. NIH Publication Number 04–5495. Available at http://privacyruleandresearch.nih.gov/clin_research.asp. Accessed March 10, 2004.

Nicoll, L. H. (2003). A practical way to create a library in a bibliography database manager: Using electronic sources to make it easy. *CIN: Computers, Informatics, Nursing, Plus, 21*(1), 48–54.

Ortiz, E. (2003). Federal initiatives. *Healthcare Informatics, 20*(1), 49–52.

Reimers, B. D. (2003). Too much of a good thing? Real-time data analysis sounds good, but not if the data is wrong or can't be absorbed by the organization. *Computerworld, 37*(15), 38.

Schuerenberg, B. K. (2003). An information excavation: Las Vegas payer uses data mining software to improve HEDIS reporting and provider profiling. *Health Data Management, 11*(6), 80.

Schleyer, T. K. L., and Forrest, J. L. (2000). Methods for the design and administration of web-based surveys. *Journal of the American Medical Informatics Association,* 7: 416–425.

Tyagi, S. (2003). Using data analytics for greater profits. *Journal of Business Strategy, 24*(3), 12.

The upside of data mining. (September 8, 2003). *EWeek,* pNA.

Van Sell, S. L., and Kalofissudis, I. (2002). Theory of nursing knowledge and practice. Extracts from their under publication work. The evolving essence of the science of nursing, a complexity integration nursing theory. Available at http://www.nursing.gr/theory/Holistic.html. Accessed March 9, 2004.

Versel, N. (2003). HHS to integrate safety data among systems. *Modern Physician, 7*(1), 3.

Wilson, R. L., and Rosen, P. A. (2003). Protecting data through 'perturbation' techniques: The impact on knowledge discovery in databases. *Journal of Database Management, 14*(2), 14.

Appendix A: Internet Primer

This primer is a supplemental reference guide designed to get you up and running on the Internet. The Internet, generally referred to as the "Net," encompasses many different methods of manipulating information and communicating, including the World Wide Web, electronic mail, news-groups, and file transfer.

TOOLS TO GET ONLINE

If you are not already online through your school or place of work, there are a few things you need to hook up to the Net:

- A computer
- A modem
- A telephone line (if you use your regular telephone line, callers will hear a busy signal when you are online; you can also get a dedicated line) or cable or wireless connection
- An Internet service provider (ISP)

Modems

A modem is a piece of equipment that changes computer information to the kind of information that can be passed over telephone or cable lines. It can be an external box or an internal card.

Modems come in different speeds. The speed of a modem determines how quickly you can download or access information from the Internet. Modem speeds keep getting faster, but as of this writing 56K is the most common speed available over dial-up connections. Faster connections can be obtained through cable TV companies, satellite connections, or DSL servers which are available from the telephone company.

Some older computers cannot provide the same level of Internet access as newer, faster computers and might not be able to handle this rate of transfer. Check with your local computer hardware store to see what modem might be right for you.

INTERNET SERVICE PROVIDERS

To access the Internet, most users go through an ISP. ISPs are companies that run the computers that enable you to get onto the Net; these computers are called servers. When you connect to the Net, your modem lights up and dials the number of your ISP. Your modem actually connects to the server's modem. Some cable and telephone companies also provide Internet access.

When choosing an ISP, you should consider:

- *Price.* There are a variety of fee structures for Internet service. It is possible to obtain Internet access at no cost, but these providers generally bombard users with advertisements and may offer little or no technical support. Some ISPs allow unlimited use for a flat fee, some offer a certain amount of time per month before they begin charging extra, and some charge by the amount of time you are online from the moment you go online.

- *Traffic.* Find out the "dial up" number (the number your modem calls to link up) of an ISP and call it at different times during the day. Some ISPs get a lot of traffic and it can be difficult to get online (particularly the larger, national companies).

ELECTRONIC MAIL (E-MAIL)

E-mail is a way of transmitting messages across a telephone line, network, or cable connection to other computers through your ISP. It works like this: You have a program called a mail browser (such as Eudora or Microsoft Mail) that enables you to send and read e-mail messages. To send e-mail, first type in the e-mail address. E-mail addresses look like this: username@servername.domainname. For example, ClaraBarton@nursingnet.com. Make sure to put what the message is about in the "subject" line. After writing your text in the "body" of the message, you can send it. The message is transmitted across telephone, cable, or network lines to the server, which sorts the mail and sends it to the correct e-mail address.

Whether you use e-mail for work or play, it is generally somewhat informal and not very lengthy. E-mail can be used for sending out memos, writing a note to a friend, and exchanging documents and files. You can even send someone your resume over e-mail (see Appendix B).

Some things to remember when using e-mail:

- Try to check your mail every day, especially if you belong to a mailing list (see section on listservs). It is amazing how quickly your mailbox can fill up with messages.
- Do not send lengthy material via e-mail.
- Know your netiquette.
- Do not send anything too confidential or sensitive over e-mail; e-mail is easily accessed by others.

- Try to proofread your e-mail before you send it; it is all too common to see typos in e-mail messages, many of which could be eliminated if the messages were read over just once.

- Most of all, have fun with it. E-mail is a good way to keep in touch, get messages out to a lot of people, and make new friends!

THE WORLD WIDE WEB (WWW)

The World Wide Web provides a way to access Internet resources by content instead of file names. Since it was launched in 1992, the Web has virtually exploded into mainstream culture.

Browsers

To get to the Web, you must to have a computer program called a Web browser. Some of the more popular Web browsers are Netscape and Microsoft Explorer. Once you are online with your server, you simply open the browser and you are ready to "surf" the Net.

Web Addresses

The Web is made up of millions of Web sites (or Web pages). Each Web site has an address, which is known as the URL (uniform resource locator). A typical URL looks like this: *http://www.prenticehall.com/health;* this is the address for the Prentice Hall Web site for the health professions. To get to any Web site, all you have to do is type the URL in the browser's "go to" box (or something similar, depending on which browser you are using).

You can dissect Web site addresses and figure out who and what they stand for:

- "http," or HyperText Transport Protocol, appears in every Web site address (with a few exceptions). You will always see "://" after "http."

- Generally you will see "www," which tells the server to get the information from the World Wide Web.

- The last two parts of the address are the domain name; in this case, prenticehall.com is the domain name. The domain indicates what kind of site it is. In our case it is ".com" (pronounced "dot-com"), which stands for "commercial." Other domains you will probably come across include: ".edu" = education, ".org" = organization, and ".gov" = government. You get the idea.

Note: Do not get http and HTML confused. HTML stands for HyperText Markup Language, the programming language that enables you to develop a Web site. Also, when you read the address for a Web site out loud, remember that every "." is pronounced "dot."

Web Sites

Web sites are generally developed around a particular topic, such as nursing or health care. The amount of information available on the Web today is staggering and continues to grow. You can use the Web for general research, as an educational tool, as a shopping mall, to find a long lost friend, to get a new job (see Appendix B), or to answer practically any question you might have.

The first page you come to is called the home page, or sometimes the splash page. This page should convey the main ideas behind the entire Web site. It generally contains a menu for the entire site.

The home page contains links to other pages. They send you into further detail by a click of the mouse. Links are generally marked by keywords or images. It's like an outline: the home page is your thesis, and each link is a breakdown of main ideas to be covered on that topic. To "follow a link" from the home page, look for highlighted text, buttons, or images and click on them with your mouse. For example, go to *http://www.prenticehall.com/health* and click on the word "nursing." This is a link to resources for nurses that includes the Prentice Hall book catalog as well as other sites of interest.

Search Engines

Now that you have a basic idea of the workings of the Web, how do you go about finding Web sites that may interest you? There are a number of popular directories on the Web called search engines. Search engines are Web sites that contain Web site information (i.e., the URL and a short description) on virtually every topic imaginable.

Some of the larger and more popular search engines are:

- Yahoo! at *http://www.yahoo.com*
- Alta Vista at *http://altavista.digital.com*
- Excite at *http://www.excite.com*
- Hot Bot at *http://www.hotbot.com*
- Lycos at *http://www.lycos.com*
- Go at *http://www.go.com*
- WebCrawler at *http://webcrawler.com*

To use a search engine, type in one of the addresses listed above. When the home page for that site comes up, you will notice a search box in which you can type a keyword or phrase. The site will then bring up all the information that it has available on that topic as a list of sites. Sometimes you will need to narrow your search; for example, if you type in "nursing," hundreds of site listings will return. On the other hand, if you are too specific, you may not have any sites returned. You may have to try a few different word combinations to find the sites you are looking for.

Bookmarks

One very useful component of your Web browser is the bookmark tool. Whenever you come to a site that you may want to return to, you can bookmark it. To bookmark a site, go to that site. After it has loaded, choose "bookmark" or a similar command, depending on your browser. Your browser will record the address of that site in your bookmark folder. Anytime you want to return to that site, you simply open the bookmark folder and click on the title of that Web site.

Patience

Have patience when using the World Wide Web. Accessing Web sites can take time, depending on how elaborate the site is (how large it is, how many pictures are on it, and so on), how fast your modem can download the information, and what time of day you are surfing. You can speed things up a bit by turning off the autoload image option in your browser.

Also, because information is generally sent via phone lines, all sorts of hiccups can occur in the transfer process. Sometimes the server of the Web site you are trying to reach may be down, there may be a lot of activity on that site, or there may be line noise. Just try a couple of more times to load the site.

Finally, because the Web is so dynamic, sites and links change every day. You might find numerous links on Web pages that go nowhere. There are many reasons for this: people move their pages to new servers, get new Web site addresses, or take the pages down. Do not get discouraged; chances are there is another site right around the corner that contains all the information that you need. You can search for a particular site by enclosing the name in quotation marks.

MAILING LISTS AND LISTSERVS

Mailing lists are electronic discussion groups that take place through e-mail. They are groups of people who "get together" online to discuss a specific topic. There are numerous mailing lists on nearly every topic imaginable.

A listserv is the software program that is used to run the mailing list. Here is how it works:

- You find out about a mailing list dealing with a subject you are interested in discussing with others (such as culture and nursing).

- To get involved in this discussion group, you have to subscribe to it. To subscribe, send an e-mail message to that mailing list's listserv.

- Most often, the listserv automatically will subscribe you to the list and send you instructions on how to post to the group. Posting means that you send out a comment to the entire mailing list that you have subscribed to.

- Once you have subscribed, you will begin to receive e-mail messages from the mailing list. Be careful: some discussion groups have a large following and you may find your mailbox filling up rather quickly.

Newsgroups/Usenet

Newsgroups, like mailing lists, are another popular way of discussing specific topics over the Internet with other people who share the same interest. Unlike a mailing list, however, newsgroups take place on an entirely different network called Usenet.

Usenet is composed of thousands of newsgroups. Individual comments that people make to one another on a newsgroup are called articles. You post an article when you want to make a comment. The lines of discussion within a newsgroup are called threads. To read the discussions on any newsgroup, you must have a software program called a newsreader.

Generally, your ISP will provide you with a newsreader program as part of the software package. When you open the newsreader, it should download any new newsgroups that have been added. You can look through the entire list and choose which newsgroups interest you. When you find one of interest, just open it up and begin reading the articles. Newsgroup addresses are called hierarchies. Listed below are some of the standard hierarchies with examples of each. There are many other categories, some of which are from foreign countries.

> alt—groups generally alternative in nature (e.g., alt.education.distance, alt.alien.visitors)
>
> bionet—groups discussing biology and biological sciences (e.g., bionet.general, bionet.immunology)
>
> comp—groups discussing computer or computer science issues (e.g., comp.infosystems)
>
> misc—groups that don't fit into other categories (e.g., misc.fitness, misc.jobs)
>
> news—groups about Usenet itself (e.g., news.groups)
>
> rec—groups discussing hobbies, sports, music, and art (e.g., rec.food, rec.humor)
>
> sci—groups discussing subjects related to the science and scientific research (e.g., sci.med.nursing, sci.psychology)
>
> soc—groups discussing social issues, including politics, social programs, etc. (e.g., soc.culture, soc.college)
>
> talk—public debating forums on controversial issues (e.g., talk.abortion, talk.religion)

One word of caution: People take newsgroups very seriously. If you want to post an article, be sure you understand the threads (lines of discussions) that have been taking place on the newsgroup. Read a number of articles and understand the threads before putting up your own opinion.

Remember that these discussion groups are frequented by people from all over the world; because of this, newsgroups can offer a wealth of information. Many field experts frequent newsgroups. There may even be groups out there that you can monitor and to which you can provide expert advice.

PORTALS AND VIRTUAL COMMUNITIES

Portals are Web sites that offer a personalized view for you based on information provided when you register. Portals organize data into a single, easy-to-use menu providing services such as e-mail, search capability, and online shopping. America Online (AOL) and Yahoo represent general portal sites. There are also special-interest or niche portals. Some examples of nursing and health care portals include Nursing Net, WebMD, HealthGate, OnHealth, and HealthCentral. Portals continue to evolve. The term virtual community refers to a group of people who share common interests, ideas, and feelings online. This may occur through bulletin boards, chat rooms, or user groups. Special interest portals may serve as a tool to create a virtual community that models the features of a neighborhood, complete with shopping and other services.

FTP

FTP stands for file transfer protocol. FTP is a means by which you can send and receive (upload and download) documents and software over the Internet. FTP sites house these documents and software. Not all sites permit two-way traffic. Look for help with the FTP process under your browser's Help button.

NETIQUETTE

Netiquette is just like it sounds: etiquette on the Internet. It is just basic, common courtesy to others. Because no single person owns or controls the Internet, it is left to the individual user to be facilitative and kind when participating in discussion groups, authoring Web pages, or sending e-mail messages.

The following list contains general netiquette standards that most people on the Net attempt to abide by:

- Do not make assumptions
- Do not be judgmental
- Do not use all capital letters; this is interpreted as SHOUTING
- Do proofread your messages carefully
- Do be facilitative

- Do be honest
- Do be timely in your replies
- Do try to make postings brief and to the point

CONCLUSION

All of this information can be overwhelming at first, but, with time, you can learn to use the many invaluable resources the Internet has to offer. Understanding the many components that make up the Internet and using this knowledge to be discriminatory in the information that you find on-line will enable you to use the Internet as a research tool, an educational source, a meeting place, and a library. Now that you have this knowledge, you are ready to start surfing the Net.

Appendix B: Career Resources on the Internet

JOB HUNTING IN THE TWENTY-FIRST CENTURY

The advent of computers and the Internet has revolutionized the job search process. If you want to maximize your chances of finding a great job, using the Internet can help. Whether you are a recent nursing school graduate or an experienced nurse, sending out a traditional resume may no longer be enough to land an interview. The Internet and other computer technologies can help you get the attention of employers, network with colleagues, and research potential new jobs.

JOB SEARCHING ON THE INTERNET

The Internet can help you with your job search in several ways. The first that may come to mind is online job listings. Literally hundreds of sites on the World Wide Web contain help wanted listings. Most have search engines, so you can enter keywords describing the job you are seeking to see whether there are any matches in that database. Looking through all the job listings on the Web can be very time consuming, so you may want to narrow your search to health care-related sites. At this point, the majority of job listings on the Web are for computer professionals. However, listings in the health care professions will likely continue to grow.

Another way to use the Internet in your job search is to post your resume to a database. Again, it is probably best to choose a database that is specific to health care or nursing. For guidelines on writing and posting an electronic resume, see the Creating and Posting an Electronic Resume section of this Appendix.

Some of the most powerful ways to use the Internet to help find a job may be less obvious. The Internet can be a great way to make contacts all over the country. Interested in getting into home health care in Florida? There is bound to be someone out there, in a chat room or newsgroup, who knows all about it. She or he may even know of a place that is hiring. Many people who spend time online are friendly and willing to help, so post your inquiry anywhere you think you may get a response. As always, be careful about divulging personal information. You can also use e-mail to network with contacts and stay in touch with former classmates, co-workers, and others who may be able to help you find a job.

The World Wide Web can be a great tool for researching careers and potential employers. Many hospitals and other employers have Web sites you can peruse. There are also sites for professional organizations, educational institutions, and other groups that may post useful information. Be inquisitive and creative.

HOW RESUME DATABASES WORK

More and more employers are turning to automated applicant-tracking systems to sort and track resumes. These systems are actually databases that allow prospective employers to use keywords to search for applicants who meet certain criteria. For example, say a health maintenance organization is looking for a pediatric acute care nurse. The employer enters words describing her ideal candidate into the automated applicant-tracking system. In this case she may type in "pediatric," "acute care," and "registered nurse" as required keywords that resumes must include to come up in her search results. She may add other keywords if she likes, such as criteria that would be helpful for the job but are not mandatory. The tracking system then searches all the resumes in its system and retrieves those with the keywords the employer specified. Some tracking systems may display a list of resume "titles" or header lines for each resume retrieved, such as "LVN/home health care/Massachusetts." The employer can then select which resumes she wants to see in full.

How do you find these resume databases? Some employers have their own in-house automated tracking systems. Employers scan resumes received by mail into the system, and when a position opens up they log onto the database to search for a candidate. Some employers are able to receive electronic applications via e-mail; these are also stored in the database.

Employers who do not have their own database may use other generic applicant-tracking systems on the Internet. Some of these encompass all job seekers in any field; others are geared to specific areas such as health care. With these systems it is up to the job seeker to enter a resume into the database. There are several ways to do this, and the available techniques vary among systems. One common way to post your resume online is to type it directly into the database once you have logged onto the site. Many systems allow you to paste your resume from your word processor onto the database. You can often send it via e-mail. Employers search these databases according to keywords, which may include information about your skills, education, or geographic area.

CREATING AND POSTING AN ELECTRONIC RESUME

The electronic resume has many things in common with the traditional resume. Both prominently display your name, address, and telephone number and list your work experience, education, and special skills. However, there are several differences. An electronic resume will be seen by prospective employers only if it contains the keywords the employers are searching for. Many electronic resumes contain a keyword summary section toward the top, listing the standard phrases that describe the applicant's skills, areas of expertise, job titles, and credentials (see Figure B–1). It is a good idea to put the keywords in ascending order of importance. Also use common abbreviations, synonyms, or acronyms for words used in the body of the resume to increase your odds of matching the employer's keyword specifications. For example, if you list "registered nurse" in the body of your resume, use "RN" in the keyword summary. To determine what keywords to use, look at the words used in the job listings and use those that describe you. If you have access to electronic resumes, either on your computer or at your library, you can see what keywords others have used as well.

Because your electronic resume may either be scanned into a computer or sent to a database via e-mail, you will need to ensure that the formatting you use will be readable to any system. Some kinds of formatting and typefaces will turn to gibberish or become unreadable in some circumstances. To make sure this does not happen, follow these rules of thumb:

- Choose a common typeface, such as Times Roman, Helvetica, or Palatino. Avoid fancy scripts, which are likely to degrade when scanned. Use 12- or 14-point type. Do not use graphics, shading, italics, or underlining; for emphasis, use boldface or capital letters.

- If you are sending your resume electronically over the Internet, check whether there are formatting specifications you must meet. Some databases require that you meet certain margins or not use tabs. And many require that resumes be sent in plain text or ASCII format.

- If you are sending a hard copy of your resume, use a printer that produces clean, easy-to-read copy. Be sure to send an original print, not a photocopy. If you must fax it, use the fine setting.

- Use plain white 8½ × 11-inch paper with no folds or staples.

ISSUES TO CONSIDER WITH AUTOMATED APPLICANT TRACKING SYSTEMS

The advantage of getting your resume into an automated applicant-tracking system is that you will maximize your exposure to employers. There are, however, some disadvantages to consider. It may be difficult for a recent graduate with little experience to shine in a database system, since qualities like independence, perseverance, and reliability are not usually entered as keywords in a search. If you are looking for your first job as a health care professional, you may not want to rely solely on an electronic resume.

There are also confidentiality issues with database resume systems. While some systems restrict access to subscribers only, others do not. Either way, anyone, including your current boss (who could be a subscriber to the database you're using), can see your resume posted there. Some services will provide

---

Mary Lou Johnson
1234 Elm Street
Springfield, MO 12345
Home: (222) 345-6789
Work: (222) 456-7890

Keyword Summary: Nursing. Health Care. RN. BSN. Manager. Home Health Care. Geriatric Extended Care. Geriatric Preventive Care. Infection Control. Psychosocial Care. Teaching. Spanish. Relocation.

Current Position

1994–present   Nursing Supervisor, Large Nursing Home, Springfield, MO. Coordinated and supervised a nursing team responsible for 24-hour care of geriatric clients at an extended care home. Expanded program of preventive care and reduced hospital-ization rate by 20%. Taught in-service programs for floor staff on geriatric care issues. Co-chaired committee on infection control and product evaluation. Effectively represented the unique interests and priorities of the nursing home staff; turnover dropped by 25%.

Previous Positions

1989–1994   Teaching Assistant, School of Nursing, Private School of Nursing, Kansas City, MO.

1983–1989   Staff Registered Nurse, Large Medical Center, Kansas City, MO.

Education

1983   Bachelor of Science, Nursing, University of Missouri.

Continuing Education Sampling

1997   Seminar: "New Perspectives on Aging"

1997   Workshop: "Care of People with Alzheimer's Disease"

1996   Evening course: "The Changing Face of Aging in America"

1995   In-service: "New Studies on Diabetes"

Professional Memberships

1984–present   American Nurses Association

FIGURE B–1 • Sample electronic résumé

users with a list of subscribers, but this is no guarantee that the information will not get back to your current employer. One way to help protect your privacy is to leave out identifying information about your current employer in your resume. For example, you could write that you work at "a university medical center" instead of "The University of Texas Medical Center."

Before you post your resume on any online system, be sure you understand the user guidelines. They will let you know any details about formatting to use or avoid, how long your resume will remain in the system, how to update it, and whether any fees are charged.

Appendix C: Case Study Exercises—Suggested Responses

CHAPTER 1

A client arrives in the emergency department short of breath and complaining of chest pain. Describe how informatics can help nurses as well as other health care providers to more efficiently and effectively care for this client.

- *Old records (including prior medical history and medications) are available quickly through the use of information systems to all parties involved in the patient's care, no matter what their location.*
- *High-quality care is readily available through telemedicine (electronically submit ECG and chest x-ray to on-call specialists off site).*
- *The latest research on the patient's drugs and presenting symptoms is available via the Internet.*
- *Expert systems and care maps guide the treatment plan.*

CHAPTER 2

You are appointed to the hospital's information technology committee as the representative for your nursing unit. The charges of the committee include the following: Identify PC software that is needed to accomplish unit work, such as word processing, spreadsheets, and databases.

- *Word processing aids the following efforts: committee minutes, writing and revising unit policies and procedures, authoring and revising patient instructions, developing care maps.*
- *A database can be used to maintain and display personnel information.*
- *The availability of a statistical package fosters unit-based research.*
- *Browser software provides access to materials housed on the intranet such as announcements, policies and procedures, institutional phone numbers, patient education materials, and programs mandated for regulatory bodies. Internet access provides the means to retrieve reference material such as literature search results, drug information, continuing education, and professional groups.*

- *E-mail provides the capability to share information with professional colleagues within the institution and in other facilities.*

Determine criteria for the selection and placement of hardware on the units. Discuss these issues and how they affect patient care and work flow.

- *Avoid high traffic zones—they are subject to multiple interruptions.*
- *Have enough devices for all users.*
- *Provide good lighting and place monitors to avoid screen glare.*
- *Consider ergonomics.*
- *Avoid placing computers in areas subject to liquid or food spills.*
- *Ensure that work surfaces are free from clutter.*

· · ·

Your committee is charged with setting up a computer system that will automate transcription of physician orders and reporting of results. Identify the support personnel that you need at this point and write job descriptions for each identified position.

- *Have staff who do the everyday work identify the current workflow.*
- *Have staff and administrators identify information needed by each level of worker.*
- *Meet with staff and information services staff to discuss screen design, information that needs to be exchanged among systems, and desired output.*
- *Get physician and medical record approval for the information displayed in online reports.*
- *Consider whether results will be reported in pending and/or final forms.*
- *Evaluate whether charges for procedures or medications will occur at the time of order, completion, or documentation (or remain a separate process).*
- *Identify a plan for training and implementing the new system.*

· · ·

The infection control nurse has traced the spread of a nosicomial infection to a computer keyboard on a hospital unit. It is located in a work area adjacent to four patient rooms. This computer is routinely used by staff for documentation and to check laboratory and radiology results and access reference materials. The infection control nurse has asked the unit director and staff to identify strategies to eliminate this problem. Identify measures that can help to eliminate this problem.

- *Identify who is responsible for routine cleaning of computer equipment.*
- *Practice good hand washing technique.*

- *Have infection control conduct mini programs with interdisciplinary staff.*
- *Replace covers of keyboards as necessary.*
- *Periodic culture of equipment to identify if one area has specific problems.*

CHAPTER 3

Agnes Gibbons was admitted through the hospital's emergency department in congestive heart failure. During her admission she was asked to verbally acknowledge whether her demographic data were correct. Ms. Gibbons did so. Extensive diagnostic tests were done, including radiology studies. It was later discovered that all of Ms. Gibbons' information had been entered into another client's file. How would you correct this situation? What departments or other agencies would need to be informed of this situation?

- *Contact all clinical parties involved in Ms. Gibbons' care to look at whether she was treated appropriately and review her records in respective ancillary systems. Look at what drugs or blood products she may have been given and potential consequences.*
- *Involve information services, registration, medical records, and the billing department to correct the records.*
- *What was the length of time to discover the error and how was it discovered?*
- *Contact legal counsel regarding the situation.*
- *Educate all staff to seek more than one means of validation of patient identity upon admission (health insurance and photo identification in addition to verbal affirmation). Have client view information to validate that it is correct.*
- *Next time have Ms. Gibbons review the printout of her information and sign it to verify that it is correct. Be prepared to read the information to her.*
- *Delete Ms. Gibbons' information from the other client's record and/or create a new medical record number for the second client.*

• • •

A non–English-speaking Vietnamese male was admitted through the emergency department with suspected tuberculosis (TB). The system carried information under his name. Mr. Nguyen nodded his head when the admitting clerk pointed to the demographic screen. Mr. Nguyen was tested and treated for TB. When the public health nurse went to Mr. Nguyen's address for follow-up, the man there was not the Mr. Nguyen who had been treated for TB. How would you address this problem? Explain your rationale.

This situation is similar to the one above. A response of "yes" or nodding the head does not ensure that the client has heard or understood what was said. Validate identity through photo identification plus name and Social Security number. Obtain a translator as necessary. Notify all departments involved in the care of this client. Review client treatment relative to chart information for potentially harmful treatments.

• • •

You volunteered to serve on a committee to identify information from prior admissions that would be helpful to staff caring for current inpatients. What information, if any, would you select for ready access, and how long would you recommend that it remain active in the system? Remember that your system has limited capacity so that items must be carefully selected and prioritized. Identify the priority assigned to each item and provide your rationale for this priority.

Useful information: demographics, medical history, present medications, allergy information, over-the-counter products and herbal or other nontraditional treatments, and advanced directives, in that respective order. Availability of information eliminates repetitious questions and improves care.

CHAPTER 4

As the representative for your medical center's Better Care Initiative, a project with the purpose of identifying ways that services can be delivered in a more efficient manner, you have suggested that the Internet be made available to clinicians at the point of care. You must develop a report listing the potential uses of the Internet, as well as potential problems that might occur.

Potential uses

- *Intranet: to access policies and procedures, telephone numbers, human resources information, institution-specific references without worry about different versions.*
- *Internet: to access online databases and research, continuing education and degree programs, full-text retrieval of articles; increased access to experts in the field due to the ease of use of e-mail.*

Potential problems

- *Internet: staff may spend more time on the Web than expected, taking them from their other responsibilities.*
- *Some staff may surf non–work-related sites.*
- *Personnel may accept information found at face value without evaluating information for quality.*

• • •

One of your clients has a rare genetic defect. The client is requesting additional information about this from you, but no reference books on the unit describe this condition. Discuss strategies for how you might obtain this information using the Internet and electronic communication.

Try a Web search looking for support groups for the client. MEDLINE or one of the other literature databases should have information, possibly in full-text form. Use e-mail to write to specialists to request information.

• • •

The e-health committee at your facility is looking at ways to provide greater client involvement in accessing their own health information. What ramifications must be considered for this to occur in terms of security, interpretation of results, and training?

- *Do an assessment of users as to their knowledge and understanding of using the Internet.*
- *Conduct client education and training on the use of the Internet.*
- *Issue access codes and provide a procedure of changing the codes according to policy.*
- *Review confidentially statements frequently.*
- *Have a two-step procedure in place to prevent accessing unauthorized information.*

CHAPTER 5

You are a nurse participating in the customization and implementation of a medication documentation system. Define the data that must be included in the medication order entry process and the medication administration record documentation process.

- *Identify the drug by generic name (and trade name if desired), route, dose, administration times.*
- *Define times associated with daily, twice daily, three times daily, four times daily, bedtime, and before and after meals medication administration times.*
- *Develop a mechanism to display medications administered as well as medications not given.*
- *Provide a means to indicate why a medication was not given as well as that it was given by another person.*

• • •

You are the physician liaison for the IS department. Recent federal initiatives call for the implementation of CPOE. You have the technology available but you need to get administrative, nursing, and physician support. How would you go about getting this?

- *Offer several informative meetings.*
- *Post flyers announcing a catchy phase that will spark some interest.*

- *Offer demos during physician meetings with food available.*
- *Be available for training at any time that is convenient for the staff.*
- *Conduct progress meetings.*
- *Be flexible and prepared to answer questions based on individual needs.*
- *Confer with others who have had a successful implementation.*

• • •

You are participating in the customization and implementation of the radiology system. Define the data that must be included in the order entry process. Define the information that the nursing staff would like to view or print from the radiology system.

- *Must include the name of the examination, any modifiers that specify the exact body part to be filmed, date for the examination, and reason for the examination during order entry for treatment and reimbursement purposes.*
- *Output should include the test preparation instructions for staff and the client, notification that the examination has been done, and online results (preliminary and/or final).*

CHAPTER 6

You are a nurse manager in a hospital that has recently merged with two other hospitals, forming a large health care enterprise. Each of the three hospitals currently uses a different nursing information system. You are a member of the strategic planning committee, which is charged with the task of selecting which of the three systems will be used throughout the enterprise. Describe the process you would use to scan the internal and external environments, as well as the types of data you would collect.

- *Consider the strategic plan for the combined and separate institutions.*
- *Determine current staff satisfaction with each nursing information system.*
- *Look at whether the system is due for major upgrades as well as associated costs. Which one would be easier to expand? Which one has the most capability for the future? What technology is used?*

• • •

Develop a tool to evaluate each of the three nursing information systems for the scenario described above.

Develop a weighted tool that considers ease of use, expandability, compatibility with other systems, ability to customize, ability to generate reports, time needed for training, timeframe for implementation, and overall costs.

• • •

Your facility belongs to one of three health care delivery systems in the city. Competition is fierce. You have been asked to serve on a committee to study and recommend the retention or deletion of certain clinical services. Develop a plan for how you would do that and for how information services might facilitate that task via the use of benchmarking.

Compare services delivered to those provided by competitors for total number of cases served, quality of services inclusive of client satisfaction, length of stay as appropriate, cost per case, and profits or loss per cost center. Commercial packages may aid this task.

• • •

Your facility recently acquired and closed a competing hospital. All paper medical records are stored at a distant site. Records are not readily accessible. Client documentation and results were online but no longer available after the hospital closure. Some physicians never received test results for clients at the time of shut down. This had a negative impact on client care and satisfaction. How might strategic planning prevent this type of situation from occurring again?

- *Start planning early by sending letters to clients about getting copies of their x-rays, especially mammograms or testing results that will be needed for scheduled surgery.*
- *Notify physician offices and clinics about the impending closure as early as possible.*
- *If results are in the process of being stored at a different site they may not be available for some time. A test might have to be repeated, who will assume the cost?*
- *Set up a hot line that physicians and office staff can call. Have IS personnel available at the old site that are knowledgeable in all system applications, who can answer questions, and produce results if necessary.*
- *Consider that the quality and continuity of the client's care is maintained.*

CHAPTER 7

You are a member of a committee that will select a clinical documentation system for nurses. Prepare a timeline for the needs assessment and system selection phases. These processes should be accomplished over a 6-month period.

- *Set the target implementation date, then work backward to set other key dates.*
- *Start with a "kickoff" meeting to provide an overview of the process.*
- *Establish an ongoing meeting schedule and develop a project plan.*
- *Anticipate change.*

- *Collect information about workflow processes from end users and administrators.*
- *Identify problems with the current process.*
- *Review the Request for Proposal requirements and compare available products.*
- *Schedule vendor demonstrations and site visits.*
- *Narrow the selection.*

.   .   .

Develop a list of "musts" and "wants" and assign a weight to each item. Define what your weighting scale will be.

- *Choose a model for the system such as care mapping.*
- *Discuss how the new system will impact affect other systems.*
- *Develop a numeric scale, say 1–10, with 10 as the most desirable.*
- *Evaluate each of the systems using this scale.*

.   .   .

Create a list of questions related to this system selection process that you will ask at site visits:

Is it easy to use? What reports and printouts are produced or may be produced? How long is needed for implementation? training? What roadblocks were encountered? What would you do differently? Can it be adapted easily?

CHAPTER 8

You are the project director responsible for creating an implementation timeline that addresses the training and go-live activities for a nursing documentation system that will be implemented on 20 units and involve 350 users. Determine whether the implementation will be staggered or occur simultaneously on all units, and provide your rationale.

This decision may be influenced by the following:

- *Whether a system is in place now.*
- *Administrative support.*
- *Staffing and training resource availability.*
- *Ability to pull staff from other areas to the pilot unit(s).*
- *Weighing the advantages and disadvantages of doing one or all units at a time.`*

.   .   .

Create the timeline for the training and go-live schedule for this implementation.

- *Start at least 1 year in advance, then work backward to get in all activities.*
- *Plan for 24-hour IS coverage for at least 1 week (from IS).*
- *Obtain administrative support and a budget.*
- *Plan for the unexpected.*
- *Choose a training system (core trainers, educators versus outside parties).*
- *Determine the number of training hours per staff.*
- *Determine training costs for equipment, trainers, replacement staffing.*
- *Provide flexibility in the scheduling. Build in extra time before implementation.*
- *Do not start training too early, because folks forget.*

• • •

Your present manual medication administration record is being replaced by an automated information system. Discuss the specifications that you would recommend for reports that the system will generate to notify the nurses when medications are due. Determine how often the reports should print and what information they should contain.

Medication administration records need to identify drug name, dose, scheduled time, route, and special instructions. The format for reminders should be one determined to be most useful for the staff nurse (i.e., shift overview or list by a particular time, patient or group of patients, items not charted or charged). Staff need to determine the most useful frequency for these reports (every 1 or 2 hours or prior to the end of the shift?).

• • •

You have been selected to develop test scripts for interface testing for a new patient care system. Develop a test script with multiple interfaces. Define the output that you should see for each system.

A nursing documentation system would have demographic information, lab results from an outside system, radiology results plus any other diagnostic results, and a monitor interface and possibly a charge interface. Output differs for each interface and function. It must be accurate, and where it should be when it is needed. For example, demographic information passes from the registration system and is displayed in the nursing system. Diagnostic results need to pass from other systems into the documentation system. In the case of a charge interface a message is sent to accounting when a service, supply, or medication is administered.

• • •

As the manager of the GI lab in your facility you are expanding the applications for your IS system. At the present it allows physicians to capture images and produce consults and referral letters in a timely fashion. You have been working with the vendor to expand its features to include the capture of patient history. Consider the pros and cons of interchanging information collected by admitting nurse and physician.

Pros

- *Eliminate redundant data entry and preserve data integrity.*
- *More convenient because clients do not have to answer the same questions over and over.*
- *Complete history including procedures and reactions that the client encountered would be readily available to all health care professionals treating the client.*

Cons

- *Who will be responsible for verifying that all information is accurate and up to date?*
- *Agreement between parties as to how information will be communicated.*
- *Who will have the ability to update the information?*
- *Drug history and reactions to medications must be kept updated.*

CHAPTER 9

Kevin Gallagher, RN, has access to all client records on his medical–surgical unit. Consider each of the following situations:

- *Kevin's mother is admitted to the unit. Is it appropriate for him to peruse his mother's electronic medical record? Why or why not? No, not unless he is doing so directly on her behalf; otherwise, it is a violation of her privacy.*
- *Kevin's unit clerk also has access to Mrs. Gallagher's record. Is it appropriate for her to view Mrs. Gallagher's record? Only on a need-to-know basis.*
- *Kevin's co-worker Kaneesha is a client on the unit assigned to another staff nurse's care. Is it appropriate for Kevin to review her chart or lab results? Only on a need-to-know basis if he is involved in her care.*

• • •

Nancy Whitehorse, RN, routinely accesses client records on her medical unit. Does she violate her confidentiality statement if she performs the following actions?

- *She reviews the information and does not discuss it with anyone else. This is a violation.*
- *She discusses information obtained from client records with other health care workers on the unit. This is a violation.*

- *She discusses clinical cases, omitting names, in social situations. This is a violation.*

$$\bullet \quad \bullet \quad \bullet$$

Grace Elizaga has been given the charge of training the RNs and unit clerks from the first three client care units slated to start automated order entry at Potter's Medical Center (PMC). The target implementation date is in 2 months. A total of 93 RNs and 11 unit clerks must receive training prior to that time. Based on information from other agencies that have the same information system as PMC, 8 hours of training time is projected for each individual. As the nurse manager responsible for those units, you have been asked to work with Grace to develop a detailed plan to accomplish this task and submit this plan to your vice-president of Client Care Services. Include the following in your plan and provide your rationale:

- *Staffing—Replacement staffing is needed while others train.*
- *Costs for your personnel—Replacement staffing is needed while others train. People also need practice time and time to apply newly learned skills.*
- *Training start and completion dates—Training must start early and be completed 1 to 2 weeks before GL to take care of last-minute stragglers and new hires and to allow practice time.*
- *Length and number of training sessions—Consider the ability of personnel and trainers to get away from the unit, the appropriateness of the training location, and the ability of personnel to learn over a longer session.*

CHAPTER 10

In the course of conversation, your nurse manager tells you that she loaded a copy of the spreadsheet program she uses on her home office PC onto one of the unit PCs so that she can work on projects at both locations. Your institution has a well-publicized policy against the use of unauthorized, unlicensed software copies. As a staff nurse, what should you do? Explain your response.

Talk with your nurse manager, telling her that this is a violation of copyright law and can result in large fines and is probably a violation of institutional policy.

$$\bullet \quad \bullet \quad \bullet$$

You notice several of the new residents playing computer games on the nursing unit. You had not been aware of these games previously. What, if any, action should you take? Explain your rationale.

Remove them. Ask the IS department to "lock" down the machines so that additional software cannot be added without authorization. Approach the residents if necessary and ask them to restrict use on this machine to clinical uses.

$$\bullet \quad \bullet \quad \bullet$$

To remember her computer system password, university nursing instructor Pat Pawakawicz taped her password to the back of her name pin. When Ms. Pawakawicz lost her name pin recently, it was turned into hospital security and subsequently the IS department with her password still attached. When Ms. Pawakawicz picked up her name pin, she expressed intent to use the same password. Is this an appropriate way to treat a password? Should she use the same password again? Provide your rationale. What, if any, legal ramifications might there be for Ms. Pawakawicz regarding use of her password by unauthorized users?

Passwords need to be kept private. When there is any question as to whether they have been compromised they should be changed immediately. This instructor's behavior may compromise someone's confidentiality. Unless she was clear when her badge was lost, she may face civil or other disciplinary action.

• • •

The administration at St. John's Hospital takes pride in their strong policies and procedures for the protection of confidential client information. In fact, St. John's serves as a model for other institutions in this area. However, printouts discarded in the restricted-access IS department are not shredded. On numerous occasions, personnel working late observed the cleaning staff reading discarded printouts. What action, if any, should these personnel take relative to the actions of the cleaning staff? What action, if any, should be taken by IS administration? Provide your rationale. If current practices are maintained, are there any additional potential risks for unauthorized disclosure of client information? If you answer yes, identify what these risks might be.

The IS department needs to practice what it preaches. Printouts should be shredded at the time that they are discarded or at the very least the housekeeping personnel should receive an inservice and sign a confidentiality statement.

• • •

The secretary on 7 Tower Oncology receives a fax transmission about a client consult. The fax was intended for a physician's office in the adjacent building. She places the fax in the out bin of her desk to be delivered later by volunteers. No in-house mailer was used. Is this action appropriate? Explain why or why not.

This action is not appropriate. All faxes should have cover sheets and be placed in a confidential mailer. Staff need an inservice and reprimand in this case.

CHAPTER 11

You have been selected as a member of the Integration Project Team, which is charged with identifying ways that system integration could improve information flow. You work on an inpatient unit that uses a stand-alone nursing documentation system that is not interfaced or integrated with any other hospital information system. Identify the implications of this situation, and suggest integration options that could improve information flow.

This situation creates extra work and can compromise data integrity, leading to several different versions of information for every patient. Data entry should occur once whenever possible at a point closest to the source. Substantial cost savings may result for the entire organization by eliminating redundant data entry.

• • •

You are working to identify elements in your health care enterprise that could be used for a master patient index (MPI). List five basic elements and describe how each could be used for an MPI.

Obvious elements for an MPI include the client's name, medical record, Social Security number, and date of birth. Name and insurance may change. Eventually, the universal patient identifier will be a crucial element. Used in combination, these elements help to ensure access to the correct record.

CHAPTER 12

You are a member of the committee charged with designing the EHRs at your facility. Identify which components of nursing documentation should be retained in the clinical data repository. For example, would you want to include all client vital signs from the current hospital admission? Explain why you would include or exclude the various components.

History and assessment, operative notes, allergies and drug reactions, medications, specific lab data such as blood type, and some diagnostic tests need to be retained. Items such as all client temperatures would clutter the record.

• • •

Identify several external sources of information that would be useful as part of the EHR for access by a home health nurse.

Ancillary test results, social history, history and assessment, operative notes, allergies and drug reactions, and medications are useful in every care setting.

• • •

Discuss the implications of providing nurses in a hospital setting with access to all electronic client information. Identify which types of information are appropriate for access by nurses.

Nurses need clinical information but generally do not require billing and payment information. In some cases, it is not necessary for a nurse to know about every aspect of the client's history. One example might be that the emergency department client who has a laceration from an automobile accident doesn't need to relate his history of abuse as a child.

CHAPTER 13

You are teaching an undergraduate course titled "Nursing Informatics." One class session is scheduled for a discussion on the protection of client record information. How would you summarize the current status of legislative safeguards in the United States? What, if anything, would you suggest that students might personally consider to improve this situation?

Traditionally, protection of client information has been patchy from state to state. HIPAA provides protection at a federal level, although many issues remain unclear. Students can uphold standards and serve as advocates for client privacy and write their legislators and senators to view their opinions on the need for additional safeguards or changes to legislation.

• • •

You have been appointed to the Clinical Information Systems Committee, which is charged with looking at ways that automation can facilitate data collection for the next JCAHO accreditation visit. List examples of how your community hospital demonstrates adherence to JCAHO information standards, and state your rationale for why you feel these examples display compliance.

Examples include:

- *The existence and use of confidentiality and privacy safeguards, such as individual log-ons, different levels of access based on a need-to-know basis, and user sign-on statements.*
- *Improved access from different locations and by different types of providers at one time for more efficient patient care.*
- *24-Hour access with protection against loss via file backup.*
- *Documentation of client education is more legible and complete than traditional records.*
- *Improved turnaround time for documentation.*
- *Collection of aggregate data to support clinical research and client care is improved.*

• • •

You are the general information systems liaison at Wilson Rehabilitation Institution. CARF accreditation is coming up. What would you do to ensure that your automated documentation is in compliance with CARF standards? Explain your rationale.

This preparation should be similar to preparation done with a manual system, although automation can be used to facilitate the process. Reports can be run to show the extent to which required data are collected and in some cases system prompts added to guarantee that those data are provided. Automation also makes it easier to review treatment plans for completeness of documentation and to determine if they are up-to-date. These practices can be used prior to accreditation as a means to pinpoint and correct problem areas.

·   ·   ·

You are instructing new health care employees during orientation regarding HIPAA. A question is asked regarding how family members receive information on a delusional client. Discuss how you would deal with the issue and how you would provide additional safeguards over the disclosure of health care information.

The client should have in his or her file a copy of Durable Power of Attorney and/or Durable Healthcare Power of Attorney and Healthcare treatment instructions. The information would be given to them to make any necessary decisions. If this is not available, Social Services will get involved and sometimes the court must appoint a guardian to handle these issues.

·   ·   ·

You are part of a research team studying CVA treatments. Discuss how you use client data and how data are de-identified.

A Research Consent Form must be reviewed and signed prior to any study. A study number maintained in a filing system separate from the name and address files of the participants identifies all studies. Most researchers have obtained a Certificate of Confidentiality from the Department of Health and Human Services (DHHS). With this certificate, the investigators cannot be forced by court order to disclose research information that may identify a person in any State or local civil, criminal, administrative, legislative or other proceedings. Disclosures may be necessary, however, upon request of NIH, DHHS, or the IRB for audit or program evaluation purposes. Sometimes studies are requested with a specific area in mind such as by ZIP codes.

CHAPTER 14

As the clinical representative for your unit on the Disaster Planning Committee, you are charged with identifying all forms in your area that require completion of a physical vital records inventory sheet. What forms would you list and why?

Look at forms that are frequently consulted, such as staff telephone and pager numbers. Consider whether unavailability to the information creates difficulties. If the answer is yes, then add these forms to the vital records inventory sheet.

·   ·   ·

Work crews at Wilmington Hospital inadvertently cut the cable connecting all terminals at the hospital with the computer center. As the on-duty nursing supervisor, what should you tell your employees, and why? Who would you contact for further information? How do you determine whether to initiate manual alternatives?

Tell employees the truth rather than giving the appearance that some-one is hiding something. Next try to get an estimate for the expected time-frame that the system will be unavailable. If the downtime is expected to be more than 2 hours, the institution needs to implement manual alterna-tives; otherwise, nonemergency procedures may be entered into the system once it is restored, rather than manually.

• • •

An early-morning train wreck near St. Luke's Hospital derailed seven freight cars carrying chemicals that can emit toxic fumes. The accident took out power lines for the neighborhood and for St. Luke's. Emergency crews evacuated a seven-block area, stopping just outside of the hospital's main entrance. Power has already been out for 12 hours and restoration is not expected for at least another 12 to 24 hours. You are on an executive ad-ministrative committee charged with determining what information will be brought online first and what will remain in paper form. What would you restore first? What records, if any, would you not restore? Explain your ra-tionale. How would you document, for record-management purposes, that part of the record is automated and part is manual?

Demographics and registration information would be restored first be-cause the client must be in the system in order to perform any action. One of the next features would be the medication administration records (MARs). Not only do MARs have the capability to minimize med errors, but in many settings, charges occur when the medication is charted as given. Beyond these areas, consideration must be given to treatments and system features that are considered as essential for care. There should be notation in record of what is in manual form. It may be far too expensive to back-load data into the system when a paper record also exists.

• • •

As IS project manager you are responsible for helping the renal depart-ment select a new database. One of the top vendors must cancel its Web-based demonstration because its server was stolen. What questions should this raise for disaster planning with the use of vendor-supported applications?

Security of client information, because information resides on the ven-dor's equipment.

• • •

You recently learned that the information services network engineer responsible for conducting backups on the server for the tumor registry database failed to ensure that regular backups occurred properly. This was discovered when the database was found to be corrupt. Approxi-mately 20,000 entries were lost as a result. As the liaison between the tu-mor registry and the IS department how would you ensure that this would not happen again?

You must implement a procedure by which backups are accounted for. Make someone in the department accountable to verify that the backups have been completed and document the date this was performed. Periodic checking of the database to verify all records is available.

CHAPTER 15

You are on the education committee at your small community hospital. Your staff development department was eliminated several years ago. You and your colleagues are charged with developing strategies to meet the educational needs of agency RNs and LPNs. Limited capital and the isolated location of your community make this a difficult assignment. Your institution does have Internet and Web access in the medical library, as well as teleconferencing capability. Develop a proposal to meet your charge using available resources. Be prepared to defend your proposal to an administration loathe to part with monies beyond those already budgeted.

Internet access to continuing education eliminates hours of travel and expenses associated with travel.

• • •

You are the client educator at a medical center in the Pacific Northwest. Your clientele are drawn from a 150-mile radius and beyond. For this reason it is difficult to have clients complete diabetic education or other classes. You have been told to improve client completion of classes or face elimination of your department. The medical center has both teleconferencing capability presently used for consults and an established Web page that provides basic information about the institution. How might you use these resources to develop alternative strategies for client education? Address budget considerations, necessary resources, target populations that might be better served, and how you propose to link distant clients with instructional offerings.

Submit a proposal to administration to provide education via the Web as well as in the traditional classroom setting. The proposal should address provisions for access for all clients that might include use of computers in local libraries, schools, and senior citizen centers as well as the possibility of submitting a grant to obtain PCs for clients who do not otherwise have access. Work with the Webmaster for assistance in placing the material on the Web. Consider low-tech options, such as videotapes and the use of the telephone, as well.

• • •

You recently joined the faculty at a small, private rural college. Because you expressed an interest in computers and are slightly more knowledgeable about computers than your faculty colleagues, you have been asked to establish a computer lab for the nursing department and incorporate computer use in all of the nursing courses. Current resources are quite limited. Provide a detailed plan of how you would accomplish this charge from start to finish. Identify potential stumbling blocks and ways that you would address them.

This type of effort needs to be in concert with the overall strategic plan for computing within the institution, school, and department. Find out what is happening. Determine your goals. Do a project plan and establish a target timeline. Conduct a needs assessment. Investigate funding, including the possibility of writing a grant. Use institutional standards when looking at equipment. Be advised that the remainder of the institution may see this as taking resources away from them, so salesmanship is important.

CHAPTER 16

You are the nurse practitioner in St. Theresa's emergency department. A client is brought in with obvious psychiatric problems. You have no psychiatrist available and the nearest psychiatric facility is a 1-hour drive away. St. Theresa is a Tri-State Health Care Alliance Member. Tri-State has telehealth links with the regional hospital, where a psychiatrist is in the emergency department. What steps would you take to initiate a productive teleconference? Justify your response.

Be prepared to introduce the situation to the psychiatrist as well as to the patient. The patient may or may not be receptive, although the same can be true without a telemedicine link. Ensure that technical support as well as emotional support is available.

• • •

Erin O'Shell, home health nurse, just set up teleconference equipment for Dr. Bobby to evaluate Mr. Richard Goldstein for possible hospitalization for congestive heart failure. Dr. Bobby and the hospital are a 1-hour drive away. Just as the teleconference started, but before Dr. Bobby could listen to Mr. Goldstein's lungs or complete other key portions of the exam, a power outage severed the teleconference link. How should Ms. O'Shell handle this situation? Provide your rationale.

The backup situation is that the nurse uses the telephone and communicates her findings to the physician. The patient is probably experiencing distress already, which will probably increase without some action. The physician and nurse must work together to determine if this patient needs to go to the hospital or may receive further treatment in the home.

CHAPTER 17

You are the staff nurse in a busy medical–surgical department at your community hospital. You and several of your colleagues have an idea that client anxiety is decreased in direct proportion to the amount of teaching that they receive preoperatively. Describe how you might use computer applications to look at this issue and prepare a proposal for funding consideration.

This issue could be addressed in a patient satisfaction survey done during or after the hospitalization. This survey might be completed via telephone or possibly online. An argument for funding this project might be twofold. First, it provides a way to improve patient satisfaction and return visits and is therefore good for business. Second, patient stay may be decreased with cost savings to the institution. The organization may fund the survey or funding may be obtained from a number of different sites that might include professional organizations or various foundations, particularly for a specific population.

.   .   .

You and your classmates are expected to conduct a health teaching project in a public high school as one of the requirements for your Community Health Nursing course. Identify and discuss resources that you might use to gather material for this project.

There are a huge number of resources that can be tapped for this project. These may include the government, sites such as the National Library of Medicine, as well as information available through other agencies and professional groups, such as the American Academy of Pediatrics. Information from all sites should be evaluated for accuracy, authenticity, and currency before it is shared with others.

.   .   .

You are working the night shift at your local community hospital. One of your clients was newly diagnosed today with a rare disorder that is unknown to you and your peers. Mrs. Prado is unable to sleep and is asking for more information about her diagnosis. None of the reference books on your unit provide information about her diagnosis. Your unit does, however, have an Internet connection. How might you use resources on hand to meet Mrs. Prado's needs?

Either access your library through your intranet connection to conduct a search and full text retrieval or access one of the online databases such as MEDLINE through the National Library of Medicine site to do a search and retrieve literature. Consider a Web search as well, although the quality of information obtained will vary greatly and should be reviewed prior to your giving it to Mrs. Prado.

GLOSSARY

Access code Unique identifier generally provided by a name and password for the specific purpose of restricting computer or information system use to persons who have legitimate authority to view or use information found in the computer or information system.

Administrative information systems Systems that support patient care by managing financial and demographic information and providing reporting capabilities.

Aggregate data Data that are derived from large population groups.

Ambulatory Payment Classification (APC) Describes new reimbursement criteria for ambulatory procedures.

Antivirus software Set of computer programs capable of finding and eliminating viruses and other malicious programs from scanned diskettes, computers, and networks.

Application security Measures designed to protect a specific set of computer programs and the information that they create or store. A common example of application security in health care information systems is timed or automatic sign-off, which prevents unauthorized access by others when users forget to sign off the system.

Application service provider (ASP) Third-party entities that manage and distribute software-based services and solutions to customers across a wide area network from a central data center.

Application software Set of programs designed to accomplish a particular task.

Architecture Structure of the central processing unit and its interrelated elements within an information system.

Arden Syntax Standard language used in the health care industry for writing rules.

Arithmetic logic unit (ALU) Component of the central processing unit that executes arithmetic instructions.

Asynchronous Transfer Mode (ATM) High-speed data transmission method suitable for voice, data, image, text, and video information. It can use fiber or twisted pair. It is faster than ISDN, but less frequently used for reasons of cost, availability, and a lack of standards.

Audit trail Electronic tool used by information system administrators that is capable of showing system access by individual user, user class, or all persons who viewed a specific client record.

Authentication Action that verifies the authority of users to receive specified data.

Authoring tools Software programs that allow persons with little or no programming expertise to create instructional computer programs.

Automatic sign-off Mechanism that logs a user off the system after a specific period of inactivity on the terminal or computer.

Backloaded Information that is preloaded into the system before the go-live date.

Backup procedure May refer to the creation of a second copy of files and information found on a computer, or information system, for the intent of restoring information when the primary copy is lost or damaged; or an alternative means to accomplish tasks normally done with an information system when that system is not available to authorized users for some reason.

Backup systems Devices that create copies of system and data files.

Batch processing Manipulation of large amounts of data into meaningful applications at times when computer demands are lowest as a means to maintain system performance during peak utilization hours. Batch processed information is not available before processing and is little used today except to run reports.

Benchmarking Continual process of measuring services and practices against the toughest competitors in the industry.

Bennett Bill Although not passed into law, the Medical Records Confidentiality Act of 1995 was a significant piece of legislation because it attempted to establish the role of health care providers in the protection of client information; fix conditions for the inspection, copying, and disclosure of protected information; and institute legal protection for health-related information.

Binary code Series of 1s and 0s.

Binary file transfer (BFT) Set of instructions that represents another standard for file transfer.

Biometrics Unique, measurable characteristic or trait of a human being for automatically recognizing or verifying identity.

Bit Smallest unit of data that can be handled by the computer.

Blog Abbreviation for web log.

Browser Retrieval program that allows the user to search and access hypertext and hypermedia documents on the Web by using HTTP.

Bulletin Board Systems (BBS) Online service that offers a computerized dial-in meeting and announcement system, allowing users to make announcements, share files, and conduct limited discussions.

Business continuity planning (BCP) Combines information technology and disaster recovery planning with business functions recovery planning.

Business impact assessment or analysis (BIA) Process of determining the critical functions of the organization and the information vital to maintain operations as well as the applications and databases, hardware, and communications facilities that use, house, or support this information.

Byte Eight bits makes up one.

Captoha Completely automatic public test to tell computers and humans apart.

Carpal tunnel syndrome Occurs when the median nerve is compressed as it passes through the wrist along the pathway to the hand. This compression results in sensory and motor changes to the thumb, index finger, third finger, and radial aspect of the ring finger.

Central processing unit (CPU) Electronic circuitry that actually executes computer instructions. The CPU reads stored programs one instruction at a time, keeps track of the execution, and directs other computer parts and input and output devices to perform required tasks.

Client server Distributed approach to computing where different computers work together to carry out a task. The computer that makes requests is known as the client, while the high-performance computer that contains requested files is known as the server.

Clinical data repository Database where information from many different information systems is stored and managed, allowing retrieval of elements without regard to their point of origin.

Clinical information systems (CIS) Large computerized database management systems used by clinicians to access patient data that is used to plan, implement, and evaluate care. Clinical information systems may also be referred to as patient care information systems.

Clinical pathway Suggested blueprint for the care of a client by diagnosis that includes specific interventions by health care professionals, desired outcomes, and even the projected length of stay of inpatient treatment.

Cold site Company that maintains electronic records and backup media in secure, climate-controlled storage so that stored information can be used to restore information system capability in the event that information and/or system functionality have been lost.

Commission on Accreditation of Rehabilitation Facilities (CARF) Health care accrediting body. Its focus is the improvement of rehabilitative services to people with disabilities and others in need of rehabilitation.

Community Health Information Network (CHIN) Organization that electronically links providers, payers, and purchasers of care for the exchange of financial, clinical, and administrative information via a wide area network in a particular geographic area.

Computational nursing Branch of nurmetrics that uses models and simulation for the application of existing theory and numerical methods to new solutions for nursing problems.

Computer Electronic device that collects, processes, stores, retrieves, and provides information output under the direction of stored sequences of instructions known as computer programs.

Computer-assisted instruction (CAI) Use of a computer to organize and present instruction primarily for use by an individual learner.

Computer-based patient record (CPR) Automated patient record designed to enhance and support patient care through the availability of complete and accurate data as well as bodies of knowledge and other aids to care providers.

Computer-based patient record system (CPRS) Components that provide the mechanism by which patient records are created, used, stored, and retrieved. These components include people, data, rules and procedures, and computer and communications equipment and support facilities.

Computer forensics Collection of electronic evidence for purposes of formal litigation and simple internal investigations.

Computer physician order entry (CPOE) Process by which the physician directly enters orders for patient care into a hospital information system.

Confidentiality Tacit understanding that private information shared in a situation in which a relationship has been established for the purpose of treatment or delivery of services will remain protected.

Connectivity Process that allows individual users to communicate and share hardware, software, and information using technology such as modems and the Internet.

Consent Process by which an individual authorizes health care personnel to process their information based on an informed understanding of how this information will be used.

Contingency planning The process of ensuring the continuation of critical business services regardless of any event that may occur.

Control Unit Manages instructions to other parts of the computer, including input and output devices.

Current Procedural Terminology (CPT–4) Commonly used classification system that lists medical services and procedures performed by physicians and is used for physicians billing and payer reimbursement.

Cybercrime Commonly refers to the ability to steal personal information stored on computers such as Social Security numbers.

Data Collection of numbers, characters, or facts that are gathered according to some perceived need for analysis and possibly action at a later point in time.

Database File structure that supports the storage of data in an organized fashion and allows data retrieval as meaningful information.

Database administrator (DBA) Person who is responsible for overseeing all activities related to maintaining a database and optimizing its use.

Data cleansing Procedure that uses software to improve the quality of data to ensure that it is accurate enough for use in data mining and warehousing.

Data collection tool Device that has been created for the purpose of accumulating specific details in an organized fashion.

Data dictionary Tool that defines terms used in a system to ensure consistent understanding and application among all users in the institution. This process may also be achieved through the use of an interface engine.

Data exchange standards Set of agreed-on rules that permit the uniform capture and exchange of data between information systems from different vendors and between different health care providers.

Data integrity Ability to collect, store, and retrieve correct, complete, and current data so that it is available to authorized users when it is needed.

Data management Process of controlling the storage, retrieval, and use of data to optimize accuracy and utility while safeguarding integrity.

Data mining Technique that looks for hidden patterns and relationships in large groups of data using software.

Data retrieval Process that allows the user to access previously collected and stored data.

Data scrubbing Same as data cleansing.

Data warehouse Provides a powerful method of managing and analyzing data.

Decision-support software Computer programs that organize information to aid decision making related to patient care or administrative issues.

Desktop videoconferencing (DTV) Real-time encounter that uses a specially equipped personal computer with a telephone line hookup to allow persons to meet face-to-face or view the same images simultaneously.

Digital cameras Means to capture and input still images with film.

Digital Image Communication in Medicine (DICOM) Standard that promotes the communication, storage, and integration of digital image information with other hospital information systems.

Disaster planning Organized approach that anticipates potential system problems, maintains security of client information under adverse conditions, and provides an alternative means to support the retrieval and processing of information in the event that the information system fails.

Disease management Multidisciplinary approach to identify patient population with or at risk to specific medical conditions.

Distance learning Use of print, audio, video, computer, or teleconference capability to connect faculty and students who are located at a minimum of two different sites.

Distributed processing Use of a group of independent processors that contain the same information but may be at different sites as a means to maintain information services in the event of a power outage or other disaster.

Document imaging Scanning paper records to convert them to files on computer disks or other media, to facilitate electronic storage and handling.

Downtime Period of time when an information system is not operational and available for use.

E-business Refers to services, sales, and business conducted over the internet.

E-care Broader term used to refer to the automation of all parts of the care delivery process across administrative, clinical, and departmental boundaries.

E-health Term that encompasses the wide range of health care activities involving the electronic transfer of health related information on the Internet.

Electronic communication Ability to exchange information through the use of computer equipment and software.

Electronic data interchange (EDI) Communication of data in binary code from one computer to another.

Electronic health record (EHR) Electronic version of the patient data found in the traditional paper record.

Electronic mail (e-mail) Use of computers to transmit messages to one or more persons. Delivery is almost instant, and attachment files may accompany text messages.

Electronic mail software Computer program that assists the user to send, receive, and manage e-mail messages.

Electronic signature Means to authenticate a computer-generated document through a code or digital signature that is unique to each authorized system user.

E-mail application Computer program that assists the user to send, receive, and manage e-mail messages.

Encryption Process that uses mathematical formulas to code messages when content needs to be kept secure and confidential.

E-prescribing Electronic transmission of drug prescriptions.

Ergonomics Scientific study of work and space, including details that affect workers' productivity and health.

Error message Computer-generated text message that warns the user when entries are missing or improperly constructed for proper processing. May appear on the monitor screen as data are entered or later via a paper printout.

Evidence-based practice Process by which nurses and other health care practitioners use the best available research evidence, clinical expertise, and patient preferences to make clinical decisions.

Expert systems Use of computer artificial intelligence to arrive at a decision that experts in the field would make.

External environment Includes those interested parties and competitors who are outside the health care institution.

Extranet Network that sits outside the protected internal network of an organization and uses Internet software and communication protocols for electronic commerce and use by outside suppliers or customers.

Fax modem Allows computers to transmit images of letters and drawings over telephone lines.

Feature creep Uncontrolled addition of features or functions without regard to timelines or budget.

File Collection of related data stored and handled as a single entity by the computer.

File deletion software Overwrites files with meaningless information so that sensitive information cannot be accessed.

File Transfer Protocol (FTP) Set of instructions that controls both the physical transfer of data across a network and its appearance on the receiving end.

Firewall Type of gateway that is designed to protect private network resources from outside hackers, network damage, and theft or misuse of information.

Frames per second (FPS) Number of still images that are captured, transmitted, and displayed in one second of time in a video transmission. The higher the FPS, the smoother the picture. Also referred to as frame rate.

Freezing Situation in which a computer will not accept further input and does not process what has already been entered.

Frequently asked questions (FAQ) Document or file, used by many World Wide Web sites, that serves to introduce the group or topic, update new users on recent discussions, and eliminate repetition of questions.

Function Task that may be performed manually or automated.

Gateway Combination of hardware and software used to connect local area networks with larger networks. A firewall is a type of gateway that is designed to protect private network resources from outside hackers, network damage, and theft or misuse of information.

Gigahertz Represents 1 billion cycles per second in processor speed.

Goal Open-ended statement that describes what is to be accomplished in general terms, and is often used in the strategic planning process.

Go-live Date when an information system is first used, or the process of starting to use an information system.

Grand rounds Traditional teaching tool for health care professionals in training that involves reviewing a client's case history and present condition inclusive of examination findings before a mutual determination of the best treatment options.

Graphical user interface (GUI) Provides a set of menus, windows, and other standard screen devices that are intended to make using a computer as intuitive as possible.

Hardware Physical components of a computer.

Header Section at the top of an electronic mail message that tells who sent the message, when, to whom and at what location, and the address to which a reply should be directed if different from the sender's address.

Health Insurance Portability and Accountability Act (HIPAA) Also known as the Kennedy–Kassebaum Bill, represents the first federal legislation to protect automatic client records.

Health Level 7 (HL7) Standard for the exchange of clinical data between information systems by means of an extensive set of rules that apply to all data sent.

Help desk Support service, rather than a specific location, for computer users. In health care institutions it is usually available 24 hours a day by calling a special telephone number. Help desk staff generally have an information system or computer background and are familiar with all of the software applications and hardware in use.

Helper program Computer application that supports a browser by providing added functionality and performs specific tasks.

Help screens Computer messages that are displayed on the monitor screen in response to a request by the user for assistance by pressing an identified key, or in response to an inappropriate entry by the user. Help screens provide specific directions that the user may follow to reach a desired outcome.

Homegrown software Developed by the consumer to meet specific needs usually because no suitable commercial package is available.

Home page First page seen at a particular Web location.

Hospital information system (HIS) Group of information systems used within a hospital or enterprise that support and enhance patient care. The **HIS** consists of two major types of information systems: clinical and administrative.

Hot site Facility located at a separate location than the health care provider that replicates the provider's information systems for the purpose of quickly restoring information system function in the event of a disaster or disruption to services.

HyperText Markup Language (HTML) Language or set of instructions that is frequently used to write home pages for the Internet, and includes text as well as special instructions known as tags for the display of text and other media. HTML also includes highlighted references to other documents that the user may choose if additional information about that topic is desired.

Hypertext Transfer Protocol (HTTP) Transfer protocol used on Internet pages that establishes a TCP/IP connection between the client and server that sends a request in the form of a command when a link or hypertext is clicked with the mouse.

Informatics Science and art of turning data into information.

Information Collection of data that have been interpreted and examined for patterns and structure.

Information privacy Right to choose the conditions and the extent to which information and beliefs are shared with others. Informed consent for the release of medical records represents the application of information privacy.

Information security Protection of confidential information against threats to its integrity or inadvertent disclosure.

Information system Computer system that uses hardware and software to process data into information in order to solve a problem.

Information system security Protection of information systems and the information housed on them from unauthorized use or threats to integrity.

Information technology General term used to refer to the management and processing of information generally with the assistance of computers.

Input devices Hardware that allows the user to put data into the computer. Basic input devices include the keyboard, mouse, track ball, touch screens, light pens, microphones, bar code readers, fax/modem cards, joysticks, and scanners.

Integrated services digital network (ISDN) High-speed data transmission technology that allows simultaneous, digital transfer of voice, video, and data over telephone lines but at higher speeds than available via modem.

Integrated video disk (IVD) Technology that uses the interactivity, information management, and decision-making capability of computers with audiovisual capabilities of videodisk or tape to enhance CAI. IVD has largely been replaced by CD-ROM.

Integration Process by which different information systems are able to exchange data in a fashion that is seamless to the end user.

Interface Computer program that tells two different systems how to exchange data.

Interface engine Software application designed to allow users of different computer systems to access and exchange information without any special effort on their part or the need to customize equipment or write specific instructions to allow several different systems to communicate.

Internal environment Includes employees of the institution, as well as physicians and members of the board of directors.

International Classification of Disease (ICD–9/ICD–10) Provides a classification for surgical, diagnostic, and therapeutic procedures.

International standard H.320 Standard for passing audio and video data streams across networks, allowing videoconferencing systems from different manufacturers to communicate.

Internet Worldwide network that connects millions of computers and serves to link government, university, commercial institutions, and individual users.

Internet service provider (ISP) Company that furnishes Internet access for a fee.

Intranet Private computer network that uses Internet protocols and technologies, including Web browsers, servers, and languages, to facilitate collaborative data sharing.

JAVA Programming language that enables the display of moving text, animation, and musical excerpts on Web pages.

Jobs aids Written instructions that are designed to be used for reference in both training and work settings.

Joint Photographic Experts Group Compression (JPEG) Standard for the compression of digital images for transmission and storage. Although not developed for use with diagnostic images, JPEG is used for that purpose.

Joystick Allows the user to control the movement of objects on the screen.

Keyboards Input devices with keys that represent those of a typewriter.

Knowledge Synthesis of information derived from several sources to produce a single concept or idea.

Laboratory Information Systems (LIS) Computer system that provides many benefits as a result of automated order entry.

Laptop computer Streamlined version of the personal computer using batteries or regular electric current.

Learning aids Materials intended to supplement or reinforce lecture or computer-based training. Examples may consist of outlines, diagrams, charts, and maps.

Legacy systems Mainframe vendor-based information systems.

Life cycle Well-defined process that describes the recurring process of developing and maintaining an information system.

Links Also known as hypertext, links are words or phrases used on Internet pages that are distinguished from the remainder of the document through the use of highlighting or a different screen color. Links allow users to skip from point to point within or among documents, escaping conventional linear format.

Liquid Crystal Display (LCD) This technology uses two sheets of polarizing material with a liquid crystal solution between them. Each crystal acts like a shutter, either allowing light to pass through or blocking the light.

Listserv E-mail subscription list program that copies and distributes all e-mail messages to everyone who is a subscriber.

Live data Actual patient and health care system data as opposed to fictitious data used for training purposes.

Mainframes Large computers capable of processing large amounts of data quickly.

Main Memory Component of memory that is permanent and remains when power is off. Also known as read only memory (ROM).

Mapping Process by which the definition of terms used in one information system are associated with comparable terms in another information system, thereby facilitating the exchange of information from one system to another.

Master patient index (MPI) Database that lists all identifiers used in connection with one particular client in a health care alliance. Identifiers may include items such as Social Security number, birth dates, and name.

Medical informatics Application of informatics to all of the health care disciplines as well as the practice of medicine.

Megahertz One megahertz represents 1 million signal voltage cycles per second in processor speed.

Memory Computer storage device in which programs reside during execution. It comprises main memory and random access memory.

Menu List of related commands that can be selected from a computer screen to accomplish a task.

Metadata Set of data that provides information about how, when, and by whom data are collected, formatted and stored.

Microcomputer Personal computer that is either a stand alone machine or networked to other personal computers.

Microprocessor chip Electronic circuits of the CPU etched onto a silicon chip.

Minicomputer Scaled-down version of a mainframe computer that is capable of supporting multiple users at the same time.

Mission Purpose or reason for an organization's existence, representing the fundamental and unique aspirations that differentiate it from others.

Modem Communication device that transmits data over telephone lines from one computer to another.

Monitor Screen that displays text and graphic images

Monitoring systems Devices that automatically monitor biometrics measurements in critical care and specialty areas.

Motherboard Microprocessor chip that contains the electronic circuits of the CPU etched on a silicon chip, mounted on a board.

Mouse Device that can be moved around on the desktop to direct a pointer on the screen.

Multimedia Presentations that combine text, voice or sound, and still or video images, as well as hardware and software that support the same.

Network Combination of hardware and software that allows communication and electronic transfer of information between computers.

News reader software Special browser program needed by individual users to read messages posted on the news group.

Notebook computer Streamlined version of the personal computer using batteries or regular electric current.

Nurmetrics Branch of nursing science that uses mathematics and statistics to test, estimate, and quantify nursing theories and solutions to problems.

Nursing informatics Use of information and computer technology to support all aspects of nursing practice.

Nursing informatics specialist Nurse with formal education and practical experience using computers, who supports the automation needs of all facets of nursing practice.

Nursing information system Information system that supports the use and documentation of nursing processes and provides tools for managing the delivery of nursing care.

Nursing Minimum Data Set (NMDS) Consistent collection of data comprising nursing diagnosis, interventions, and outcomes that attempts to collect data that is comparable across different health care settings, to project trends, and to stimulate research.

Objective Statement that describes how a goal will be accomplished and the time frame for this activity.

Offline storage Form of data storage that uses secondary storage devices for data that is needed less frequently, or for long-term data storage.

Off-the-shelf software Commercially available, someone else has bore the cost for its development and testing.

Online Term indicating a connection to various computer resources, including information systems, the Internet, and the World Wide Web.

Online storage Form of data storage that provides access to current data. An example is a high-speed, hard disk drive.

Online tutorials Detailed instructions available to a user while he or she is using a computer, software application, or information system that show or tell how a particular software application or feature can be implemented.

Open architecture Information system architecture that uses protocols and technology that follow publicly accepted conventions and are employed by multiple vendors, so that various system components can work together.

Open system See open architecture.

Operating system Collection of programs that manage all of the computer's activities.

Optical disk drives They write data to a recording surface media and read it later.

Order entry systems Method by which physician's orders for medications and treatments are entered into the computer and directly transmitted to appropriate areas.

Output devices Hardware that allows the user to see processed data. Terminals or video monitor screens, printers, speakers, and fax/modem boards are types of output devices.

Outsourcing Process in which an organization contracts with outside agencies for services.

Password Alphanumeric code required for access and use of some computers or information systems as a security measure against unauthorized use. Password does not appear on the monitor display when it is keyed in.

Peripheral Any piece of hardware attached to a computer.

Personal computer (PCs) Known as desktop computers. This category provides inexpensive processing power for an individual user.

Personal digital assistants (PDAs) Specialized handheld devices used primarily to keep appointments, calendars, addresses, and telephone numbers.

Picture archiving communications systems (PACS) Storage systems that permit remote access to diagnostic images at times convenient to the physician.

Plug-in programs Computer applications that have been designed to support browsers by performing specific tasks. Plug-in programs require the browser to be running.

Point-of-care devices Computer or terminal located at the actual worksite, which is at the patient's bedside with the delivery of health care.

Point-to-point interface Interface that directly connects two information systems.

Portal Term that refers to some Web sites. Portal sites require registration and collect information from the user that can be used to personalize features for individual users.

Printer Produces a paper copy of computer generated documents.

Privacy Freedom from intrusion or control over the exposure of self or personal information.

Production environment Point at which a planned information system is actually used to process and retrieve information and support the delivery of services.

Public key infrastructure (PKI) Provides a unique code for each user that is embedded into a storage device.

Radiology information system (RIS) Provides scheduling of diagnostic tests, communication of patient information, generation of patient instructions and preparation procedures, and file room management.

Random access memory (RAM) Component of memory that can be accessed, used, changed, and rewritten repeatedly while the computer is turned on.

Read-only memory (ROM) Component of memory that contains startup instructions for each time the computer is turned on. ROM is permanent and remains when power is off.

Real-time processing Entry and access to information occurs almost as soon as it is provided.

Redundant array of independent disks (RAID) Duplicate disks with mirror copies of data.

Refresh rate Term used to refer to the speed with which the screen is repainted from top to bottom.

Remote access Ability to use the resources contained on a network, or an information system, from a location outside of the facility where it is physically located.

Remote backup service (RBS) Company that provides backup services for customers from an off-site location to an on-site location.

Repetitive stress injuries (RSIs) Results from using the same muscle groups over and over again without rest.

Request for Information (RFI) RFI is a letter or brief document sent to vendors that explains the institution's plans for purchasing and installing an information system. The purpose of the RFI is to obtain essential information about the vendor and the system capabilities in order to eliminate those vendors that cannot meet the organization's basic requirements.

Request for Proposal (RFP) Document sent to vendors that describes the requirements of a potential information system. The purpose of this document is to solicit proposals from many vendors that describe their capabilities to meet these requirements.

Resolution Term used to refer to the sharpness, or clarity, of an image on a computer monitor. Resolution itself is determined by the number of pixels, or tiny dots or squares, displayed per inch on a monitor screen.

Response time Amount of time between a user action and the response from the information system.

Rule Predefined function that generates a clinical alert or reminder.

Sabotage Intentional destruction of computer equipment or records to disrupt services.

Scan Gather information from external and internal environments.

Scanner Input device that converts printed pages or graphic images into a file.

Scope Statement in an organization's mission that defines the type of activities and services that it will perform.

Scope creep Unexpected and uncontrolled growth of user expectations as the project progresses.

Search engines Tool to help users find information on the World Wide Web. Each search engine maintains its own index or list of information on the Web and uses its own method of organizing topics.

Search engine unifier Programs that search servers and databases, such as the World Wide Web, and can shorten search time by looking at several search engines at one time, often yielding more comprehensive data in less time.

Search indexes Automated programs that search the Web when general information is requested.

Secondary storage Format of computer memory that retains data even when the computer is turned off. Any one of the following devices can provide secondary storage: hard drives, CD-ROM discs, redundant array of inexpensive disks (RAID), optical disks, magnetic disks, magnetic tape, and floppy disks.

Serial Line Internet Protocol (SLIP) Protocol that allows passage of data through communication lines and is used to access the Internet and World Wide Web.

Server Any type of computer that stores files.

Site license Agreement between the computer lab and the software publisher on the terms of use.

Smart card Storage device for patient information that resembles a plastic credit card. The card is kept by the client and presented to health care providers when services are rendered, eliminating redundant data entry and the need to store this information on a network.

Software Computer programs, or stored sequences of instructions to the computer.

Software shredder Set of computer programs that prevents recovery of deleted, or discarded, computer files by writing meaningless information over them.

Spam Unwanted or "junk" mail.

SPYWARE Detection Software Data collection mechanism that installs itself without the user's permission.

Standardized Nursing Languages (SNLs) Common set of terms that have been reviewed and accepted by the American Nurses Association.

Strategic planning Development of a comprehensive, long-range plan for guiding the activities and operations of an organization.

Strategy Comprehensive plan used by an organization that states how its mission, goals, and objectives will be achieved.

Structured data Data that follow a prescribed format, often presented as discrete data elements.

Supercomputers Largest, most expensive type of computers. They are complex systems that can perform billions of instructions every second.

Superuser Staff person who has become proficient in the use of the system and mentors others.

Switched multimegabit data service (SMDS) High-speed data transmission service that uses telephone lines, also known as a T1 line. SMDS is faster than ISDN but slower than ATM.

System check Mechanism provided by a computer system to assist users by prompting them to complete a task, verify information, or prevent entry of inappropriate information.

Systemized Nomenclature of Human and Veterinary Medicine (SNOMED) Classification system that includes signs and symptoms of disease, diagnoses, and procedures and is meant to represent the full integration of all medical information in an electronic medical record.

T1 lines High speed telephone lines that may be used to transmit high-quality, full-motion video at speeds up to 1.544 Mbps.

Tablet PC Smaller and lighter than a notebook computer but can be carried in a hand like a clipboard.

Tape drive Copies files from the computer to magnetic tape for storage or transfer to another machine.

Technical criteria Hardware and software requirements needed to attain a desired level of overall computer or information system performance.

Teleconferencing Use of computers, audio and video equipment, and communication links to provide interaction between two or more persons at two or more sites.

Telehealth Provision of information to health care providers and consumers as well as the delivery of services to clients at a site separate from the health care professional through the use of telecommunication and computer technology.

Telemedicine Use of telecommunication technologies and computers to provide medical information and services to clients at another site.

Telenursing Use of telecommunications and computer technology for the delivery of nursing care to clients at another location.

Terminal Used to input data and receive output from a mainframe computer. It consists of a monitor screen and a keyboard.

Test environment Separate software program like that used for the actual application or information system, which permits trial of programming changes prior to their implementation in the actual system, thereby protecting the "real" system from unwanted alterations.

Thin client technology Computing model that allows PCs to connect to a server using a highly efficient network connection.

Touchpad Pressure and motion sensitive surface.

Trackball Contains a ball that the user rolls to move the on-screen pointer.

Training environment Separate software application that mirrors the actual information system but permits learners to practice skills without fear of harming the system or data contained in it. In the case of health care information systems, the training environment consists of fictitious clients and scenarios that can be used for instruction and practice.

Training hospital Collection of simulated, or fictitious, client data assembled and stored in a database separate from the actual information system for the purposes of instruction and practice. Most, if not all, features available on the actual information system are available for use with the fabricated database.

Training plan Organized approach for the delivery of instruction that should include a philosophy; identification of instructional needs, approaches, and persons responsible for instructional design and delivery; a target date for completion; a budget; and methods for evaluation.

Unified Medical Language System Attempt to standardize terms used in health care delivery.

Unified Nursing Language System Attempt to standardize and link nursing databases as a means to extend nursing knowledge.

Uniform Hospital Data Set (UHDS) Most commonly used data set in the United States, even though it does not include data on nursing care and outcomes.

Uniform resource locator (URL) String of characters that provides an address that identifies a document's World Wide Web location and the type of server it resides on.

Unique patient identifier Single, universal identifier for client health information that ensures availability of all data associated with a particular client.

Unstructured data Data that do not follow a prescribed format such as may be seen in narrative charting.

Usenet news groups Popular Internet feature similar to listservs in content and diversity, with each newsgroup dedicated to a different topic. These groups provide a forum where any user can post messages for discussion and reply.

User class Group of individuals who perform similar functions, and for the purpose of information system training and use, require instruction in how to access and use the same set of system features.

Vendor Company or corporation that designs, develops, sells, and/or supports a product, which in the context of this book is generally a computer, peripheral device, and, more often, an entire information system.

Videoconferencing Face-to-face meeting of persons at separate locations through the use of telecommunications and computer technology.

Virus Malicious program that can disrupt or destroy data.

Web-based instruction (WBI) Uses the attributes and resources of the World Wide Web, such as hypertext links and multimedia, for educational purposes.

Webcam Small camera used by a computer to send images over the Internet.

Webcast Format that allows multiple learners to access a Web site.

Webmaster Person responsible for creating and maintaining a World Wide Web site.

Wide area networks (WANs) Large expansive network systems.

Wireless modem Communication device that sends and receives information via access points provided with a subscription to wireless service.

Work breakdown structure (WBS) Plan to develop the project timelines or schedule a hierarchical arrangement of all specific tasks by using project-planning software.

World Wide Web (WWW) Information service for access to Internet resources by content instead of file names. The World Wide Web uses a graphical user interface (GUI) and supports text, images, and sound, as well as links to other documents.

Zip drive High-capacity floppy disk drive.

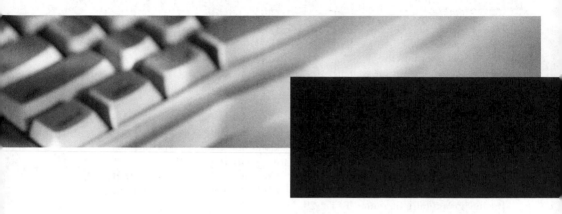

Index

Psychiatric facilities, 284–85
PsychINFO, 384, 386
Publications, online, 100–101
Public health informatics, defined, 9
Public key infrastructure (PKI), 85, 222–23
PubMed, 384, 386, 388

Qualitative analysis, 391–92
Quality, consumer demand for, 19–20
Quality assurance systems, 136
Quality information, characteristics of, 73–75
Quality initiatives, 281–82
Quantitative analysis, 390–91

Radiology information systems (RISs), 130–31
Random access memory (RAM), 37
Reader software, 95
Read-only memory (ROM), 37
Real-time processing, 239
Real-time research, 396
Recovery, 302–6
  backup and storage for, 303–6
Redundant array of inexpensive or independent disks (RAID), 44, 70
Referral, for telehealth, 367–68
Refresh rate, 42
Registration criteria, 167
Registration systems, 136–317
Regulation, of telehealth, 371
Reimbursement, 280–81
Relational databases, 68
Remote access, 216–17
Repetitive stress [motion] injuries (RSIs), 49
Request for information (RFI), selecting HISs and, 169–70
Request for proposal (RFP), selecting HISs and, 170–74
Research, 20, 383–402
  collaborative, 396–99
  data analysis for, 389–92
  data collection tools for, 386–89
  data presentation graphics for, 392, 393
  dissemination of findings of, 399
  HIPPA implications for, 399–400
  identification of topics for, 384

impediments to, 394–99
literature searches for, 384, 386, 387, 388
multi-institutional, 396
online access to databases and, 392–94
in real time, 396
student computer use for, 400–401
unified language efforts and, 395–96, 397–98
Resolution, 42
Response time, 165
Restarting system, 312–13
Results reporting criteria, 167
Resume databases, 414
Resumes, electronic, 414–15
Risk management systems, 136
Rules, in laboratory information systems, 129

Sabotage, 213–14, 301
Safety, of patients, 17–18, 371
Scanners, 45
Scanning environments, 149–50
Schedules, for training, 196–97
Scheduling systems, 137
Scope, of organizational mission, 143
Scope creep, 184
Search engines, 94, 408
Search engine unifiers, 94–95
Search indexes, 93–94
Search tools, 93–95
Secondary storage, 38, 43–44
Security, 216–20
  administrative and personnel issues in, 220–27
  antivirus software for, 220
  for applications, 219–20
  of electronic health record, 259
  firewalls for, 105, 219
  Internet and, 105–6
  passwords and other authentication methods for, 217–19
  physical, 216–17
  spyware detection software for, 220
Security officers, 58
Security risks, 212–16
  errors and disasters, 214
  sabotage, 213–14